The Care and Wellbeing of Older People

Older People

A Textb

01726 226787

The Care and Wellbeing of Older People

A Textbook for Health Care Students

Edited by Angela Kydd, Tim Duffy and F.J. Raymond Duffy

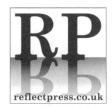

reflectpress.co.uk

First published in 2009

ISBN: 978 1 906052 15 7

British Library Cataloguing in Publication Data
A catalogue record for this book is available from the British Library

The authors and publisher have made every attempt to ensure the content of this book is up to date and accurate. However, health care knowledge and information is changing all the time so the reader is advised to double-check any information in this text on drug usage, treatment procedures, the use of equipment, etc. to confirm that it complies with the latest safety recommendations, standards of practice and legislation, as well as local Trust policies and procedures. Students are advised to check with their tutor and/or mentor before carrying out the procedures in this textbook.

Production project management by Deer Park Productions, Tavistock, Devon
Cover design by Oxmed
Typeset by Kestrel Data, Exeter, Devon
Printed and bound in the UK by Bell & Bain Ltd, Glasgow
Distributed by BEBC, Albion Close, Parkstone, Poole, Dorset BH12 3LL
Published by Reflect Press Ltd
11 Attwyll Avenue
Exeter
Devon EX2 5HN
UK
01392 204400

www.reflectpress.co.uk

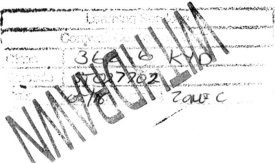

Contents

Foreword

Priscilla Ebersole

This much needed text meets the needs of many professionals caring for the aged in a way that has not been done before. The basic premise running through the entire text is that the caring, compassionate approach to care makes a decided difference in response and recovery, or dignified death. Interviews with a number of elders, recipients of care, show how important it is to approach their care with respect and individualised responses. Nurses are always busy but a few minutes well spent in approaching an elder is of critical importance, perhaps more important than their treatment regimen. In addition, interactions often are so rewarding for the caregiver.

The structure of the text supports the various backgrounds of the authors with sophisticated information when needed and information applicable to all. The book contains 20 chapters including: strategies for care, assessment, medications, communication, homelessness, life transitions, health and illness prevention all within the framework of person-centered care. In addition, for those wishing to study any of these topics in more depth, there are, at the end of each chapter, current websites and literature sources suggested. All chapters have been written by professionals who have extensive experience of caring for the aged. I would highly recommend this text for all persons involved in the care of the aged.

Priscilla Ebersole, RN, PhD, FAAN, Professor Emerita, San Francisco State University, San Francisco, CA, USA

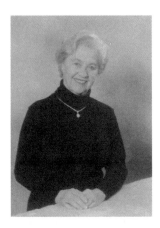

Introduction and Author Biographies

This book has been compiled for health care students who are training for a career in nursing or social work, or professionals allied to health and social care who may be new to the field of gerontology. It has also been compiled for any staff working with older people who seek to further their knowledge on issues concerned with the health and wellbeing of older people who may be in their care. We hope that this generic book will provide a useful reference for the reader and will inspire some to read further to explore in greater depth the topics of interest to them.

The process of ageing and old age is now everybody's business. The population of the Western world is both ageing and shrinking. Older people are at the fore of policy initiatives. 'Older people', sometimes viewed as a drain on an economy's resources, are in actual fact essential to an economy. Many older people provide unpaid care for their parents, grandchildren, friends and neighbours. They make up a large percentage of voluntary staff working for large organisations. A large proportion of retired professional older people continue to work at consultancy level for major and minor organisations. Such people happen to be old and contribute to society. However, there are a proportion of older people who are in need of care and care services. This population are usually quite vulnerable and have little say in their futures. Confusion occurs because both groups of older people are classed as 'old', which is often synonymous with 'in need of care'.

We wanted to create a book that would encompass issues in ageing, growing older and making life transitions. We wanted to address the misconception that as people age they automatically become dependent. We wanted to show readers that, while the ageing trajectory will lead ultimately to death, no one has ever died of 'old age'. We wanted to help the reader explore interventions and initiatives that help older people actively to stay healthy, maintain their health and manage health problems.

In designing the layout of the book we chose to employ a uniform format, which we hope the readers will find useful. Every chapter starts with learning outcomes, includes a literature review, a case study, exercises, the user's perspective and implications for joint working. A short list of useful websites and recommended further reading are provided for those readers who wish to examine the topic in greater depth.

Chapter 1 starts by reporting on consultation we carried out with 35 older people (selected from family, friends and older people's forum members). This consultation aimed to identify what they want from the people who care for them. The ages ranged from 74 to 93 and the responses were made available to the authors who had agreed to contribute to the book. Without doubt, the most sought-after attributes that were seen as important in health care professionals were those of kindness, thoughtfulness and respect.

Chapter 2 on demography outlines the importance of studying the art and science of caring for and enabling older people. Due to demographic changes that show that there are more older people than younger people, policy makers have to address the challenges and issues of such changes. We acknowledge that many people stay fit and well following retirement and into their old age and one of the many reasons for this is due to timely interventions with health care promotion and illness prevention. Chapters 3–20 address current issues in the health and social care provision for healthy older people and frail older people. The topics aim to cover the transition from healthy ageing into frailty. Topics included are sociology, person-centred care, communication, promoting dignity and compassionate care for older people in hospital, assessment and care planning, involving relatives and carers, advocacy and rights of individuals, protecting older vulnerable adults, interprofessional working, lifestyle choices, promoting mental health and wellbeing, promoting physical health, transitions, palliative care, death and bereavement, medicines and concordance, homelessness, life in care and social networks.

The authors were selected for their knowledge on the subject areas and were instrumental in deciding what topics to select and what to discard. The group decided on a multi-disciplinary, interprofessional approach to the content. We believe this book contains all the essential ingredients for a generic textbook on the key aspects of good quality health and social care in the UK, with a strong emphasis on the perspective of older people who need to use services. We hope to foster an empathetic approach to the client group and provide a knowledge base for those who are involved, or are thinking of becoming involved, in a career in older people's services.

This book focuses on policy, practice and research in the United Kingdom. Readers from England, Wales, Scotland and Northern Ireland are encouraged to follow their own country's policies on health and welfare provision and standards of care. The authors have attempted to include major policy initiatives from each country, where appropriate, but readers are urged to think about their own practice in relation to the client group, rather than the underpinning policy initiatives.

AUTHOR BIOGRAPHIES

Angela Kydd

Dr Angela Kydd is a senior lecturer in gerontology within the School of Health, Nursing and Midwifery at the University of the West of Scotland. She is a qualified general and mental health nurse and specialised in working with older people in both acute and long-term care settings. She worked in a clinical capacity for ten years post-qualifying and then moved into higher education in 1995. She set up degree modules and workshops in gerontology for post-registered nurses. In 1998 she started a Gerontology Interest Group for all staff in clinical, academic and research settings. The group meets regularly three times a year and has grown in numbers to include older people. In 2000 she took on the role of programme leader for the BSc Specialist in Gerontological Nursing programme.

In 2002 Angela took on the project management of an Erasmus Intensive Programme for students from Scotland, Finland and Sweden to study together. She has also undertaken research in attitudes to health care professionals working with older people, self care beliefs of women with diabetes and her PhD thesis was on delayed discharge from a policy and patient perspective. She has also undertaken evaluations of clinical areas. She is currently working on a Masters module on frailty.

Tim Duffy

Dr Tim Duffy is Director of Distance Learning within the School of Health, Nursing and Midwifery at the University of the West of Scotland. He is a qualified social worker and specialised in working with people with alcohol and drug related problems. For six years he was National Training Officer with responsibility for training social work and health care personnel to develop strategies to help motivate clients and patients of all ages to reduce problems related to alcohol and drug use. During this time he regularly delivered training programmes focussing on assisting older people to change using Motivational Interviewing, problem solving and goal setting. He evaluated the effectiveness of this training and also the effectiveness of a minimal intervention treatment package for people with alcohol problems.

Since 1995 he has supported the development, delivery and evaluation of a range of undergraduate and post-graduate distance learning programmes including the BSc in Nursing Studies (with Gerontology). In this role he has supported academic staff to develop and deliver distance learning teaching materials for students in 28 countries.

Tim's PhD study evaluated the impact of a *S*elf *A*dministered *M*otivational *I*nstrument (the *SAMI)* in a UK Higher Education setting. He is currently researching student learning styles and approaches to study, student motivation, methods of supporting students online and student retention.

F.J. Raymond Duffy

Raymond is currently a Nurse Lecturer in Gerontology at The University of the West of Scotland. He first became interested in nursing older people as a mental health nursing student and has continued this interest. He has been a Nurse Lecturer since 1995 initially teaching pre-registration adult nursing. Since 2001 he has been teaching post-registration gerontology courses. He is also an experienced distance learning and online learning tutor who has developed and written a number of eLearning and Distance Learning modules for his current employers. He is a member of the Higher Education Academy and also the Royal College of Nursing Older People's Forum and Respiratory Nurse Forum. Since 2002 he has been a Member of Alzheimer's Scotland NHS and Community Health Care Committee. He is also a Committee Member of the British Computing Society Nursing Specialist Group (Scotland).

Mike Danson

Mike Danson is Professor of Scottish and Regional Economics and Associate Dean of Research and Commercialisation in the Business School at the University of the West of Scotland. He has over 30 years' experience teaching and researching in higher education, as well as an established reputation in policy advice and analysis. This is recognised in his position as an Academician of the Academy of Social Sciences, where he is also Treasurer and Scottish Convenor, and as elected Fellow of the Institution of Economic Development. An economist and social scientist with broadly-based interests, he has collaborated with colleagues in many disciplines, institutions and countries. In recent years, Mike has written widely on ageing, demographic change, migration and policy interventions. He has published extensively in these areas and presented keynote addresses at a number of international conferences and symposia. Among many other activities around ageing and demographic policy, Mike was an invited member of Scottish Government's 'Talent Management of Older Workforce Project Team', and a member of the Scottish Executive Strategy for a Scotland with an Ageing Population Advisory Group. He has also established an expertise in volunteering and contributed the research and policy advice for the Government's 'Volunteering Strategy for Scotland'.

Anne Llewellyn

Anne Llewellyn is a Senior Lecturer in the Faculty of Health at Leeds Metropolitan University, where she has worked for the past six years. She originally trained as a nurse and worked in a number of clinical areas, before taking a degree in Social Policy and Administration at the University of Leeds.

Anne has worked in higher education for the last 18 years, specialising in teaching social sciences as applied to nursing and social work practice. She has particular teaching interests in social theories and policies in working with older people and people at the end of life and recently undertook research to evaluate a multi-agency project to enable older people to live more independently. Her publications include *Sociology for Social Workers* and *Fundamentals of Nursing Care: A Textbook for Students of Nursing and Health Care* (Exeter: Reflect Press).

Anne is currently researching effective methods of teaching and active learning, with particular emphasis on the engagement of students and development of personal knowledge and values for interpersonal communication.

Margaret Brown

Margaret Brown is a lecturer in Mental Health Nursing within the School of Health, Nursing and Midwifery at the University of the West of Scotland. She is a Registered Nurse in mental health and has worked in the full spectrum of mental health care settings, finally specialising in the care of the older person with mental health care needs. She set up and was the team leader of a community mental health team for older people for 12 years before entering a career in education.

In addition to teaching in both pre- and post-registration mental health programmes, she developed and led the older person's pathway for a specialist nursing practice qualification leading to MSc.

She has been involved with a variety of research projects in older people's care including a needs assessment of older people with severe mental health care needs and a palliative care in dementia learning needs project. Her current research interest is quality of life for the person with severe dementia.

Susan Royce

Sue Royce is a lecturer in the pre-registration nursing programme within the School of Health, Nursing and Midwifery at the University of the West of Scotland. She also teaches on the post-registration programme specifically the gerontology, rehabilitation and respiratory modules. She has been a qualified nurse since 1982. She has worked in a variety of clinical settings, culminating as senior sister on a medical admissions ward for the over 60s. She has also worked at the University of Salford, where she ran the diploma and BSc gerontology specialist programmes, and taught on the MA in gerontology. She has been a community health council member for four years and assisted in the planning and transferring of two care of the older adult units in Lancaster and Morecambe.

She has commenced her PhD studies with the University of Manchester in the history of nursing. She is looking at the role of the cottage hospital in Scottish rural society.

Michelle Walters

Michelle Walters is an Adult Nurse Lecturer within the School of Health, Nursing and Midwifery at the University of the West of Scotland. Michelle's nursing career began in the 1980s at James Paget University Hospitals NHS Foundation Trust formerly known as Great Yarmouth Royal Infirmary. On qualifying, she worked in Birmingham for several hospitals, including Birmingham Heartlands & Solihull NHS Trust, and Sandwell General Hospital within Intensive Care. In 1997 Michelle moved to Scotland to take up the post of Clinical Co-ordinator at the Royal Infirmary of Edinburgh within the Practice, Research and Development Unit.

Michelle has a keen interest in nurse education and in 1997 completed a Postgraduate Certificate in Education in Further, Adult and Higher Education at the University of Wolverhampton and is a Registered Nurse

Tutor. She has a BA (Hons) in Sociology and Social Policy and a Masters of Social Science in Health Care Policy and Management, and is currently studying through the University of Liverpool to attain a Masters of Public Health.

Austyn Snowden

Austyn is lecturer in mental health nursing, School of Health, Nursing and Midwifery at the University of the West of Scotland. He has 23 years' international mental health nursing experience, mostly in care of older adults and is a qualified non-medical prescriber. The difficulty of operationalising prescribing within his community mental health team in 2005 led to his current research interest, a PhD studying the impact of mental health nurse prescribing in Scotland. He is widely published on the topic and is also on the editorial board of *Nurse Prescribing* as well as being a peer reviewer for various other nursing journals. His book *Prescribing and Mental Health Nursing* was published by Quay Books, MA Healthcare in June 2008.

Rick Henderson

For the past seven years Rick has been Chief Executive of Action for Advocacy, the lead resource and support agency for the advocacy sector in England and Wales. He has over 15 years' experience of managing and developing advocacy services. Rick started work as a nursing assistant at Darenth Park Hospital in Kent in the 1980s and became involved in the movement to resettle ex-hospital patients into the community. His first book, *Prisoners, Patients or People?* with Mark Wallis (Freedom into Action, 1992) was a reflection on his experience of working in an institutional environment and the lessons learned. After that Rick worked in residential care services in Kent and London and studied for his MA in the Management of Community Care at the University of Kent. His dissertation was on improving access to advocacy services for Black and Minority Ethnic communities.

More recently, Rick was responsible for the development and delivery of training for the new Independent Mental Capacity Advocacy (IMCA) service across England and Wales.

Rick is the co-author of *A Right Result? Advocacy, Justice and Empowerment* (Policy Press, 2001), which is one of the key texts on independent advocacy in the United Kingdom.

Joy Gauci

Joy Gauci is Senior Lecturer at the University of Worcester and Course leader for the Masters in Social Work programme. Joy is a qualified and registered social worker with 20 years' of post-qualifying experience working as a statutory social worker with vulnerable adults in a range of community contexts. Joy holds an MA in Applied Ethics for Welfare Practice, and undertook her MA Dissertation on the Protective Rights of Vulnerable Adults. This included an evaluation of the value, and impact, of *No Secrets* (2000) for community welfare practice with vulnerable adults. Joy lectures in key areas relating to social work and social welfare practice, including vulnerable adults and safeguarding, applied ethics, law and policy for welfare practice. She has a particular interest in alternative and therapeutic responses to victimhood.

Joy also holds a Practice Assessor and Mentor Award for Social Work practice education and is committed to the promotion of quality in practice learning and consistency in accountable social work practice.

Michelle Cornes

Dr Michelle Cornes is a Research Fellow in the Social Care Workforce Research Unit at King's College London. Her main area of interest is the integration of health and social care services for older people. She has published widely on a range of topics, most recently on the impact of the controversial reimbursement policy on delayed hospital discharge. She has worked on behalf of the Healthcare Commission to ensure the involvement and engagement of older people in the review of the National Service Framework for Older People (NSFOP) and works closely with many local older people's groups and forums to support campaigning and user-led research. Prior to joining King's College, Michelle was Intermediate Care Programme Manager at Help the Aged.

Billy Mathers

Billy Mathers is a lecturer in mental health nursing at the University of the West of Scotland. After qualifying as a mental health nurse he then trained in counselling. Thereafter he worked in forensic units for several years and later as a community psychiatric nurse (CPN) in east London. In his early research he studied the changing role of the CPN in newly formed community mental health teams and the role of the CPN in community depot clinics. This research has been presented at conferences in both national and international locations.

He commenced working in higher education in 1995 and was for many years module leader for both pre-registration and post-registration mental health nursing programmes at City University, London. Billy's Doctor in Education study evaluated a training programme for acute mental health nurses and examined ways to increase their therapeutic clinical involvement. He is currently campus lead in the pre-registration mental health nursing programme, campus mental health lead in the mentorship programme and is liaison lecturer for several older adult wards.

Graham Harris

Graham Harris is both a Registered Nurse and Registered Nurse Tutor. He has worked in a variety of roles in the NHS and Higher Education sector – including as a Charge Nurse in an acute elderly care ward, Clinical Teacher for an older people's unit and more recently as a Senior Lecturer within a health faculty. Currently he is working as a Community Nurse for Suffolk Primary Care Trust.

Graham's professional interests are broad but principally surround the care of older people, men's health, and the protection of vulnerable adults. He has undertaken research into mentorship for pre-registration nursing students and more recently into nurses' perceptions of their role in the prevention and management of cases of elder abuse. He has contributed to the development of a variety of educational programmes, led the adult branch programme of an undergraduate degree in nursing and participated actively in the delivery of numerous professional courses, study days and workshops.

Graham's publications include papers related to men's health and end of life care. He is currently planning for the publication of a chapter within a communication book for pre-registration nursing students.

Dr Stuart Milligan

Stuart Milligan is lecturer in Palliative Care at the University of the West of Scotland and Education Facilitator at Ardgowan Hospice, Greenock. He qualified as a nurse in 1988 and has held a number of posts in hospital, hospice and community settings. His current responsibilities include delivering a range of palliative care modules at both graduate and postgraduate level. He is also involved in supporting the learning and development of hospice staff and volunteers and providing an outreach education service for health and social care practitioners in the Inverclyde area.

He gained his PhD during a previous career in plant physiology, and has retained an interest in research, publishing papers on symptom management and spirituality. He is particularly interested in how professional carers provide spiritual care for people living with life limiting illnesses or nearing the end of life.

Stuart is committed to 'spreading the message' about the importance of palliative care, not only at the end of life but throughout the course of life-limiting illnesses. To this end he regularly gives talks to groups and organisations ranging from high school pupils to retirement clubs. He is also interested in patient empowerment and leads workshops on 'Finding a spiritual path through illness'.

Elaine Stevens

Elaine Stevens holds a joint appointment between The Ayrshire Hospice and the University of The West of Scotland. She manages the education service at the Hospice and is the programme leader for the palliative care named award at degree level within the University. Elaine's main interests are loss, grief and bereavement, decision making at the end of life, pain management, communication issues and palliative day care. Before this Elaine held a number of nursing posts in hospices, including managing palliative day services. She remains lead for education and research for the Association of Palliative Day Care Leaders. Elaine is also the current chair of the Palliative Nursing Forum of the Royal College of Nursing. This forum has over 8 000 members and the steering group acts as a voice for palliative nurses within the United Kingdom. The steering group is regularly involved in commenting on palliative care guidance at international, national and local levels to ensure nurses influence new policies, protocols and standards.

Jennifer Stewart

Jennifer Stewart is a Day Centre Senior Project Worker with Churches Action for the Homeless (C.A.T.H.) in Perth. Within this role she responds to the varying needs of service users through the provision of both practical and emotional support. C.A.T.H. is a progressive charitable organisation supporting anyone 16+ who is either homeless or at high risk of homelessness across Perth and Kinross. Its mission is 'working together to end homelessness' and it currently runs ten individual projects including two hostels, tenancy support, literacy support, an outreach service and a rent deposit scheme. Further information about the organisation and the work carried out by Jennifer and her team can be found at **www.cath-org.co.uk**.

Jennifer graduated from Stirling University with a BA (hons) in Sociology and Social Policy in 2003. Her fourth year dissertation was an exploratory study of Traveller Children's experiences and perspectives of mainstream education. Jennifer's education and vocational experience has strengthened her three key areas of interest which are older people, volunteering and violence against women.

Eveline Kearney

Eveline Kearney is a Nurse Lecturer in gerontology at the University of the West of Scotland. She is an RGN, has a BSc(hons) in Health Studies and is a Specialist Practitioner in Gerontology Qualification (SPGQ). Her nursing background has mainly been in palliative care and care of the older person. Before taking up the role of lecturer, she was a Care Home manager for several years. During this time her client group comprised mainly people over the age of 65 who had a learning disability, dementia or dementia requiring specialist care. This background has provided a wealth of practical experience in dealing with older people and their carers and insights into the social, psychological, spiritual and physical challenges facing older people, particularly in a care home setting.

Eveline has a particular interest in quality of life issues for older people such as autonomy, the recognition and position of spirituality in older people's lives and the role played by ageism.

Her current role allows her to develop and deliver education and training to nurses and social care workers, with the aim of changing their practice and improving the quality of life for older people they look after in care settings and beyond.

Catherine Rae

Catherine Rae has an Honours Degree in Sociology and a Masters Degree in Applied Social Research from Stirling University. She is at present an associate researcher with the Dementia Services Development Centre [DSDC] at Stirling University.

Part One

Chapter 1

Values: What Older People Told Us

Angela Kydd

Learning outcomes

Reading this chapter will enable you to:

- explain possible reasons why service care provision does not match consumer requirements;

- examine some views held by older people on what they would like from service care provision;

- explore issues that lead to older people feeling let down by the care provided;

- discuss the role of the older person as a consumer in the design and delivery of care services.

INTRODUCTION

This book has been compiled for health care students who are training for a career in nursing or social work, or a profession allied to health and social care. It has also been compiled for professionals who are working with older people and who seek to further their knowledge on issues concerned with the health and wellbeing of older people who are in their care.

There is currently a drive to include the user's voice in health care planning and delivery. Of course, issues seen as important to policy makers and service providers are not always the issues seen as important to the people who actually use the service(s). However, by including the user's perspective, a greater sensitivity can be brought to bear in the provision of services and the delivery of care. Therefore, with the user perspective in mind, when writing this book it was necessary not only to think about what future and current professionals deemed necessary in the content, but to also think about what older people expected from the professionals. To achieve this, a scoping exercise was carried out in September 2007. This was done by sending out a questionnaire to individual older people, and taking the questionnaire, for discussion, to several groups for older people. The questionnaire was simple; it posed two questions:

1. What six things would you expect from a health care professional?

and

2. What six things detract from your ideal for a health care professional?

The only personal detail asked for was the respondent's age.

The response to this small exploratory exercise was excellent. Fifty people were asked and a total of 35 people responded. Nineteen respondents were part of an older people's forum and 16 were individual older people who were family and friends of the authors. The ages ranged from 74 to 93 and the responses were made available to all the authors who have contributed to this book.

This exercise was carried out purely as a starting point for this book. The aim is to provide you with some of the thoughts of good and poor care from a variety of articulate older people. This chapter addresses what we were told by the older people we asked and then goes on to briefly explore the advent of the user's voice in the design of services. It also raises some of the issues surrounding the problems involved with representing users' views in service provision.

THE QUESTIONNAIRE RESPONSES

1. What six things would you expect from a health care professional?

There were seven main attributes that the respondents wanted from a health care professional and the majority of people asked mentioned at least four of these attributes in their responses. The attributes have been listed below with quotes from some of the responses.

A caring, understanding and kind person

The human nature of caring was seen as the most important attribute in a health care professional by the older people we asked. To be caring, understanding and kind took priority over the need for a skilled practitioner. The older people we asked stated that they wanted someone who cared; someone whose time was dictated by a patient's needs and not by a schedule. One person wrote:

> Whilst caring, talk to me, even though you may feel I may not be able to reply. It isn't always possible to know what people can still understand.

Another person had stated that a caring attitude was important, 'even towards someone who is so ill that he/she has become fractious and difficult to deal with'. Others spoke of a need for a practitioner who 'above all showed understanding and compassion and a genuine regard for the welfare of their client and their family'.

Two people gave examples of why a caring attitude was necessary. The first wrote:

> Many difficulties old people experience are a cause of embarrassment, for example, incontinence. A person who had sympathy and understanding of this condition would make a wonderful health care professional.

The second person wrote:

> An understanding of the difficulties of coping with having to travel distances for appointments, minor treatments at hospitals, or clinics, when having to rely on public transport, which can be infrequent and difficult to get to.

Many people simply wrote that they wanted to feel cared for and valued as a person. They looked for a person who would understand their need for comfort and several mentioned having their pillows straightened. One person pointed out:

> The vulnerability of a sick, elderly person is immense and needs to be handled with great sensitivity.

While training was not often mentioned in this section, four people had linked a well-trained professional with someone who was willing and able to help with what was termed basic requirements, and these included things such as straightening bedclothes and carefully checking for bed sores.

In essence, older people told us that they wanted a person with a caring attitude, someone who showed understanding and kindness and a real commitment to the patient and the patient's family.

A professional attitude to older people

The second attribute the older people in our scoping exercise wanted was a health care professional who had a positive attitude to working with older people. Many of the older people in the scoping exercise tended to give advice on how to treat older people in care. Examples of the desire for individual care are given in the quotes below:

> An understanding that age or infirmity does not necessarily mean an inability to participate in informed decisions concerning health care or where one should reside.

> I value a health care professional who can understand the problems of old people and appreciate their valuing of independence.

> An understanding that in general a 70-year-old cannot do what a 30-year-old can, even when they are essentially fit.

Some older people remarked on ageist attitudes among professionals and the quote below illustrates this point:

> Some people are 'old' at 50 while someone may still be 'young' at 90. An older person's needs depend not so much on their chronological age as on their apparent age.

Some older people pointed out the need to see the person behind the age:

Remember that each older person is an individual; this is not lost on reaching retirement. Individuality and dignity are equally important to the old as to the young.

Although one part of a person may not function as well as when they were young they may still have an appetite for doing something else.

One person stated that health care professionals needed:

The realisation that I was once able to do all the things the health professional does now without thinking. I wasn't always like this.

A patient person who will listen

Patience and taking the time to listen were seen as very important attributes. One person wrote that they wanted professionals to:

Take more time to listen to my expectations and requirements and discuss what is and what is not possible.

Another older person pointed out that tests can help diagnose illnesses, but the person themselves has knowledge of their own body and should be able to contribute to their programme of care. Several older people commented that they wanted to be treated as equals and not idiots. One stated:

Professionals need to remember that although you are old you can still think.

Another stated:

It is important to remember I am a person with a past life, I have not always been old.

Some people acknowledged that patience was needed when looking after older people. One remarked:

I know it can be difficult when always dealing with the old.

Another stated:

Remember that age can bring a certain slowness and confusion resulting from loss of hearing, sight or movement which requires extra patience and tolerance.

It was interesting to note that the older people we spoke to wanted professionals to remember that the deleterious effects of ageing on a person can be just as frustrating for the older person as they are for those who are looking after them.

A respectful person

Respecting the dignity of individuals was another sought-after attribute. The older people we consulted told us that they wanted professionals to find out how they would like to be addressed. Many people stated that health and social care professionals frequently referred to them by their first names and they found this disrespectful. One person stated:

> All people should be treated with courtesy, including not using Christian names without permission. There is a lack of appreciation among the younger generation that 80/90/100-year-olds grew up in an age when there was a greater formality than today.

They had also experienced patronising attitudes and several stated the need to 'remember I have not always been like this'.

Another wrote:

> There needs to be a realisation that age, frail health or limited mobility may still be accompanied by an active and interested mind which welcomes normal conversation.

Respect included manners and several older people felt that they had been kept waiting for treatment or appointments unnecessarily and without apology. Given that they had struggled to keep an appointment, they would have appreciated some form of explanation and apology for the delay.

A skilful, knowledgeable practitioner

The older people we consulted wanted to have confidence in the skills of the professional. They stated that they needed to know that professionals kept themselves up to date and had experience in caring for older people. They also wanted to know that the health and social care professional would refer a case onto another professional should they feel they lacked the experience to handle their problems.

The people we consulted also wanted a practitioner who made the effort to find out what suited each individual's needs with regard to their illness, their social circumstances and their rehabilitation. They also wanted someone who could provide them with answers to their questions and advise them on how to cope when they returned home.

Continuity of care

It was apparent that some of the older people we talked to had received fragmented care and this was viewed as poor practice. One person wrote:

> I would like the same carers to come on a regular basis as far as possible so that I can learn to be comfortable with them. This will make it easier for me to talk to them about my family and the outside world. This will help to give me something else to think about.

Another wrote:

> Professionals need to realise that older couples no longer able to cope at home should not be placed into separate accommodation, sometimes miles apart.

Some people gave reports of excellent care they received, due to services being in place following discharge from hospital, and acknowledged that because they had received good continuity of care, they were able to make a full recovery.

A cheerful person

Several people wanted to see a happy, cheerful and willing health care professional. One person stated:

> A nurse must have a sense of humour – even if mine is lacking a bit at the time!

Others wanted to see cheerfulness in mundane tasks, such as help in arranging any necessary walking aids, day care centre visits and help with form filling for allowances. One person stated that a bright and happy attitude when dealing with general day-to-day queries was a very special quality. Several people gave examples of how therapeutic they found cheerful health care professionals. One wrote:

> I remember when I was in [names hospital], there was this one cheery little nurse, she always had a smile for everyone and it brightened up my day. I used to look forward to her coming on duty.

Another stated:

> You feel like you're a nuisance, so when someone looks happy it doesn't make you feel so bad.

2. What six things would detract from your idea of a health care professional?

We posed the above question to the 35 older people we consulted. While we had written responses, this question prompted people to tell stories of their experiences of poor care. One of these stories has been selected for the case study in the next section of this chapter. The responses we received from this second piece of work were much shorter. There are several possible reasons including:

- the first question covered negative as well as positive responses;
- this was the second piece of work asked for and respondents had spent a considerable amount of time on the first question;
- older people in general do not like to complain; an issue raised in the penultimate section of this chapter.

It is unsurprising that there is overlap between the two pieces of work. The attributes the older people wanted in a health care professional directly correlated to what would detract from their ideal for a health care professional. Similar headings have therefore been used to show the responses. It is interesting to note that only a few older people worried about the lack of skills a professional may have; their main focus was on the professional's attitudes and behaviour towards the patient.

A professional who does not care, lacks understanding and shows no kindness

The older people we consulted did not want to see professionals who were:

> Uncaring, or had a slipshod attitude to care of their patients.

Caring, or lack of it, was one of the main themes of this section. Many people told us that they knew looking after older people was 'a difficult job'. One person stated:

> I would not like to be cared for by someone who was actually unkind, despite allowing for the difficult job to be done.

An unprofessional attitude to older people

The negative attitudes of professionals towards older people were well documented in the responses we received and many people reported on the poor attitudes they or their loved ones had encountered. Several quotes below serve to sum up how people felt:

I hate an off-hand attitude, it just belittles the patient.

One person stated:

I don't like it when arrangements are made without full knowledge and permission of patient.

Another person wrote:

I really don't want someone who will not talk to me, or my family, about what is going on and then end up arranging things without proper discussion.

The quote from the person below was one of several that mentioned a person's past capabilities:

It's awful to know that people don't see you and realise that you were once fit and active.

Other comments stated that patronising attitudes were most unhelpful and several people spoke of health and social care professionals working with excessive speed, which serves to make the patient feel a nuisance and a burden.

An impatient person who will not listen

The older people all had something to say on being heard. The quotes below give a flavour of what people did not wish to see in a professional:

Someone who doesn't take the time to understand the problems me or my family have.

Someone who lacks understanding that patients often do not like to ask for help.

And more tellingly:

Someone with an erratic temperament with a tendency to air her/his problems instead of the patients'.

9

A disrespectful person

Pseudo-friendliness, for example using the Christian names of the patients on first meeting them, and using the word 'we' was found to be both patronising and presumptuous. One person wrote:

> I don't want false bonhomie and I don't want to be treated as though I am deliberately slow, when the spirit is willing but the body is weak.

Many other points were made about the need for a respectful practitioner and this frequently came with stories of how older people and their relatives had been treated in the past. One person told us:

> It is awful when someone talks over the top of an older person as if they weren't there; this particularly annoyed my 94-year-old mother when the treatment she was to have was told to me. I was even given her eye drops to take home when she was sitting there as well.

One person told us of the treatment their sister had when she was coming round after an operation:

> There was over-familiarity for her post-operative treatment, but most of the time she was ignored on that ward. I hate to see the staff congregating in the ward, discussing their social affairs, when patients are in need.

Other points made were poor time-keeping by practitioners who were visiting people at home. Four people commented that it would be courteous for a professional to phone to say they would be late, because everything has to go on hold at home until after the visit. Many felt that one indication of a poor practitioner was:

> Someone you can't rely on to be punctual and consistent.

Respect for the patient and his/her feelings and tact with relatives were mentioned many times, and several points made were accompanied by stories of disrespectful staff.

An unskilful practitioner

There were only a few comments on this type of practitioner. People told us:

I don't want to be cared for by an untrained carer unsupervised.

Others remarked that poor professional care was:

Failing to seek senior advice if any problem should arise outwith the health care professional's remit or capability. People who lack the humility to say they do not know what to do.

And:

Someone who does not take the time to understand the difficulties age can bring.

Another wrote:

Failing to give patients a feeling of safety that all aspects are dealt with efficiently, promptly and with understanding and kindness and respect.

One person remarked on the lack of time professionals have:

Sometimes the health care professional's workload does not enable them to remain long enough with a seriously ill person who can feel abandoned after too short a visit.

Lack of continuity of care

Three people wrote of the need for agencies to co-ordinate services. One person had several services coming to the house and the individual never knew when a member of the services was due to call. The person felt that health care professionals should make an appointment because of the worry an individual might have about leaving the house for fear they should miss a call. One person noted that there was rivalry between some agencies. This person remarked that some staff spoke about other teams in derogatory ways. The person wrote:

Sometimes Health and Social Work do not co-operate to the benefit of the patient.

A bad-tempered person

Several people said that mood and attitude were very important attributes. The older people told us that bad temper, offhand manners, impatience, indifference and intolerance are not acceptable in professional practice.

Activity 1

In reading what older people think about good practice and poor practice in the section above, it is clear that much of what was told comes from first-hand experience. Take some time to complete the exercise below, which has been designed to make you think about your perceptions of good and poor practice. It needs to be carried out in practice ideally, but if you don't work with older people, think of a time when you have been working with older people. If you do work in this area you could take notes next time you are on duty.

- What do you see as good care in your area of work?

- What do you see as poor care?

- Do you think your perceptions of good care match what your client(s) see as good care?

- Talk to one of your clients and ask what qualities they like to see in a health care professional.

Activity 2

Think of a person you love who is over the age of 65. This person may be a relative, a friend or someone whom you know well locally. Now imagine that person in a hospital or a care home.

- What concerns, if any, would you have on the way this person might be treated?

- Can you think of anything that would make their stay in a hospital or care home a good or bad experience for them as an individual?

- Would anything concern you about the fact that they have had to leave their homes for a while? For example, would they have concerns about a pet, their garden, losing their routines?

Compare the answers you have with those of the answers you gave for Activity 1.

Activity 3

One of the respondents in the survey carried out for this chapter said that when they were in hospital they were longing to tell the nurses that they needed to know that they were liked. Read the following extract from what this person said they wanted to say to the night nurse:

> When you have finished putting me to bed, please say goodnight and try to show me that I mean something to you by taking hold of my hand or giving me a kiss on my forehead before you leave me. You might be the only caring contact I have had today.
>
> Respondent aged 73

- Do you think that, if you held this person's hand and kissed them, your actions might be interpreted as patronising?

- How do you know when someone would like to be treated in this manner and when someone would see this as patronising?

GOOD QUALITY CARE PRACTICE

The answers to these exercises may show you that every action and interaction you have with any client is as individual and unique as the person they are. The skill of practising good quality care is in knowing what type of responses will be appreciated, and what type of responses will be seen as patronising. Such interactions are intuitive, will usually feel right in the circumstances and cannot easily be taught.

It is interesting to note that, within the present climate of health and social care, there has been a shift from a 'cared for' paradigm to one of 'enablement'. While the enablement model is good, in that it fosters a culture of empowering clients, this should not be at the exclusion of a 'caring' model. There are some times in people's lives when they need to be 'cared for', times when they do not have the strength, energy or motivation to be 'enabled'. It is the skill of the practitioner to intervene at such times. Such a skill involves an empathetic approach to the client and knowledge of when to 'care for' and when 'to enable'.

Individual responses to human needs are unique. To be in a professional position to respond to another's need is a privilege that comes with responsibility, and that is either to address that need or refer it on to a health or social care professional who can.

Case study

Many of the older people had stories of good and poor experiences they had encountered within the health and social care arena. The story selected here clearly illustrates the need for careful care. One 75-year-old person told the story of their mother's death in hospital. The incident took place when the person was 68 and their mother was 94. The incident has been related below.

I think they [staff] just don't care any more when you are old. I know this because of the way my mum was treated, the way we [her sister and brother] were treated. It was how my mother died, and I will never forget it. This [incident] was six years ago now, I will never forget it. My mother was always very independent. She had lived a full life and went into hospital because she could not eat. We all came to see her [her three surviving children]. There was just me and my sister at first. My brother came up from Newcastle and that was hard for him as his wife is not keeping well. Mum was bad, we knew she was dying. The staff had put her in a side room, but in the move they had lost her teeth. She was clean and all that, but she hated to be seen without her teeth, she was proud and she always looked good. She looked awful, and what made it so bad was that we couldn't understand what she was trying to say to us. It still upsets me now. Mum was trying to talk to us, she was trying to tell us something, but to this day I do not know what that was.

Respondent aged 75

The person who was speaking was clearly upset. They were haunted by not knowing what their mother's final words were and no-one in the group had any words of comfort for her. The moment had gone. Nothing could change what had happened and nothing could be said to make them feel better. The loss of that last message was unresolved and caused the person much fresh grief each time they remembered the event.

HEARING WHAT PEOPLE HAVE TO SAY ABOUT SERVICES

Historically, people in receipt of health and social care services were rarely asked for their opinions of those services. Using members of the public for consultancy purposes is a relatively new concept. Up until the 1970s users of services had very little say in their experience of using health and welfare services. Most studies focussed on the professionals' perceptions of client care or satisfaction surveys, which collected a great deal of interesting data from clients, but gave no indication of their individual experience (Seltzer and Kullberg, 2001).

In the 1970s a publication by Mayer and Timms (1979) entitled *The Client Speaks: Working Class Impressions of Casework* heralded the start of long overdue research into the narratives of users of services. However, it was not until the 1990s that consumer rights and citizens' charters (Department of Health, 1992) became buzz words and service designers wanted to involve users in decisions about their treatment and care. A major change occurred to address the paternalistic approach of service provision to passive recipients (NHS Executive, 1999) and service users were encouraged to become involved in the provision of care (Richards, 1999). In 1998, The Health Advisory Service 2000 (HAS, 1998) published a document entitled *Not Because They are Old* and the first recommendation from this document was that:

> Older people and their families must be more involved with their care at every stage, and in relation to every decision made about their care.
>
> (HAS, 2000: iii)

However, while this change appeared to put the consumer or user at the forefront of services, making a reality of the rhetoric was not always easy to put into practice. With regard to hearing the opinions of older people, Wertheimer (1993) suggests that the way forward in terms of older people is via citizen advocacy. She suggests that as older people are often reluctant to complain and often have low expectations of services, the only way their views can be heard is through the support of an advocate.

A recent piece of research commissioned by the Scottish Executive (Dewar, Jones and O'May, 2004) explored older people's involvement in planning, delivering and monitoring services throughout Scotland with a view to identifying barriers and informing community planners about how to address such barriers. This work was important as, even after many years of public consultancy, there is still evidence that conventional services do not provide what is usually at the top of the users' and carers' wish lists and that some sections of the community are very hard to access. Copperman and Morrison (1995) point out that there are a variety of constraints to user involvement and these receive scant attention in the current drive to involve users in decisions about their care. In addition, there remains a resource issue in that services are provided 'as available' rather than 'as required' by the client (Crompton, 2004).

At the heart of many statutory documents and standards, there is usually a section that now encompasses the views of users of services. User involvement by older people can take on many forms and a useful publication outlining the levels of involvement is that by Carter and Beresford (2000). Additional reading can also be found in an excellent research review entitled *Addressing What Older People Want* by Clark and Raynes (2006). This review summarises findings from some of the research and policy literature that focusses upon older people's views of the help they say they want in order to continue an independent life.

CONCLUSION

There is a shift from a paternalistic stance on what constitutes good care. Users of services are becoming increasingly more involved in consultations, user groups and evaluations of services. However, it is still difficult to access hard-to-reach older people, those in care homes, the housebound, homeless, etc. and ascertain their views. Given that satisfaction with services is highly individual and bound by the context of that situation at that time, it is the duty of health care professionals, particularly those dealing with hard-to-reach groups, to check with their clients/patients that their needs are really being met. Obtaining such feedback can be done sensitively and quietly, using cues provided by both the client and their loved ones.

In using the voices of a small number of older people to inform this book, we have demonstrated that many perceptions of good care come from positive attitudes and sensitive interactions with patients/clients and their families. The people we spoke to wanted to feel cared for and respected. This is not a new concept and can be seen in many government publications and standards on good care. We therefore highlight the point that fundamental good manners and respect for an individual are at the forefront of good professional practice. These qualities require no extra funding, resources or time. It is simply the way that you, the professional, interacts as a human being with the individual older person in their time of need.

FURTHER READING

Carter, T. and Beresford, P. (2000) *Age and Change: Models of Involvement for Older People*. York: Joseph Rowntree Foundation
A useful text looking at the ways older people can be involved in contributing to service design and delivery.

Ebersole, P., Hess, P., Touhy, T., Jett, K. and Luggen, A. (2008) *Toward Healthy Aging: Human Needs and Nursing Response* (7th edn). St Louis, MI: Elsevier Mosby
An excellent all purpose gerontology textbook from American authors. It is beautifully written and places the individual at the centre of care delivery.

Foote, C. and Stanners, C. (2002) *Integrating Care for Older People: New Care for Old – A Systems Approach*. London: Jessica Kingsley Publications
An insight into the change in welfare provision for older people which helps individuals to live as independently as possible.

Raynes, N., Clark, H. and Beecham, J. (eds) (2006) *Evidence submitted to the Older People's Inquiry into 'That Bit of Help'*. York: Joseph Rowntree Foundation
The Joseph Rowntree publications are an excellent source of up-to-date information. This book examines supporting people in the community.

Useful websites

www.jrf.org.uk
The Joseph Rowntree Foundation.

www.bgop.org
This site is from the 'Better Government for Older People' initiative and informs good practice.

www.who.org
The World Health Organisation site is essential to most student studies for information on demographics, trends and good practice.

www.doh.co.uk
The Department of Health website contains the relevant English White Papers.

www.scot.gov.uk
The Scottish Executive website contains the relevant Scottish White Papers.

www.new.wales.gov.uk
The Welsh Assembly website contains the relevant Welsh White Papers.

REFERENCES

Carter, T. and Beresford, P. (2000) *Age and Change: Models of Involvement for Older People*. York: Joseph Rowntree Foundation

Clark, H. and Raynes, N. (2006) 'Addressing what older people want', in Raynes, N., Clark, H. and Beecham, J. (eds) *Evidence Submitted to the Older People's Inquiry into 'That Bit of Help'* (pp. 23–62). York: Joseph Rowntree Foundation

Copperman, J. and Morrison, P. (1995) *We Thought We Knew . . . Involving Patients in Nursing Practice*. London: King's Fund Centre

Crompton, S. (2004) 'New help for dementia is lost in a fug'. *The Times*, Body and Soul News, Saturday 1 May, pp. 4–5

Department of Health (1992) *The Patient's Charter*. London: HMSO

Dewar, B., Jones, C. and O'May, F. (2004) *Involving Older People: Lessons for Community Planning*. Social Justice Research Programme. Research Findings No. 9/2004. Edinburgh: Scottish Executive

Health Advisory Service 2000 [HAS] (1998) *Not Because They are Old: An Independent Inquiry into the Care of Older People on Acute Wards in General Hospitals*. London: HAS 2000

Hickey, G. and Kipping, C. (1998) 'Exploring the concept of user involvement in mental health through a participation continuum'. *Journal of Clinical Nursing*, 7 (1): 83–8

Mayer, J. and Timms, N. (1979) *The Client Speaks: Working Class Impressions of Casework*. New York: Atherton Press

NHS Executive (1999) *Patient and Public Involvement in the New NHS*. Leeds: NHS Executive

Richards, T. (1999) 'Patients' priorities: need to be assessed properly and taken into account'. *British Medical Journal*, 318: 277

Scottish Executive and NHS Health Scotland (2004) *Mental Health and Well-being in Later Life: Older People's Perceptions*. Edinburgh: Scottish Executive

Seltzer, M. and Kullberg, C. (2001) 'Foreword: Listening to Talk at Work in the Nordic Welfare Systems', in Seltzer, M., Kullberg, C., Olesen, S. and Rostila, I. (eds) *Listening to the Welfare State*. Aldershot: Ashgate

Wertheimer, A. (1993) *Speaking Out: Citizen Advocacy and Older People*. London: Centre for Policy on Ageing

Chapter 2

Older People: Economic and Demographic Challenges

Mike Danson

Learning outcomes

Reading this chapter will enable you to:

- explain some of the issues caused by changing demographic trends in the developed world, Europe and the UK;

- examine the challenges facing policy makers in the economic and labour market at regional and national level;

- explore strategies used to address demographic changes within the UK;

- discuss what policy changes may need to be implemented to address the shift in 'potential support ratio' in relation to the workforce and to carers.

INTRODUCTION

Many nations are considering strategies for a declining and ageing population, with policies and actions proposed around public and private concerns including pensions, the size of the workforce, the capacities of the health and social services, and so on. This chapter sets out to explore the issues of a declining and an ageing population, and goes on to consider the economic and labour market opportunities and potential advantages of these forecast changes as well as the problems and difficulties. A shrinking and an ageing workforce are discussed, and ageism and the older carer's role are addressed. The chapter then goes on to examine some of the proposed direct policy responses in the United Kingdom to these demographic developments, and takes Scotland as a case study in order to illustrate to students the importance of taking different national and indeed regional demographic variations into consideration. Active ageing is addressed, with discussion on how older people can and should be encouraged to continue to play full and active roles in society and the economy, and the chapter includes some specific lessons learned from elsewhere. This approach is deliberate as too much of the debate to date has been couched in terms of the negative affects of ageing, as if greater longevity and better health are not to be welcomed and celebrated. Finally, comparisons with European countries and developed countries are made throughout the chapter.

THE DECLINING POPULATION

By the middle of this century, virtually all the countries of Europe are expected to decrease in population size. The population of the geographical continent of Europe is set to decline by 100 million from 730 million. These changes will impact more strongly on some countries than others so, for example, the population of Italy, currently 57 million, is projected to decline to 41 million (United Nations, 2007).

By the year of the most recent Enlargement (2004), the European Commission was recording general patterns of underlying decline across the 15 EU member states, with only large-scale in-migration into the largest four countries offering some apparent stability; but all these member states were to have entered an era of falling populations by the third or fourth decade of the century. Similarly, six of the ten Accession countries were already in decline on entry and these falls were set to continue into the foreseeable future. The only exceptions across Europe would be the microstates, and to an extent England, which would face decline later than elsewhere because of in-migration from outside the continent. The declining population is also affecting countries outside Europe. Japan, for example, currently has a population of 127 million – projected to fall to 105 million by 2050 and the Russian Federation is expected to decrease from 147 million to 121 million between 2000 and 2050 (United Nations, 2007).

THE AGEING POPULATION

In addition to the decrease in population size, then, the countries of Europe are undergoing a relatively rapid ageing process. Indeed, all of the developed world is having to face the challenge of populations that are ageing as well as declining and these twin developments 'will require comprehensive reassessments of many established policies and programmes, including those relating to international migration' according to the United Nations (United Nations, 2007). They forecast a doubling in the proportion of people over 60 from 11 per cent to 22 per cent in the world as a whole, with a rise in numbers from 688 million in 2006 to 1968 million in 2050. The developed countries should expect an increase from 20 per cent to 32 per cent, though all regions of the world would see rising numbers and the ensuing significance of the over 60s. Much of the increase in developed countries would be among the eldest with a rise from 19 per cent to 32 per cent in the proportions of those over 60s who are 80 years or more. In Europe, there would be a rise from 21 per cent to 34 per cent in the over 60s, and eventually 28 per cent of these would be over 80. Southern European countries should anticipate over 40 per cent of their people being over 60 by 2050, with other European regions following these trends (United Nations, 2007).

Life expectancy at 60 does not vary greatly across the continent and is not expected to go up much in the near future but the median ages of all European countries are forecast to increase as a result of these various changes, typically rising from just over 40 to close to 50 years old.

THE WORKFORCE

The shrinking workforce

The ratio of the population aged 15 to 64 years to the population aged 65 or older, the 'Potential Support Ratio', is one way to measure the dependency of those over a particular age on those of working age – which itself is not necessarily stable nor fixed. Given expected ageing of these national and continental populations, this ratio would fall from four to two between 2006 and 2050, with little variation across Europe.

While there has been much attention on barriers to recruitment into work, perhaps more significance and attention should be on retaining workers in the labour market. It is clear that for all age groups a period of detachment from the field of work can generate negative behaviours, such as negative attitudes from employers and the loss of self esteem and confidence in individuals plus the erection of other barriers to re-engagement.

The older workforce

Part of the solution to poverty and financial distress for older people is greater flexibility over retirement. This would mean that older people would be able to continue to lead active and involved lives and to contribute to society and the economy across several dimensions of life. Already, a significant proportion of the labour force is now working beyond State Pension Age and this is likely to be encouraged in the future as people enjoy longer, healthier lives. Often financial hardship is an important reason to continue working, with those groups of men and women with the highest probability of labour market participation being those with outstanding mortgages on their properties. This is one of the main reasons that the UK has higher rates of working among older men and women than most of continental Europe. Working past state pension age has become more prevalent in other countries such as the USA and Japan and is likely to be a future trend in the UK. By contrast, one half of men and one third of women now retire before state pension age and this is likely to be progressive: each cohort of men appears less likely to remain in employment at older ages so these trends cannot simply be explained as a consequence of the downturn in the economy during the 1980s and 1990s but rather part of an ongoing process. Because older people are becoming embedded into the economy and culture of the workforce, not least within public sector employment, there is a greater imperative to proactively reverse these trends before the higher participation rates are a necessity. Scotland has addressed this issue and the Scottish Government's Talent Management Taskforce (Economic and Social Research Council, 2008) has been considering the effects of an ageing workforce over 2007–08.

Although industrial restructuring can partly explain the current low rates of employment in many regions and rural areas, the shrinking employment share of those over 50 has taken place in both growing and declining industries, confirming that this problem will not disappear as the workforce moves into newer sectors over time. So, age discrimination against older workers appears to be deeply embedded in the cultures, policies and practices of many organisations and industries. However, service sector employers generally exhibit a more positive orientation to older workers, and this should increase the range of employment opportunities for older people both now and progressively into the future. Getting it right early rather than panicking in the decades to come should offer a better solution in the long run (Scottish Executive, 2007). Indeed, generally, those countries such as Scotland which are facing significant population changes have tended to react early. Others with continuing population growth have been less active in seeking strategies to address an ageing society. There are differences in the preparedness of different countries, therefore, to population decline and ageing.

Age discrimination

Within wider European Union priorities for inclusion, the UK government have legislated against age discrimination in employment and vocational training, with acts to address both age and disability discrimination (EHRC, 2008). In a flexible labour market, lifelong learning has become increasingly important but there are a number of barriers to older people gaining training. Examples of such barriers include:

- previously interrupted learning;
- lack of current opportunities;
- lack of local provision;
- cost of courses;
- accessibility and transport;
- confidence about ability;
- perceived lack of necessary qualifications;
- and a lack of relevant and interesting courses.

Employers often perceive older workers as not in need of training and are sometimes disinterested in personal development opportunities. As a result, older workers (who tend to have fewer formal qualifications in the first place) can be less likely to be provided with training opportunities. Some of these barriers will diminish over time as the proportion of graduates – who have a much higher propensity to be offered and to gain from training throughout life – increases in the workforce, but this will threaten to deepen divides between those with further and higher education qualifications and the 50 per cent of the population who do not have such qualifications. Other barriers will still affect most older workers, however, and these will require specific attention.

OLDER PEOPLE AS CARERS

In the future, caring responsibilities are likely to have an ever increasing impact on the working lives of many older workers. Already one in six employees have carer responsibilities and of the six million carers in the UK, it is thought that half are aged between 50 and 64. Of course, many carers are over 65 and they are critical to the efficient functioning of the labour market for many younger workers. However, there is particular pressure on those close to the 'traditional retirement ages' to withdraw themselves from active paid work in favour of this unpaid caring whether it is for grandchildren or older relatives. As parents and older relatives live longer, average family size reduces and fewer young people are available for recruitment into the caring sectors, so these demands will increase. The role of care giver impacts more on women and results in a barrier to paid employment.

There are strong reasons based on inclusion and cohesion for ensuring that markets are open and free from both age and gender discrimination and all barriers to participation in the work place should be removed. Future demographic time bombs should be an excuse for accelerating the importance of this. Each developed nation has to confront these issues and most are anticipating comparable transformations. In doing so, many countries are conducting policy initiatives to address the projected demographic changes.

STRATEGIES TO ADDRESS DEMOGRAPHIC CHANGES IN THE UK

The United Nations set out the international priorities for older people with the aim 'to add life to the years that have been added to life' (United Nations, 1999). The aim is to ensure that priority attention will be given to the situation of older persons. The UN Principles address the independence, participation, care, self-fulfilment and dignity of older persons. Many countries and regions have based their strategies on the contents of this document.

Notably, within the UK, it can be seen that while the UK-wide, but effectively English, treatment of many of the issues has been dominated by the caring agenda (see 'With Respect to Old Age: Long-term Care – Rights and Responsibilities. A Report by the Royal Commission on Long Term Care', CM4192), there have been initiatives since devolution in 1999 which are more innovative and more broadly-based. These divergences in practice and policy between the different nations are briefly addressed below.

- In England, *The National Service Framework (NSF) for Older People* (Department of Health, 2001) consists of ten priorities for older people and there is also the more recent *New Ambition for Old Age: Next Steps in Implementing the National Service Framework for Older People* (Department of Health, 2006).
- Northern Ireland has undergone a restructuring of health and social services between 2006 and 2008 and has an inclusive strategic

approach for its total population, the 'Priorities for Action' strategy sets out a planning framework for health, social and public safety services in 2006–2008 (Department of Health, Social Security and Public Safety, 2006).

- The publication of *The Strategy for Older People in Wales* in 2003 by the Welsh Assembly Government (Welsh Assembly Government, 2003), with the establishment of a Commissioner for Older People (the first in Europe), has been widely acknowledged for its progressiveness. There is also the *National Service Framework for Older People in Wales* (Welsh Assembly Government, 2006), which addresses health and social care services for older people across primary, secondary and community care.
- The Scottish strategy *All our Futures: Planning for a Scotland with an Ageing Population* (Scottish Executive, 2007) is similar to the Welsh strategy, in that the data and analysis that informed these strategies and subsequent implementation demonstrate the advantages of cohesive and integrated approaches within smaller nations.

The involvement of older people in the development of strategy in the UK is also consistent with the Joseph Rowntree Foundation's view that 'older people are themselves major providers of support to other older people, as well as active supporters of families and communities', tellingly reported in the *Older People Shaping Policy and Practice* publication (Joseph Rowntree Foundation, 2004).

Activity 1

How and why do the strategies for older people vary across the nations of the UK? Which are best suited for the needs of the economy and society and how well informed are they by good practice elsewhere in the world?

SCOTLAND AS A CASE STUDY

One of the advantages for Scotland is that demographic changes tend to happen slowly and so reasonable plans can be put in place to address the challenges (Scotland's Futures Forum, 2007). This allows the Scottish Government and civic society to consider what politics and strategies are suitable for the future health and wellbeing of the Scottish economy and people (Scottish Executive, 2007). Also, as Scotland is not alone in exploring these issues, knowledge exchange and good practice can be transferred between countries.

Key issues relating to Scotland's population

Scotland can be regarded as a typical small European country and therefore can learn from the experiences and strategies of comparable nations, and the issues and challenges facing this nation illustrate what is developing elsewhere. Scotland is not like England, however. England's population is expected to continue to expand by another 6 million to reach almost 57 million by 2031, and then to continue to grow to be 61.4 million by 2074. Scotland is also unlike the USA, whose population is forecast to grow from 290 million now to 354 million in 2031 and to 477 million in 2074. Yet these countries are the two sources of much of Scotland's social and economic policies and interventions. It is therefore imperative for all countries that the needs of the economy and society are based on analyses of sensible and reasonable comparisons and not on those of countries facing such markedly different demographic futures.

Population forecasts tend to be fairly stable over time, especially with regard to the numbers in age groups over 30–35. There is therefore a good deal of confidence in the projections for the next few decades of the actual numbers of those over statutory retirement age. The challenges in meeting their demands can be addressed in the context of adequate forewarning of the dimensions of their likely caring needs. Similarly, better policies and attitudes towards the more able among them can help with potential supply problems in the labour market. However, both these aspects of society and the economy require proactive interventions now to ensure desirable outcomes.

The paths of development of Scotland and the Nordic countries and Ireland in particular have diverged markedly over the last century, confirming that significant population shifts are nothing new and reflect long-term differentials in economic growth rates. Demographic and economic change are inextricably linked – improve economic performance in the latter and some of the population issues can be revised to the mutual benefit of the country, migrants and all age groups, as will be discussed below. Scotland was one of the first countries to recognise the implications of demographic change and has a long history of living with emigration and local depopulation. Critically, as a society, Scotland may be more willing than most to embrace some quite radical measures to overcome issues raised by population decline and ageing.

Scotland in line with the rest of the UK is part of a number of wider political organisations. The European Union and United Kingdom Parliament both reserve significant powers over relevant policy and strategic matters, so discussion on policy change has to recognise changes and concerns elsewhere. Importantly for Scotland, however, the evolving demographic issues it faces are quite different from those in the rest of the UK and are much closer to those being experienced by some of our other European neighbours. Policy initiatives and lessons from the Nordic countries especially are of interest here, but experiences and lessons appear relevant from across the globe. Therefore, while there are some general points of principle and lessons to be shared across borders and boundaries, the specific circumstances, policies and issues facing particular countries need to be considered carefully.

In the following section the population changes expected to happen in Scotland are discussed, and they are compared and contrasted with changes in the world, Europe and the UK.

Demographic change in Scotland

What is most remarkable about the evolution of the population profile of Scotland over the last century is that it is unremarkable! It is almost the same now as it was in 1951, has hardly varied since and is not expected to change much till the 2030s. Underneath this apparent stability there have been some very interesting flows and structural changes at work, and many of these will shape the next half-century or more. The last 80 years have seen major improvements in health and wellbeing for all ages. This has led to people living longer, as their general standards of living have risen over the decades. These long-term and well-established trends in birth and death rates are set to continue into the foreseeable future.

For much of the twentieth century Scotland lost significant numbers of people through migration to England and overseas. However, during the last decade this has been gradually reversing with both return migration and, recently, migrant workers from central and eastern Europe – especially Poland. What will happen over the next 20–25 years will be dependent on further economic changes – in-migration is driven by job opportunities. Although the population will eventually start to fall slowly, there will continue to be more households being created than disappearing.

Given what has been encouraging migration into and out of Scotland in recent times, the best estimates of demographic changes (GROS, 2007)

27

show a gradual rise in population from 5.09 million in 2006 to reach the highest ever levels of 5.37 million in 2031 before slowly declining to fall below 5 million in 2076. These changes illustrate, firstly, the significance of migration in reversing short-term trends and secondly that, even in the long run, falls do not point to a crisis. As migrants are encouraged by economic potential and policy to come to Scotland then stability looks assured for the coming decades. However, below these totals are some significant structural developments. The proportion of children (under 16) will fall from 18 per cent now to 16 per cent in 2031, with 64 thousand fewer than today. As family sizes have been reducing from the early 1960s there have been impacts on succeeding generations so that the proportions in the working age cohorts will decline from 62.8 per cent in 2006 to 60 per cent in 2031. This will mean 14 thousand fewer potential workers than now, but with an ageing workforce. The most dramatic changes will be felt in terms of the older groups. Most of the increase (by 31.1 per cent or 306 thousand) in those of 'pensionable age' (which is 65 for men, 60 for women until 2010; between 2010 and 2020 pensionable age for women increases to 65) will be among the over 75s; their numbers will rise by 81 per cent to reach 692 thousand. Therefore, by 2031, one in eight people will be over 75.

Considering these changes in terms of the projected numbers of dependants versus population of working age, these are expected to remain fairly stable until 2021 and then to increase from 60 to 67 per hundred. While the ratios of children and of those between pensionable age and 75 to working age adults should be between 48 and 45 per hundred for much of this period, the numbers of those over 75 will almost double from 12 to 21 per hundred. This is widely perceived as representing the greatest challenge to the economy and society. While there is a long period of grace ahead, when Scotland can seek to raise economic activity rates by addressing the barriers to employment faced by many older workers, by those in successive NEET (not in employment, education or training) groups and by others disadvantaged in the labour market, and can encourage new migrant workers and return migrants, there are both limits on these strategies and outstanding issues with the position and status of the very old in society.

Households

A critical but often neglected dimension of demographic change concerns the formation, dissolution and evolution of households. Smaller family sizes, the enhanced mobility of people within and outwith Scotland, as well as the ageing of society all impact on the development of households. So while the number of people is expected to be hardly changed by 2024, current predictions suggest there will be 11 per cent or 300 thousand more households than in 2004. The starkest change is the predicted rise by 47 per cent for men and by 33 per cent for women in the proportion of one-person households. One implication of these changes will be that the average size of a household will have fallen from 2.22 to 1.97, with the cities, islands and remote rural areas tending to have household sizes even lower than this average. Behind these changes are the ageing of the population and other social developments. The number and proportion of households headed by all groups over 55 are expected to increase, and someone over 'pensionable age' will be head of almost a third of homes by 2024 and those aged over 75 will be head of one sixth. These forecasts imply that substantially higher proportions of those over 75 and especially women (70 per cent of the over 85s) will be the only persons in their households. These changes will have profound implications for individuals and families, whether they are living together or not, and for society and service providers alike.

In 2007, the Scottish Government introduced a national debate on demographic change, encouraging immigration and continuing residence by students (through the Fresh Talent Initiative) and migrant workers (through active participation in UK-wide recruitment of labour from Poland and other EU countries) and addressing ageing through strategic developments (including the 'Strategy for an Ageing Scotland', Scottish Government, 2007). It was reacting to projections of population decline and ageing that were extreme if not unique in Europe. The reality, it has become clear, is that Scotland is in fact absolutely typical of countries throughout Europe and the developed world.

Participating in society

The most recent poverty estimates (New Policy Institute, 2007) suggest the proportion of Scottish pensioners living in low income households is almost one in five (average of 18 per cent for both singles and couples) in the years 2003/04 to 2005/06. However, relatively, pensioners are now less likely to be living in low income households than non-pensioners. Of those pensioners on low incomes, about a fifth were more than £50 per week below the low income threshold at that time. The incidence of pensioner poverty is similar to the rest of the United Kingdom, but within Scotland those on guaranteed Pension Credit (a good proxy for low incomes) in Glasgow, Eilean Siar and West Dunbartonshire are more than double the rates in East Dunbartonshire and East Renfrewshire. Links between poverty and deprivation during childhood, working age years and ill health are well-established, and these carry over into later life. The high incidence of multiple deprivations in the cities, old industrial communities and some remote rural areas affect all ages but can impact heavily on old vulnerable members of the community. Those living alone and in disadvantaged neighbourhoods are particularly at risk of poor health, morbidity and shortened life expectancy.

Over the next quarter century Scots are likely to experience even more changes in their family circumstances and, in particular, live a greater part of their life alone. Although they may be living longer, the real threat is that more years of ill health will be experienced. Rather than a healthy active later life, the additional years are more likely to be a time of suffering from chronic disease and mental ill-health problems. With divided communities and with many still trapped in the outfall from the deindustrialisation and worklessness of the 1980s and 90s, an even wider gap is developing in terms of health outcomes and behaviours depending on where in Scotland people are born and grow up. There is a direct link between the achievement of a long, active and healthy working life and a happy and lengthy retirement. Looking to how these can be promoted for all and so how an inclusive and cohesive society can be realised for all citizens presents the greatest challenge facing Scotland in the twenty-first century, and this issue is more than a simple focus on the size of the working population.

At the end of 2008 economic activity rates were at an all time high, there is still a strong declining trend after 50 with increasing numbers of workers taking early retirement or spending several years on incapacity benefits before retiring. As older workers become progressively higher proportions of the potential workforce so this exclusion will become critical to the ability of the Scottish economy to provide services to all its population, raise sufficient public finance to fund health and education for all, to improve its productivity and performance, etc. Also, if men and women in Scotland in the future could attain the traditional levels of labour force participation of men over 50, then it would go a significant way to closing the demographic gap in the size of the workforce after 2030. Removing the barriers to continuing economic activity therefore becomes the priority, and removing poor employer attitudes and (mis-) information regarding older workers is an essential element of this.

As well as lower levels of economic activity the potential effects of workforce ageing should not be exaggerated and are relatively small, but do include:

- increased employer costs – though these are neither inevitable nor without society compensations;

- reduced labour mobility and reduced voluntary levels of staff turnover – again there are often compensations to employers in savings on recruitment costs, retention of skills and experiences;
- ageing of the stock of knowledge and skills – which can also be interpreted as retaining and enhancing embedded knowledge and experience;
- ill health and disability within the labour force – though the data on this are not as conclusive as might appear, with the encouragement of older workers on to incapacity benefits distorting figures and analyses.

(Scotland's Futures Forum, 2007)

A healthy working life

Reflecting good practice elsewhere, the UK and Scottish Government are supporting a general approach of promoting a healthy working life. They appear to limit this, however, to the period up to the statutory pension age. Removing this qualification would go much of the way to confirming that the UK was progressing towards a society which discounted age, as well as gender, race, disability, religion, skin colour, as reasons for exclusion. So, revising their philosophy by replacing 'work' with 'activity[ies]', the pursuit of a healthy working life comes to mean 'continuously providing . . . people with the opportunity, ability, support and encouragement to *be active* in ways and in an environment which allows them to sustain and improve their health and wellbeing. It means that individuals are empowered and enabled to do as much as possible, for as long as possible, or as long as they want, in both their working and non-working lives' (Scottish Executive, 2005).

Active ageing

A healthy life depends upon far more than the absence of disease or infirmity. It demands that individuals maximise what is sometimes called 'functional capacity' – the physical, mental and social capacity to make a positive contribution to society and gain the maximum satisfaction and consequent benefit from our life. This involves improving people's fitness for the activities they choose, equipping them to undertake such activities and adjusting expectations of fitness, as the activities available or personal circumstances change. This is as much about having appropriate skills, knowledge and being able to be active in a safe and supportive environment that does not cause unnecessary stress or strain, as it is about physical wellbeing.

Then addressing the needs of people as workers, volunteers, tourists, consumers and pensioners becomes the objective of the strategy for an ageing population by making age irrelevant to considerations of inclusion.

LESSONS FROM ABROAD AND OTHER CULTURES

The economy and community have a common interest, therefore, in ensuring that people are able to live healthy and active lives for as long as possible. Wellbeing and happiness are both promoted by better access to opportunities for volunteering, leisure, caring, domestic duties, civic responsibilities and work. Such an approach to healthy and active living is increasingly promoted throughout Europe through a number of strategies and means (see Ilmarinen, 2006 for a very good survey and proposed strategy (CEC, 2005)). Lessons can be learned from these without disrupting the underlying culture that has given the smaller UK countries their own capacities to adapt to the massive changes of the last 25 years. In the case of Scotland, it was to welcome migrants, refugees and asylum seekers and, over a much longer period, to retain its own identity and nationhood which have made the rest possible.

Transnational work demonstrates that the standard model of later years implies reaching a statutory retirement age (if not being given redundancy before this), giving up work completely and then progressively withdrawing from other areas of life entirely. This contrasts with the now preferred model where flexible working, retirement, volunteering, and other activities are stressed and encouraged so that involvement and inclusion are prolonged for as long as the individual and community consider reasonable. Such a pattern should lead to a healthy life expectancy beyond the usual model, avoiding the 'cliff edge' or 'guillotine' retirement, where the scrap heap beckons regardless of personal or economic capacities, experiences or needs.

The idea of flexible lifestyles has been embraced readily within the Nordic countries, where economic activity rates are already high, work–life balance appreciated, women's participation and involvement in civic life better established, inclusion and a cohesive society promoted. These are among the most successful economies and societies in the world; they have a clearer social contract between state, citizen and enterprise with a public fiscal and expenditure philosophy to achieve coherence and inclusion. Addressing the demographic issues of ageing and decline, and the not unrelated dimensions of potential spatial divides, is much easier in that context than in an unbridled market system or one dominated by the needs of a state with a population that is forecast to continue expanding for many decades.

Proposals from Finland based on multinational studies and dialogues are designed to establish such approaches more deeply within society (Ilmarinen, 2006). Finland was faced with similar problems to those Scotland is confronting so it made promoting health and functional capacity and raising the retirement age their first priorities. Demonstrating what can be achieved, even within a fairly short time scale, 'employment among the ageing population was successfully improved and the retirement age began to rise as a result of legislative amendments and improved efficiency for action programmes' (Lehto, 2006). Nevertheless, the dependency ratio continues to deteriorate, globalisation and international competition is growing and even the regional and social differences are increasing. However, and reflecting the position in Scotland because of a common awareness of the challenges, 'after ten years of hard work, [they] are better prepared to cope with the challenge of an ageing population. Nevertheless, work in this area must continue' (Lehto, 2006). In particular, 'implementation problems have come to the fore'. Strategies and policies are being developed which address the same challenges as are faced in Scotland, as the demographic and economic contexts are comparable these offer solutions that can be modified for Scottish circumstances. That they are based on international studies and dialogues strengthens the power of their significance for Scotland.

STRATEGIES FOR THE FUTURE

In setting out a strategy acceptable to the private and public purse, moving *Towards a Longer Worklife* (Ilmarinen, 2006), which is both healthy and without functional limitations, is an objective which can be pursued through a number of changes to society, the workforce and the workplace. First, all stages of life once again should be seeking to support parallelism of life's phases so that training, work, leisure time, building families and solidarity between the generations becomes the norm rather than being undertaken at different ages. Second, more attention needs to be paid to the future demands of mental and social wellbeing, including what is required for the workplace. This means providing part-time work where this is compatible with individuals' financial requirements, support for those for whom their working life has not been without physical and mental stress, and the opportunity for shorter careers for those who have shorter life expectancies. In many ways this suggests that a flexible retirement system is required that recognises that life has not been fair to some and those who are best able to continue working should be encouraged to do so, for the sake of the community.

Third, working hours are already very long in the UK while, for many, incapacities, unemployment and early retirement have reduced their employment activities to an undesired zero hours. Reduced work hours should be pursued more aggressively including for those where 'exclusions' have been agreed as longer hours often lead to negative long-term impacts on health and wellbeing. Age management is part of this, with shortening hours being an element of the package towards a flexible retirement. Justice in retirement planning and entitlements is vital to the social acceptance of change, with consideration of the needs for sectors and small and medium enterprises (SMEs) especially important. Given that the government has identified the demographic challenge as critical to UK development, the interests of all social partners need to be addressed. The Finns propose adjusting the indirect workforce costs of older employees accordingly. Similar actions to include others disadvantaged in the economy should be introduced at the same time so that one group of workers or the inactive are not substituted for another.

Unlike in many other areas of economic and social policy, it is to Europe rather than North America that such lessons and good practice can be and are being looked for. The NHS, social security and welfare regimes in all parts of the UK are still closer to the rest of the European Union than to the private and market-driven regimes of the US (see Taylor, 2006; Vickerstaff *et al.*, 2007).

CONCLUSIONS

Many developed countries are beginning to face challenges from an ageing and declining population. Poverty and ill health in old age are an increasing issue for many communities in societies such as the UK where there are significant levels of inequality. Proposals and strategies have been constructed by the UK government and each of the devolved countries that are informed by the experiences of other EU countries and elsewhere. These cover health and wellbeing, shift work and ageing, public policy programmes, actions for new talent management at workplaces and for a better work life for all ages. Flexibility and appropriate actions that are consistent with the needs of the UK economy and society are being identified, but their utility across the whole of the UK continues to be debated.

Activity 2

Write a short summary on the latest policy/strategy for an ageing population in your country. Then go on to look at any strategies that are available locally to address the issues concerning an ageing population within your district/region. Does national policy reflect the regional policy? Give reasons why there may be differences.

Websites are given below to help you access the data available at national level.

FURTHER READING

CEC (2005) *Confronting Demographic Change: A New Solidarity Between the Generations*. 94 final. Brussels: Commission of the European Communities

Ilmarinen, J. (2006) *Towards a Longer Worklife! Ageing and the Quality of Worklife in The European Union*. Helsinki: Finnish Institute of Occupational Health and the Ministry of Social Affairs and Health

Joseph Rowntree Foundation (2004) *Older People Shaping Policy and Practice*. **www.jrf.org.uk/knowledge/findings/foundations/044.asp** (Accessed 3 December 2008)

Scotland's Futures Forum (2007) *Growing Older and Wiser Together: a Future's View of Positive Ageing*. **www.scotlandfutureforum.org/sff/forum%20age. pdf** (Accessed 9 August 2008)

Websites

Centre for Policy on Ageing (England)
www.cpa.org.uk/policies_on_ageing.html

EHRC (2008) Equality and Discrimination webpages
www.equalityhumanrights.com/en/yourrights/equalityanddiscrimination/ Pages/EqualityHome.aspx

Scotland's Futures Forum (2007) 'Growing Older and Wiser Together: A Future's View of Positive Ageing', Scottish Parliament
www.scotlandfutureforum.org/sff/forum%20age.pdf

Scottish Government (2007) 'All Our Futures: Planning for a Scotland with an Ageing Population', Edinburgh
www.scotland.gov.uk/Resource/Doc/169342/0047172.pdf

UN Principles for Older Persons (1999)
www.un.org/esa/socdev/iyop/iyoppop.htm

Welsh Assembly Government 'The Strategy for Older People in Wales'
http://new.wales.gov.uk/about/strategy/strategypublications/strategy_olderpeople/?lang=en
http://new.wales.gov.uk/docrepos/ 40371/288363/571684/1043756/1043768/OP(06-07)06-Annexes_A_and_B.doc?lang=en
http://new.wales.gov.uk/strategy/strategies/2166490/strategyphaseII.doc?lang=en

Information for Northern Ireland
www.ark.ac.uk/services/olderpeopleni.html
www.ageconcernni.org/pdf/Policy%20Booklet.pdf

REFERENCES

CEC (2005) *Green Paper* 'Confronting Demographic Change: A New Solidarity Between the Generations', 94 final. Brussels: Commission of the European Communities

Department of Health (2001) *The National Service Framework for Older People*. London: DoH

Department of Health (2006) 'New ambition for old age: next steps in implementing the National service framework for older people'. London: DoH

Department of Health, Social Security and Public Safety (2006) *Priorities for Action*. Belfast: DHSSPS

Economic and Social Research Council (2008)
www.esrcsocietytoday.ac.uk/ESRCInfoCentre/Images/Talent%20management%20and%20the%20older%20workforce_tcm6-26383.pdf (Accessed 15 August 2008)

EHRC (2008) Equality and Discrimination webpages,
www.equalityhumanrights.com/en/yourrights/equalityanddiscrimination/Pages/EqualityHome.aspx (Accessed 9 August 2008)

Future Skills Scotland (2007) *Labour Market Projections 2007–2017*. Glasgow: FSS.

GROS (General Register Office for Scotland) (2007) *Projected Population of Scotland (2006-Based)*. Edinburgh: GROS

Ilmarinen, J. (2006) *Towards a Longer Worklife! Ageing and the Quality of Worklife in the European Union*. Helsinki: Finnish Institute of Occupational Health and the Ministry of Social Affairs and Health

Joseph Rowntree Foundation (2004) *Older People Shaping Policy and Practice.* York: JRF

Lehto, M. (2006) *Strategies for Social Protection 2015 – Towards a Socially and Economically Sustainable Society*, Ministry of Social Affairs and Health's publications 2006:16, **stm.teamware.com/Resource.phx/publishing/ documents/8284/index.htx** (Accessed 14 October 2008)

New Policy Institute (2007) 'Older people in lower income households', London, **www.poverty.org.uk/S38/index.shtml** (Accessed 9 August 2008)

Scotland's Futures Forum (2007) *Growing Older and Wiser Together: A Future's View of Positive Ageing.* Scottish Parliament, **www.scotlandfutureforum.org/ sff/forum%20age.pdf** (Accessed 9 August 2008)

Scottish Executive (2005) *Healthy Working Lives: A Plan for Action,* **www. scotland.gov.uk/Resource/Doc/924/0034156.pdf** (Accessed 14 October 2008)

Scottish Executive (2007) *All Our Futures: Planning for a Scotland with an Ageing Population.* Edinburgh: Scottish Office, **www.scotland.gov.uk/ Resource/Doc/169342/0047172.pdf** (Accessed 9 August 2008)

Scottish Government (2007) *Strategies for an Ageing Population.* Scottish Government: Edinburgh

Taylor, P. (2006) *Employment Initiatives for an Ageing Workforce in the EU15.* European Foundation for the Improvement of Living and Working Conditions, **www.eurofound.europa.eu/pubdocs/2006/39/en/1/ef0639en. pdf** (Accessed 9 August 2008)

United Nations (1999) *Principles for Older Persons,* **www.un.org/esa/socdev/ iyop/iyoppop.htm** (Accessed 9 August 2008)

United Nations (2007) *World Population Projections 2007.* New York: United Nations.

Vickerstaff, S., Loretto, W. and White, P. (2007) *The Future for Older Workers: New Perspectives.* Policy Press: Bristol

Welsh Assembly Government (2003) *Strategy for Older People in Wales.* Cardiff: WAG

Welsh Assembly Government (2006) *National Service Framework for Older People in Wales.* Cardiff: WAG

Chapter 3

Sociology and Ageing

Anne Llewellyn

INTRODUCTION

The sociological understanding of old age is concerned with understanding and explaining the social construction of ageing, as well as the diversity of subjective experiences of older people themselves. Traditionally, old age has been conceptualised as a transition within the life course, where the life cycle is divided into a number of different periods, related to chronological age. Thus, old age is a social construction, based on the notion of belonging to a distinct phase of the life course at a given age. However, there has been a tendency within traditional approaches to see older people as a homogenous group, sharing similar characteristics and experiences.

Social gerontology is a relatively new sub-discipline of sociology and offers a more critical approach to the understanding of old age. It is concerned with three inter-related issues: people's experiences over their life course, the impact of age-related social structures and institutions on the personal experience of ageing and the dynamic interplay between people and structures, as they both influence each other (Riley and Riley, 1999). Within this perspective, there is an acknowledgement of the diverse range of experiences of older people, based on location within the social system, as well as the impact of institutional processes.

> . . . the variability of the ageing process is one of the few truly universal social principles.
>
> (Riley and Riley, 1999: 125)

The aim of this chapter, therefore, is to explore the different sociological theories of ageing and discuss how they can contribute to an understanding of old age and developments in clinical practice with older people.

Learning outcomes

Reading this chapter will enable you to:

- explain a range of social definitions of ageing;
- describe the social processes and factors that impact on experiences of ageing;
- explain the relationship between stereotypes of older people and ageist practices;
- reflect on how an understanding of sociological perspectives can aid reflection on our own personal values and attitudes to older people.

AGE STRATIFICATION THEORY

Age stratification theory assumes that people can be grouped according to chronological age, and it can be assumed that they will have similar experiences and age-related abilities. Therefore, within this theory, social context is important for understanding the meaning of old age and the relative position of old people in relation to other age groups in that society. In Western industrial societies, the period of old age is related to the social construction of the category of retirement, and the processes of allocation of resources are based on social definition and the construction of relative worth of age cohorts.

Chronological age as an indicator of old age is associated with the institution of pension provision in the UK under the 1908 Pensions Act, providing pensions for those over 70 who were deemed eligible (Thane, 1982; Laybourn, 1995). Pensions were further developed under the Beveridge blueprint for Social Insurance in 1942, providing provision through an insurance system and establishing the age of entitlement at 65 for men and 60 for women. This system was based on the ideology of the male breadwinner model of the family, making assumptions that women would be provided for by their husbands (Baldwin and Falkingham, 1994). The different ages of eligibility for men and women were also based on the patriarchal ideology of the male breadwinner family, based on the assumption that, on average, women marry men two years their senior and therefore setting different ages for eligibility would allow for more equal timing of the access to pension provision (the age at which men and women are eligible to receive the state pension was equalised to 65 in 1995).

There is no clear rationale for the choice of age of eligibility for pensions, which has largely been adopted as the retirement age in the UK and other industrialised societies. Predicating the category of old age on this basis can therefore be seen as a social construction. There is limited evidence of people's reduced ability to work as they age, depending on the nature of the work, but increasingly the age of 65 or 60 has been seen as the norm for withdrawal from the labour market for most men and women (Phillipson, 1998).

Within age stratification theory, there is an assumption of homogeneity among older people, where they are assumed to display the same characteristics and have similar experiences and circumstances. Nevertheless, the theory is useful for exploring the power that underpins social definitions and it helps to explain the relative value of different social groups within a divided society. Evaluation of the worth and status of each group is based on dominant social values, with power being used to marginalise certain groups economically, politically and socially. However, age stratification theory poses problems when trying to make cross-cultural comparisons. Age is not calculated according to annual birthdays in some countries (for example, Bangladesh) and therefore population structures look quite different from Western models (Wilson, 2000).

While all societies base the notion of old age on a social construction, the experience of old age varies between societies. In simple terms, it can be generalised that pre-industrial societies see old age as a period of value and status within the society where older people are revered by younger generations. Yet, in industrialised societies, old age is seen as a period of denigration, decline and low status (Hunt, 2005). As an illustration of this, Fischer (1978) identified four significant historical periods of attitudes to older people in the USA (which are mirrored throughout other industrialised countries):

1. A period of veneration, where older people were valued and revered (approximately 1607–1820 in the Western world).
2. A period associated with industrialisation in the Western world, with increasing emphasis on the values and virtues of the young (from 1750s onwards). Older people started to be denigrated, which is reflected in the fact that pejorative terms for older people started

to enter into the languages of USA and Europe (e.g. the term 'fogey' first entered American language in this period).
3. Consolidation of the increased emphasis on the values and virtues of youth. Fischer argued that this encompassed the period from the 1800s to approximately 1970, although many would argue that it is still manifest today (see below).
4. From the 1970s onwards, older people have increasingly been seen as a burden, requiring welfare intervention.

The age of 65 as a chronological indicator of old age has become firmly embedded in institutional practices within health and social care in the UK. For example, the specialism of geriatric medicine developed in the 1930s and 1940s with the pioneering work of Marjorie Warren (Bernard and Philips, 1998) and mental health services are structured around people of working age, with an additional category for the over 65s. The impact of this has been to see the over 65s as a distinct category of the population, with different needs to other groups, rather than seeing ageing as part of a normal transition within the life course.

FUNCTIONALIST THEORIES OF AGEING

Functionalist sociologists are concerned with social roles and how these roles inter-relate and contribute to the smooth functioning of society and the maintenance of equilibrium. Early sociological theories of old age focussed on social roles and, in particular, withdrawal from the labour market (disengagement theory). Cumming and Henry (1961) said that it was natural for older people to withdraw from society as this helped to protect the stability of society, as younger people are able to take on the relinquished social roles. The process is seen as natural and mutual, as society also withdraws its commitment from older people. The process is seen as advantageous, as older people disengage from the roles of adult life in order to embark upon personally fulfilling activities.

In contrast to disengagement theory, Havighurst's (1963) activity theory argued that normal ageing does not necessitate the relinquishing of roles, but that successful ageing requires a substantial amount of social activity and formal and informal social actions. Havighurst suggested that personal wellbeing is dependent on social activity, rather than disengagement.

Functionalist theories can be criticised for the assumptions that are made and for their lack of analysis of power and political and economic distribution of resources. There is no universal pattern of disengagement from the labour market, nor is there a norm of social activity, and rather than being a time of personal fulfilment and social activity, for a significant number of older people, older age is a time of impoverishment and declining health. Levels of engagement and disengagement will therefore depend on previous life experiences, and the pattern of economic and health inequalities and access to opportunities in working age life will continue into retirement.

Disengagement theory has been criticised as it portrays old age as a period of inevitable negative experiences and fails to acknowledge the increased levels of activity that some older people may experience (Tanner and Harris, 2008). While some roles may be lost, new roles and activities may be engaged with (see later discussion about caring roles, grandparenting and older consumers). In their research into older people's perceptions of quality of life, it was found that the opportunity to engage with new hobbies and activities was not only valued by older people, but was also an important factor in life satisfaction. Disengagement theory has been further criticised as it provides the justification for policies and practices that segregate older people, contributing to the isolation and marginalisation of older people (Tanner and Harris, 2008).

In addition, the retirement age creates a category of dependence. As people are required to leave the labour market, they become dependent on other sources of income, including state provided pensions, funded through public expenditure. This leads to concerns about the increasing burden on the treasury and the rising cost of providing for a growing number of pensioners. Phillipson and Walker (1986) have argued that structural and institutional processes have led to categorisation of older people as dependent and with the increasing numbers of older people, and the growing longevity of the population, increasing numbers of older people have become reliant on welfare provision to meet these culturally created needs (for example, state pensions). Within this perspective, the state has three important functions:

- the allocation of scarce resources;
- mediation between different groups in society;
- addressing the conditions that threaten social order.

(Estes, 2001)

Phillipson and Walker (1986) refer to this as the burden of dependency thesis, where older people have come to be viewed as a problem for the welfare state, due to the rising costs of sustaining this provision, which contributes to the negative image of older people. This may, in turn, lead to intergenerational conflict, as groups become segregated and compete against each other for resources (Attias-Donfurt and Arber, 2000). In particular, concerns have been raised about the relationship between workers and pensioners and the priorities for different groups (Phillipson, 1998).

Although the burden of dependency thesis has been criticised for failing to acknowledge the diversity of old age and its positive aspects, it does reflect a dominant view that old age has come to be seen as a social problem at an economic and societal level. However, this is not a universal view of ageing, with older people being integrated within many societies across the globe (Wilson, 2000).

Nevertheless, in the industrialised world, old age is seen as a social problem for individuals. The understanding of old age as a social problem derives from a biological model of ageing, which views old age as a period of inevitable physical decline and increasing dependency (Victor, 2005). Biological theories are reductionist and tend to make the assumption that these processes are universal and occur in a uniform way as we age, failing to acknowledge diversity and the impact of social, environmental and psychological factors on the processes and experiences of ageing.

Sociologists have argued that chronological age is a poor indicator of old age, as it is based on social constructions of 'normal' retirement, and fails to take account of the diverse experiences and subjective accounts of older age, as well as the structural and social context within which ageing takes place (Victor, 2005).

POLITICAL ECONOMY THEORY

Political economy theory challenges both biological and functionalist approaches to ageing. Exponents of this theory argue that experiences of ageing are structured within a given political and economic context. In advanced capitalist societies, old age is seen within the context of the division of labour and the income inequalities that are structured through this and which persist into retirement. Globally, experiences of ageing can be evaluated within the global division of labour. The most rapid increases in population ageing can be seen in developing countries, and poverty and disadvantage among older people in sub-Saharan Africa and Asia is widespread (Help the Aged, 2008).

As discussed above, retirement is a social construction, but it also creates a structured dependency in the UK as people are forced out of the labour market (Walker, 1981), irrespective of their ability to continue to work. Estes (1979) referred to this as 'structural lag' as retirement constructs age barriers to work leading to a mismatch between older people's resources and abilities and affecting their opportunities in the capitalist economy. In addition she referred to the 'ageing enterprise' of capitalist society, where older people are treated as commodities to be cared for, which is reflected in social policies that segregate older people from other adults, leading to social divisions and stigmatisation. Means and Smith (2003) have argued that the health and social care of older people has been based on a dominant medical model of care to manage 'social problems' within an institutional context, with power concentrated in the hands of welfare professionals. This process of institutionalisation may lead to loss of liberty, stigmatisation, lack of autonomy, poor material resources and loss of dignity.

Activity 1

Read the following account of an older woman's experience of residential care.

> Nothing quite prepared me for the shock of entering residential care. Most of the staff are incredibly patient and kind – and I appreciate their help – but it is the constant bustle and ringing of bells from which one cannot escape . . . and the limited choice about food, activities or even companionship, which I find so hard to take. Then I am not allowed to do anything considered the least bit risky, one understands it is to keep one safe . . . but it's pretty galling at my age, after a life of independence, to find oneself so powerless and constrained.
>
> (cited in McClymont, 1999: 33)

- What features of institutionalisation are evident within this account?
- What features of structured dependency can be identified here?
- What do you think is the impact of this experience on self-esteem and self-worth?
- Are there elements of this account that you can identify in your own experiences of working in health and social care settings?

Critical Gerontology

While the political economy perspective can help to explain older people's relative economic disadvantage and the institutionalisation of care practices, it has been criticised for the over-emphasis on class as the basis for divisions and inequalities. In addition, there is an over-emphasis on the structural context of older people's experiences, and a lack of exploration of subjective experiences for individuals, which is concerned with meanings, interpretations and interactions within society. In response to this, a critical gerontology has developed, which aims to integrate structural and subjective theories to provide a more comprehensive analysis of old age (Phillipson, 1998). Estes (2001) has been particularly influential here through the development of a theoretical approach to ageing that explores the intersection of multiple roots of oppression in old age, based on class, gender and ethnicity. This offers opportunities for exploring a plurality of sources of power and oppression for older people but, at the same time, explores how old age can have meaning or lack meaning for older people and can offer opportunities for empowerment. Old age is therefore not conceptualised as a homogenous experience. While disadvantages of income and status may affect the experiences of some older people, they also need to be seen in relation to other variables, such as gender and ethnicity.

Gender and ageing

Arber and Ginn (1995) argue that ageing is gendered, in that it operates differently for men and women. It is only recently that mainstream sociology has looked at the relationship between gender and ageing, where it is acknowledged that women are disadvantaged in terms of chronological, physiological and social ageing.

> Western societies are ageing and later life is dominated by women, yet gender and age relations have been traditionally ignored by mainstream sociological theory, both separately and in terms of their intersection.
>
> (Arber and Ginn, 1995: 13)

From a chronological point of view, the institutional practice of retirement disadvantages women, as financial distribution in later life is based on the patriarchal assumptions inherent in labour market practices and in the tax-benefit system based on contributory benefits. Two thirds of men receive non-state pensions, whereas three quarters of women do not. This is significant as non-state pensions offer a better income than state pensions, so the incidence of poverty and social exclusion among older women is much higher (Department of Work and Pensions, 2005).

Older people with low levels of material resources were over-represented by women, those living alone, people who are widowed, divorced or separated, in poor health, with lower education and living in deprived neighbourhoods.

(Joseph Rowntree Foundation, 2006)

From a physiological point of view, women are also disadvantaged. On average, women outlive men and outnumber men in older age groups (Bernard and Phillips, 1998). This is related to the different morbidity and mortality patterns of men's and women's lives, where women are less likely to suffer premature mortality through life-threatening diseases, but are more likely to experience poorer health and functional disabilities through life-limiting illnesses (although there is evidence that gender inequalities in health are decreasing as lifestyle practices and behaviours change – Annandale, 1998). The age differentials are significant, as they also contribute to the poverty of older women and the greater incidence of life-limiting illnesses (Arber and Cooper, 1999).

Social ageing is related to transitions in the life course and the cultural expectations of normal gendered behaviour. In this respect, there is a double standard of old age (Sontag, 1978), as women are seen to be past their sell-by-date when they are no longer able to reproduce, as this is the norm of women's primary role, whereas historically men are seen to have the primary role of breadwinner and provider. Although there are changes in labour market organisation, and traditional gender roles are less evident, the ideological underpinnings of the patriarchal society remain. Thus women's power is concentrated in their physical appearance, which will diminish over time in a society that sees beauty within youth and youthful appearances. This sexualisation of women's value leads to differential experiences of ageing for men and women (Ginn and Arber, 1993). Once past the age of reproductive capacity, women's contribution to society becomes devalued as women are judged in terms of physical appearance and their procreative function. Men's physical appearance is less important, as they are valued as the breadwinner in the paid labour market of the capitalist economy. Age-related appropriate behaviours are constructed in terms of the body and fashion and can affect both genders, but have particular resonance for women, where appearance is commodified in consumer markets through the availability of cosmetic surgery and anti-ageing products.

Advertising, feature articles and advice columns in magazines and newspapers ask individuals to assume responsibility for the way they look. This becomes important not just in the first flush of adolescence and early adulthood, for notions of 'natural' bodily deterioration and the bodily betrayals that accompany ageing become interpreted as signs of moral laxitude. The wrinkles, sagging flesh, tendency towards middle-aged spread, hair loss, etc. which accompany ageing should be combated by energetic body maintenance of the part of the individual with help from the cosmetic, beauty, fitness and leisure industries.

(Featherstone and Hepworth, 1991: 178)

This may change, as women's roles change, with increased participation in the labour market and greater choices about childbirth (Equal Opportunities Commission, 2006).

The dual standard of ageing is not just about appearance, but further contributes to women's experiences of ageing and oppressive practices. In a non-participant study of people caring for older people, Evers (1981) found that nurses behaved differently towards older women and older men. They were far more likely to depersonalise older women and knew less about them as individuals than older men. In addition, older women tended to be labelled as more difficult than older men, perhaps reflecting ideological constructions of normal gendered behaviour, where women are expected to be passive and subservient (Ehrenreich and English, 1978).

Ageing and ethnicity

There are also significant trends in relation to minority ethnic groups and the ageing population. There is, historically, a paucity of literature about ethnic elders (Ahmad and Walker, 1997), and one of the explanations for this is that ethnic elders constitute a very small percentage of the total aged population and of the total minority ethnic population. However, minority ethnic elders constitute one of the fastest growing groups of the population, and as those who migrated to the UK in the 1960s and 1970s reach retirement age, the numbers of black and minority ethnic elders will dramatically increase (Blakemore and Boneham, 1994). This is starting to be reflected in a growing body of research and literature (PRIAE, 2005) exploring inter-agency approaches and solutions to the problems that ethnic elders may face.

Like other social groups, the experiences of minority ethnic elders will be varied, and need to be understood in the context of wider social practices and ideologies. Retirement income may be affected by the structural position of ethnic minority populations during working life and the impact of direct and indirect racism throughout the life cycle.

One third of older Black Caribbeans, half of older Indians and three-fifths of Pakistani and Bangladeshi older people are in the bottom fifth of income distribution compared to just over a fifth of white and a quarter of Irish older people.

(Evandrou, 2000: 11–18)

Ethnic elders may be particularly disadvantaged in accessing services and are more likely to suffer discrimination (King's Fund, 2002). Norman (1985) refers to the triple jeopardy for ethnic elders of ageism, cultural and racial discrimination and the perception of a lack of access to health, housing and social services. There may also be a fourth jeopardising factor of not having English as a first language, thus further reducing the accessibility of the services. A significant number of ethnic elders across Europe have unmet needs because of a lack of understanding by service providers or a perception about the appropriateness of services by ethnic elders themselves (PRIAE, 2005). The King's Fund Report (2002) concludes that most black elders would prefer to access mainstream services rather than specialist service provision, but may have difficulties because of a lack of awareness among service commissioners and providers.

Ageing and disadvantage

It can be seen therefore that ageing and the experience of ageing is, in part, based on access to resources, and that income and health inequalities of working-aged life persist into older age. Thus, for a significant minority of older people, old age is a period of disadvantage, poverty and social exclusion.

Phillipson and Scharf (2004) have explored the impact of Government policy on social exclusion among older people. They identified four important groups of conditions that cause social exclusion.

1. **Age-related characteristics**. – in older age, people may be disproportionately affected by losses and restrictions, such as loss of income through retirement, loss of health through chronic disabling conditions or the loss of home or partner, leading to adjustments to living alone and increased potential for social isolation. There are 2.2 million people (over one in five pensioners in Great Britain) living below the poverty line and 33 per cent of homes occupied by older people in England fall below acceptable standards of decency (Help the Aged, 2008). Although this means that four out of five people do not live in poverty, a significant minority suffer from the

disadvantage and exclusions associated with poverty and this age-related disadvantage is not unique to industrialised countries. More than 100 million older people in developing countries live on less than $1 per day (Help the Aged, 2008).

2. **Cumulative disadvantage** – this refers to the accumulation of disadvantage over the life course, so that the inequalities of income or health are perpetuated into old age, as discussed above. In addition, people may have limited access to resources such as health care and social services, due to their lack of understanding or awareness about the available services. Nearly 10 per cent of older people have lived in poverty for most of their lives (Scharf *et al.*, 2003) and although three quarters of people accessing NHS health and social care services are aged 65 and over, only two fifths of total expenditure is spent on this group (Seshamani and Gray, 2002).

3. **Community characteristics** – older people may have strong attachments to their locality and community, and this may make them vulnerable if there is a loss of this community. In a recent study, ten per cent of Britain's older citizens felt that there had been a breakdown in community life and community cohesion (Cunningham and Cunningham, 2008). This may result in a perception of increased vulnerability to crime and social disorder, leading to social isolation and exclusion from participation in society (Scharf *et al.*, 2003). Fifty per cent of all people aged 75 and over live alone and 13 per cent were lonely and socially isolated. As an example of this, over one million older people spent Christmas Day alone in 2004 (Help the Aged, 2008).

4. **Age-based discrimination** – ageism exists within economic and social policies and contributes to the divisions in old age. Seventy-three per cent of older people felt that they had experienced age discrimination on a daily basis (Help the Aged, 2008).

AGEISM

The generalisation of old age as a social problem has contributed to the negative stereotyping and ageist practices in relation to older people. Ageism is defined in terms of the sets of ideas that are based on biological variations over the life course, where the process of ageing is used as the basis for discrimination (Bytheway and Johnson, 1990).

Bernard (1998) argues that ageism is rife in industrialised societies and it is one of the most pervasive and pernicious forms of discrimination. Ageism also exists among those who care for older people.

Age discrimination remains rife in our national health service, despite a government pledge as far back as 2001 to root it out. All too often, older people must resign themselves to a poorer standard of health care than their younger counterparts, simply because of their age.

(Help the Aged, 2008)

McCormack (2003) suggests that ageist attitudes are manifest in health and social care in the assumptions that older people are dependent and unable to participate in the decision-making process. This may be further compounded as older people themselves internalise these dominant social attitudes and lose the confidence to express their needs. Nurses and other health and social care professionals are in an ideal position to empower older people, through partnership working and promotion of inclusion and involvement (Toofany, 2007). However, this requires a critical understanding of the sources of oppression and discrimination.

Thompson (1998) has identified that discrimination operates at three levels in society: personal, cultural and structural.

- Personal oppression or discrimination occurs at a micro level between individuals. An example of this oppression would be a care worker who makes derogatory comments about older people, based on stereotypical assumptions of ageing.
- At a structural level, institutional practices discriminate against and oppress older people. For example, health and social care policies can directly discriminate against older people through the use of explicit age criteria for services (for example, breast screening) or indirectly discriminate through referral and commissioning practices (King's Fund, 2002).
- At a cultural level, it is the sets of ideas of a society (ideology), which contribute to the denigration of a group of individuals. In particular, the stereotyping of individuals and the language that permeates discussions about older people are evidence of this ageist ideology.

  Ageism generates and reinforces a fear and denigration of the ageing process, and stereotyping presumptions regarding competence and the need for protection.

(Bytheway and Johnson, 1990: 11)

Stereotypes

Stereotypes are characteristics that are deemed to be universally applicable and obscure the interpersonal differences between people. They affect interpersonal behaviours and interactions by obscuring the visibility of an individual's uniqueness. Many of the stereotypes associated with older people are based on the assumption of inevitable and universal physical and mental decline as part of the ageing process (Hazan, 2000) and stem from a biomedical approach to ageing. Of particular concern in health and social welfare are the assumptions about the relationship between ageing and increased levels of dependency, the pervasiveness of senility as people age and the inability to learn new things or process information. In addition, there is a pervasive stereotype of asexuality in older age, inhibiting older people's ability to engage in intimate and sexual relationships (Pickard, 1995).

Discourses are important in shaping dominant sets of ideas, and constructions of power are reflected in the language we use (Foucault, 1979). In particular, the media is a dominant social institution that has the power to construct symbols and images through language and discourse (Habermas, 1989). From this perspective, the pervasiveness of negative language in relation to older people reflects the negative stereotyping and contributes to the marginal status of older people.

Activity 2

- Make a list of terms that are used when referring to older people.
- Look at the way that popular media portrays older people (newspapers, television programmes, etc.).
- Divide them into positive and negative features.
- In what ways do these portrayals reflect stereotypes of older people?

Featherstone and Hepworth (1991) refer to the mask of ageing, which relates to the observable physical processes associated with ageing (wrinkles, greying or thinning of hair, loss of physical stature, decline in sensory perceptions). The physical characteristics and outer signs of ageing tend to conceal the inner self and the experience of ageing, which may be very different. The person may feel quite youthful, but they physically appear to be ageing. This is not the same as saying that people attempt to disguise ageing but is a reflection of the stereotyping of ageing, associated with the biological process of physical decline.

Ageism and stereotyping are therefore important in shaping both perceptions of ageing and experiences of ageing. However, ageing is not necessarily a period of dependency, decline and unhappiness, and a critical questioning of ageist practices allows us to look at more diverse and enabling experiences of ageing. Contemporary gerontological theory places increased emphasis on a life course perspective, where the experience of ageing needs to be located within the context of the whole life journey (Binstock and George, 2001). Instead of focussing on the structural or context of ageing or the subjective experience of ageing, it integrates the two. Thus the experience of old age is, in part, dependent on other experiences throughout the life course, such as racism, sexism or other forms of discrimination and the discourses that may affect people's perceptions and experiences in old age, as well as the social divisions that contribute to people's income and health status in older age. Thus old age is a period of heterogeneity, with people having very different experiences.

Phenomenological and biographical approaches – user perspectives

Biographical approaches shape the way that people age from within and people's narratives are important for understanding the richness and complexities of lived experiences. Seeing beyond the mask of ageing, through a phenomenological understanding of the meaning of ageing to individuals, helps us to see beyond the negative experiences and engage with individuals as unique human beings. A focus on the structural context of ageing or the moral panic in relation to the burden of dependency thesis fails to account for 'normal' or non-problematic ageing. Rather than older age being a period of depression, isolation and dependency, the core of inner self persists for most older people (Biggs, 1999). Furthermore, old age does not necessarily involve disengagement and relinquishing of roles, but may be a period of personal fulfilment and engagement with new roles. For example, in older age people may take on volunteering roles, giving them a sense of purpose and fulfilment (Baldock, 1999) and grandparents are increasingly playing a part in the care of pre-school children and in after-school care of older children (Thompson, 1999).

Laslett (1989) argues that old age can be a period of liberation and personal fulfilment. In his theory of the third age he states that the life course can be divided into four ages. The third age is often associated with the period of retirement, where people are no longer engaged with work roles or childcare responsibilities, and may pursue goals of personal fulfilment. Although the theory has been criticised, as the pursuit of personal fulfilment may depend on access to income and health resources, the theory does nevertheless identify old age as a positive experience for some.

Consumption processes and older people

Sociologists have argued that social class is no longer a useful term for explaining societal divisions (Crompton, 1998) as it fails to account for the multiple variables that structure societies. Access to consumer markets and products is seen as a more reliable indicator of different social groupings.

Consumption processes are important for integrating people into the political economy (Vincent, 1995). Rather than older people being seen as a burden on the capitalist economy, there is a growing commercial interest in the increasing numbers of affluent older people, with the recognition of the importance of the 'grey market' (Featherstone and Wernick, 1995). Consumption of social goods can be an important aspect of social identity (Hockey and James, 2003) and fashion is an important aspect of consumer practices. Although there is evidence of a cultural domination of youth and youthful styles within consumer markets, with the promotion, for example, of products to defy the ageing process, increasing attention is being paid to older people as active consumers. Travel companies, insurance companies and the fashion industry have all recognised the importance of this grey market. Thus consumer practices offer opportunities for the expression of personal identity and personal fulfilment. However, consumption patterns vary between different social groups and reflect their relative economic standing and power.

Consumption processes are also relevant in health care. The introduction of direct payments and individual budgets has the potential to empower older people as active consumers of health and social care services and shift the balance of power between welfare professionals and older people (Care Services and Improvement Partnership, 2008). How can sociological perspectives help us to understand clinical situations?

Case study

Michael is a 76-year-old man who was recently admitted to hospital with acute hypothermia, having fallen in his bathroom. On admission, Michael is slightly confused, unkempt, malnourished and seems quite withdrawn. He has lived on his own since his wife died five years ago. He has three grown-up children, all of whom have their own families. They visit when they can, but do not live locally and, as Michael explains, all have their own busy lives. While in hospital, Michael often wakes at 4 a.m. and finds it difficult to get back to sleep. He is also emotionally vulnerable and, at times, nursing staff have found him in tears, although he insists that everything is OK. When Michael's son visits, he informs staff that his father does not eat properly and has found it increasingly difficult to cope at home, and wonders whether he should be discharged to a nursing or residential home.

If we employ a political economic perspective here, the fact that Michael is malnourished and unkempt might be due to lack of income. If, during his working life, Michael was on relative low pay, then this will have left him with low pension income and he may be finding it difficult to afford to feed himself adequately. In addition, he may be living in poor quality housing, which is damp and cold and may have contributed to the hypothermia. This may be further exacerbated by fuel poverty, where, although there is heating in the house, Michael is either unable to afford to use it or the home is energy inefficient. According to statistics from the Department of Trade and Industry (2005) 49.2 per cent of households in fuel poverty are occupied by people aged over 60. Michael may therefore be eligible for a grant or additional funding to alleviate fuel poverty.

A functionalist perspective might help us to understand Michael's withdrawn state and malnourishment. Arber and Ginn (1995) argue that older people are more likely to adopt traditional gendered roles within a marital relationship than other generations, where gendered boundaries may be more blurred. If this is the case, it may be that Michael's wife was the one who was responsible for cooking throughout their married life, and he does not really know how to cook a balanced and nourishing diet. The loss of his traditional working role may have left Michael with a lack of purpose. He may also be mourning the loss of other roles, such as husband or grandparent. In addition, his emotional lability may be explained by the socialisation of traditional gendered roles, where men are expected to be emotionally strong, which may have led to unresolved grief (Martin and Doka, 2000). Perhaps Michael could therefore be offered the opportunity to go to a luncheon club run by one of the voluntary agencies, which would have the dual purpose of providing better nutrition and an opportunity for socialisation.

A biographical approach would help us to locate Michael's current context within the broader context of his life course. His early waking and wandering, for example, might be explained by the fact that he worked as a milkman, and this pattern of early waking is part of a norm for him, rather than an indicator of depression. He may also fear the loss of his home, as it is not only a roof over his head, but houses precious memories of his life with his wife and his growing family. This understanding is important in terms of person-centred care, so that Michael can be offered choices in order to maximise his independence.

CONCLUSION

Social gerontology is of direct relevance to health and social care practice in a number of ways. Firstly, structural theories help to explain the social disadvantage that may be experienced by older people, in particular the poverty of old age, social exclusion and social isolation and the impact of negative stereotyping and ageist practices on older people. Assessing and understanding the social circumstances of care recipients is an important aspect of holistic care. Secondly, sociological perspectives can inform anti-discriminatory practice and promotion of positive ageing as identified in Standards 1 and 8 respectively of the National Service Framework for Older People (Department of Health, 2001). Thirdly, an understanding of subjective and biographical approaches to ageing can help in the planning of person-centred care in collaboration with the service user and their carers and can help us to understand different coping strategies and responses to health, illness and health care. Finally, an understanding of ageism and ageist practices can help individuals to personally reflect on their own values and the impact of this for practice with older people.

FURTHER READING

Hockey, J. and James, A. (2003) *Social Identities Across the Life Course*. Basingstoke: Palgrave Macmillan
   This book focusses on the processes of ageing and the impact on social identities. It explores structural and institutional influences on identity,

as well as individual subjective experiences. There is also some critical discussion of the body and social identity.

Hunt, S. (2005) *The Life Course: A Sociological Introduction*. Basingstoke: Palgrave Macmillan
This text is an accessible exploration of theories of ageing across the life course, incorporating traditional and contemporary sociological theories.

Tanner, D. and Harris, J. (2008) *Working with Older People*. Abingdon: Routledge in association with Community Care
Although this is primarily aimed at social work students, this book provides some important debates about the nature of ageing and provision of care and support for older people and their carers, which are relevant to nursing practice. In particular, it has useful discussions on the nature of positive ageing and combating ageism, and explores the importance of working in partnership with users and carers.

Victor, C. (2005) *The Social Context of Ageing: A Textbook of Gerontology*. Abingdon: Routledge
This text is an accessible read that provides a good overview of social theories of old age, as well as issues about social disadvantage and discrimination.

Walker, A. and Hennessy, C. (eds) (2004) *Growing Older: Quality of Life in Old Age*. Buckingham: Open University Press
This text is based on material from an ESRC funded project that looks at ageing as a positive experience. A major focus of the different chapters is the experiences of older people themselves.

Useful websites

www.ageconcern.org.uk
Age Concern is a voluntary organisation that campaigns on issues that affect older people, conducts research and produces information sheets for older people and carers.

www.britishgerontology.org
This is a site that brings together papers and discussions from a range of academic disciplines, with the aim of promoting an understanding of ageing and later life.

www.csip.org.uk
The Care Services Improvement Partnership works with communities and organisations to improve outcomes for users of health and social care service.

www.helptheaged.org.uk
Help the Aged is a voluntary organisation that conducts research, produces information leaflets and campaigns on behalf of older people to influence government decision-making.

www.priae.org.uk
The Policy Institute for Research on Ageing and Ethnicity brings together relevant stakeholders with older people from minority ethnic groups to identify solutions to issues that they might encounter.

REFERENCES

Ahmad, W.I. and Walker, R. (1997) 'Asian older people: housing, health and access to services'. *Ageing and Society*. 17 (2): 141–66

Annandale, E. (1998) *The Sociology of Health and Medicine: A Critical Introduction*. Cambridge: Polity Press

Arber, J. and Cooper, H. (1999) 'Gender differences in health in later life: the new paradox?'. *Social Science and Medicine*. 48 (1): 61–76

Arber, S. and Ginn, J. (1995) *Connecting Gender and Ageing: A Sociological Approach*. Buckingham: Open University Press

Attias-Donfurt, C. and Arber, J. (2000). *The Myth of Generational Conflict*. Abingdon: Routledge

Baldwin, S. and Falkingham, J. (eds) (1994) *Social Security and Social Change: New Challenges to the Beveridge Model*. Harvester Wheatsheaf

Baldock, C.V. (1999) 'Seniors as volunteers: an international perspective on policy'. *Ageing and Society*. 19 (5): 581–602

Bernard, M. (1998) 'Backs to the future? Reflections on women, ageing and nursing'. *Journal of Advanced Nursing*. 27 (3): 633–40

Bernard, M. and Phillips, J. (eds) (1998) *The Social Policy of Old Age*. New Romney: CPA

Beveridge, W. (1942) *Social Insurance and Allied Services*. Cmnd 6404. London: HMSO

Blakemore, K. and Boneham, M (1994) *Age, Race and Ethnicity*. Buckingham: Open University Press

Biggs, S. (1999) *The Mature Imagination*. Buckingham, Open University Press

Binstock, R. and George, L. (eds) (2001) *Handbook of Ageing and Social Sciences*. San Diego, CA: Academic Press

Bytheway, B. and Johnson, J. (1990) 'On defining ageism'. *Critical Social Policy*. 27: 27–39

Care Services Improvement Partnership (2008) *High Impact Changes for Health and Social Care*. London: DoH. **www.csip.org.uk** (Accessed 30 May 2008)

Crompton, R. (1998) *Class and Stratification: An Introduction to Current Debates*. (2nd edn). Cambridge: Polity Press

Cumming, E. and Henry, W.E. (1961) *Growing Old*. New York: Basic Books

Cunningham, J. and Cunningham, S. (2008) *Sociology and Social Work*. Exeter: Learning Matters.

Department of Health (2001) *The National Service Framework for Older People*. London: HMSO

Department of Trade and Industry (2005) *The UK Fuel Poverty Strategy. 3rd Annual Progress Report, 2005*. London: Department of Trade and Industry, Department for Environment Food and Rural Affairs

Department of Work and Pensions (2005) *Women and Pensions*. London: HMSO

Ehrenreich, B. and English, D. (1978) *For Her Own Good: 150 Years of the Experts' Advice to Women*. London: Pluto Press

Equal Opportunities Commission (2006) *Sex and Power: Who Runs Britain?* Available at **www.eoc.org.uk** (Accessed 26 November 2008)

Estes, C. (1979) *The Aging Enterprise*. San Francisco, CA: Jossey-Bass

Estes, C. (2001) *Social Policy and Aging*. London: Sage

Evandrou, M. (2000) 'Social inequalities in later life: the socio-economic position of older people from ethnic minority groups in Britain'. *Population Trends 101*, Autumn, 2000 11–18

Evers, H. (1981) 'Care or custody? The experiences of women patients in long-stay geriatric wards' in Hutter, B. and Williams, G. (eds) *Controlling Women: The Normal and the Deviant*. London: Croom Helm

Featherstone, M. and Hepworth, M. (1991) 'The Mask of Ageing and the Postmodern Life Course' in Featherstone, M., Hepworth, M. and Turner, B.S. (eds) *The Body, Social Process and Cultural Theory*. London: Sage

Featherstone, M. and Wernick, A. (eds) (1995) *Images of Ageing: Cultural Representations of Later Life*. Abingdon: Routledge

Fischer, D.H. (1978) *Growing Old in America*. New York: Oxford University Press

Foucault, M. (1979) *Discipline and Punish*. London: Penguin

Gabriel, Z. and Bowling, A. (2004) 'Quality of Life from the Perspectives of Older People'. *Ageing and Society* 24: 675–91

Ginn, J. and Arber, S. (1993) 'Ageing and Cultural Stereotypes of Older Women' in Johnson, J. and Slater, R. (eds) *Ageing and Later Life*. London: Sage

Habermas, J. (1989) *The Structural Transformation of the Public Sphere: An Inquiry into a Category of Bourgeois Society*. Cambridge: Polity Press

Havighurst, R. (1963) 'Successful Aging' in Williams, R.H., Tibbitts, C. and Donohoe, W. *Processes of Aging*, Vol 1. Chicago, IL: University of Chicago Press

Hazan, H. (2000) 'The Cultural Trap: The Language of Images' in Gubrium, J. and Holstein, J. (eds.) *Aging and Everyday Life*. Oxford: Blackwell

Help the Aged (2008) *Older people in the UK*. **www.helptheaged.org.uk** (Accessed 26 September 2008)

Hockey, J. and James, A. (2003) *Social Identities Across the Life Course*. Basingstoke: Palgrave Macmillan

Hunt, S. (2005) *The Life Course: A Sociological Introduction*. Basingstoke: Palgrave Macmillan

Joseph Rowntree Foundation (2006) *The material resources and well-being of older people*. **www.jrf.org.uk** (Accessed 26 September 2008)

King's Fund Report (2002) *Age Discrimination in Health and Social Care*. London: King's Fund

Laslett, P. (1989) *A Fresh Map of Life: The Emergence of the Third Age*. London: Weidenfeld & Nicolson

Laybourn, K. (1995) *The Evolution of British Social Policy and the Welfare State*. Keele: Keele University Press

McClymont, M. (1999) 'Hearing Older Voices'. *Elderly Care*. 11 (6): 8–12

McCormack, B. (2003) 'Researching nursing practice: does person-centredness matter?'. *Nursing Philosophy*. 4 (3): 179–88

Martin, T.L. and Doka, K.J. (2000) *Men Don't Cry . . . Women Do: Transcending Gender Stereotypes of Grief*. Philadelphia, PA: Brinner/Matzel

Means, R. and Smith, R. (2003) *Community Care: Policy and Practice* (3rd edn). Bristol: Policy Press

Norman, A. (1985) *Triple Jeopardy: Growing Old in a Second Homeland*. London: Centre for Policy on Ageing.

Phillipson, C. (1998) *Reconstructing Old Age*. London: Sage

Phillipson, C. and Sharf, T. (2004) *The Impact of Government Policy on Social Exclusion Among Older People: A Review of the Literature*.London: Social Exclusion Unit, Office of the Deputy Prime Minister

Phillipson, C. and Walker, A. (eds) (1986) *Ageing and Social Policy: A Critical Assessment*. Aldershot: Gower

Pickard, S. (1995) *Living on the Front Line*. Aldershot: Avebury

PRIAE (2005) Black and Minority Ethnic Elders in the UK: Health and Social Care Findings. **www.priae.org.uk** (Accessed 30 May 2008)

Riley, M.W. and Riley, J.W. (1999) 'Sociological research on age: legacy and challenge'. *Ageing and Society*. 19 (1): 123–33

Ruth, J.E. and Kenyon, G. (1996) 'Biography in adult development and aging' in Birren, J.E., Kenyon, G.M., Ruth, J.E., Schroots J.J.F. and Svensson.T. (eds) *Aging and Biography: Explorations in Adult Development*. New York: Springer

Scharf, T., Phillipson, C., Smith, A. E and Kingston, P. (2003) *Older People in Deprived Neighbourhoods: Social Exclusion and Quality of Life in Old Age*. ESRC Project

Seshamani, M. and Gray, A. (2002) The Impact of Ageing on Expenditures in the NHS. *Age and Ageing*. 31, A, 297–94

Sontag, S. (1978) 'The double standard of ageing' in Carver, V. and Liddiard, P. (eds) *An Ageing Population*. Buckingham: Open University Press

Tanner, D. and Harris, J. (2008) *Working with Older People*. Abingdon: Routledge in association with Community Care

Thane, P. (1982) *The Foundations of the Welfare State*. Harlow: Longman

Thompson, N. (1998) *Promoting Equality – Challenging Discrimination and Oppression in the Human Services*. Basingstoke: Macmillan

Thompson, P. (1999) 'The role of grandparents when parents part or die: some reflections on the mythical decline of the extended family'. *Ageing and Society*. 19 (4): 471–503

Toofany, S. (2007) 'Empowering older people'. *Nursing Older People*. 19 (2): 12–14

Victor, C. (2005) *The Social Context of Ageing: A Textbook of Gerontology*. Abingdon: Routledge.

Vincent, J. (1995) *Inequality and Old Age*. London: UCL Press

Walker, A. (1981) 'Towards a political economy of old age'. *Ageing and Society*.1 (1): 73–94

Wilson, G. (2000) *Understanding Old Age: Critical and Global Perspectives*. London: Sage

Chapter 4

Person-Centred Care

Margaret Brown

Learning outcomes

Reading this chapter will enable you to:

- explain the term person-centred care;

- examine the literature on person-centred care with the older person;

- explore some of the benefits of adopting a person-centred approach;

- discuss the challenges involved in the person-centred approach.

INTRODUCTION

The term person-centred care is used widely in both health and social care settings. What is not widely understood is what this term really means. It has been used interchangeably with individualised care or holistic care and it can have different meanings in different settings. The term has been applied to any person, of any age and with a variety of health and social care needs. It has been described as trying to have the ideal in the real everyday world (Morris, 2004). Planning person-centred care includes actively listening to the person's needs and wishes. It should explore with them their beliefs, values and preferences in the light of their culture and history. It endeavours to build on their strengths and puts them at the centre of the planning and the processes of care.

This chapter is about the application of the concept of person-centred care related to the older person, including the older person with dementia. The term 'person-centred care' is explored from a variety of perspectives and theories. The relevant literature is examined and discussed and studies of care and reflective exercises are used to help you clarify and explore the benefits and challenges of this approach to the care of the older person.

THEORIES AND FRAMEWORKS

Research on person-centred care is limited but it is an area rich in theory. The term 'person-centred' derives from the work, in the 1950s and 1960s, of the American psychotherapist Carl Rogers. His was an approach to therapy that emphasised the need to understand the whole person and to explore issues from their perspective. The standpoint in this approach is about the person's right to choose how they wished to 'be' (Wilkins, 2003). Such an approach includes these principles:

- having respect and being non-judgemental and accepting of the person;
- seeing them as a whole person and having a positive approach that focusses on their strengths;
- recognising the value of emotions and feelings and understanding the impact of interpersonal relationships that are truthful and honest;
- in caring for the person, 'doing with' them rather than 'doing to' them.

This human, person-centred approach is in contrast to the medical model of care that can be seen as one that reduces the person to clinical symptoms and treatment, focussing on the disease process and its cure. Kelly *et al.* (2005) found that this curative model was perceived to be dominant in older people's health care services. However, in the field of dementia care Morton (1999) suggests that this view was challenged very effectively by the work of Tom Kitwood, who developed a theory of person-centred dementia care. He challenged what he called the 'standard paradigm' of the prevalent disease-oriented approach to dementia that saw the condition purely in terms of an organic brain disorder. Instead, he developed his theories about person-centred care, influenced by the work of Carl Rogers.

Tom Kitwood was the first person to use the term 'personhood' and he defined this as 'a standing or status that is bestowed upon one human being, by others in the context of relationship and social being; it implies recognition, respect and trust' (Kitwood, 1997: 8). He shows in this definition how important relationships with others are in this area of care. Indeed, the concept of personhood, as described by Kitwood and related to the person with dementia, can also be understood and applied to the care of the older, vulnerable person with care needs. In particular, the suggestion that the promotion of personhood was the main aim of person-centred care and that key to this was respect and trust.

The field of person-centred dementia care has been further developed by Brooker (2007) who uses the acronym VIPS to define the elements needed for care to be considered person-centred:

- **V** is for valuing the person in all their diversity;
- **I** is for individualising the approach taken in order to recognise that everyone is different – she considers individualised care to be only one element of person centred care;
- **P** is for perspective, that is seeing the world from the older person's standpoint, in other words being empathetic when caring for them;
- **S** is for providing a social environment that is supportive and rich in opportunities to maintain relationships.

She suggests that, for some people, person-centred care is the same as individualised care, which may simply mean ensuring the person has a choice of, for example, diet or personal hygiene. However, Brooker (2007) intimates that individualised care by itself is not enough and only when all these elements are present can care truly be described as person-centred. Although Brooker's work is related primarily to the person with dementia, she considers that it applies equally to any vulnerable person who needs care, including the older person.

McCormack's (2001) study explored the challenges to the autonomy of the older person and the opportunities for person-centred care in the hospital setting. A key theme from this study was that of 'speaking for you or speaking for me' (McCormack, 2001: 161). This explored the efforts of nurses working with the older person to make decisions about their care. At the same time as trying to be person-centred the nurses were constrained by the policies, rules and limited resources in the ward, all of which created tensions for them in their daily work. The routines that were described in this study militated against a person-centred approach. One example of this was their assessment processes, which involved a set of questions where nurses were simply to record the patients' answers. This seriously affected the patients' ability to talk about their own priorities.

This is in contrast to an approach that sees the person's narrative or story as very important when gathering information. The person with care needs is likely to have these in the forefront of their minds and these will naturally spill into their narrative with minimal prompting. This is in contrast with the person being faced by a barrage of questions about their health care needs and lifestyle where they may simply answer the questions asked, resulting in a formal communication process and very limited amount and quality of data (Barker, 2003a). Therefore, a key to person-centred care seems to be the narrative or story people tell about their past and present, their life experience, their current care needs, their perception of the care provided and the place and position they find themselves in.

Definitions of person-centred care

There are obvious difficulties in researching a concept such as person-centred care, as can be seen from the previous discussion of the meaning of this term. As it is so difficult to have one definition of this, it makes investigation more complex. Indeed there are few published studies of person-centred care with older people and, as McCormack (2004) has identified, fewer still that measure outcomes or the results of such an approach to care.

This lack of research has also been commented upon by Kelly *et al.* (2005) who make the point that just having person-centred principles and values may not make a difference to care and that studies that look at the outcome of such an approach for older people would make a valuable contribution.

Person-centred care is a much-used term and perhaps we need to break it down to fully understand what it means. The concept of being a person involves having a will that allows us to deliberate on our actions (Ford and McCormack, 2000). The concept of autonomy or self determination is central to this. However, for those older people in care, and particularly for those with dementia, they may not be allowed to deliberate and make choices. Often they are considered not capable of doing so.

Barker (2003b) discusses the idea of the word 'care' as reflecting the sensitive, cautious and delicate approach you would use handling a piece of fragile china; indicating and reflecting concern and respect.

Despite the difficulty defining person-centred care, participants in a Scottish study (Kelly *et al.*, 2005), who were all experienced older people's nurses, came together to provide a definition of person-centred care as:

Understanding and acknowledging the needs and wishes of the older person and ensuring that these underpin the planning and delivery of care. Promoting continuity of care that values the older person's unique past, present and future individuality and recognising and respecting the person's role and contribution to family and wider society.

(Kelly *et al.*, 2005: 23)

McCormack and McCance (2006) have developed a framework for nurses working within a person-centred framework. This framework consists of four elements:

1. The nurses' attributes, such as being committed to the work with older people, having good interpersonal skills, having clear values and knowing themselves.
2. The context where care is delivered; this includes systems in place that support staff and encourage innovation, positive staff relationships and leadership within the team.
3. Person-centred processes that allow nurses to work with patients' values and beliefs, to negotiate and support them in decision making and to form appropriate interpersonal relationships.
4. Outcomes of the person-centred approach in practice including satisfaction with care, providing a therapeutic environment and creating a feeling of wellbeing in patients.

(Adapted from McCormack and McCance, 2006)

Person-centred care, then, is a complex and diverse set of ideas that are difficult to research but seem to include the following principles:

- the older person's life story;
- respect for the older person's autonomy;
- good interpersonal relationships;
- valuing and respecting the older person;
- negotiation and reciprocity.

BIOGRAPHY

One way to explore the older person's values is to use a biographical approach that can give them the opportunity to share their life experience with you. Listening to the story of a person's life gives them the message that they are important to you (Clarke, Hanson and Ross, 2003). Life story books developed by the older person and their carers and family can also be helpful and the construction of these can forge deep and meaningful relationships between older people and their carers. These provide a narrative of the person's history and can bring this to life for those caring for them.

McCormack (2003) agrees that these values, beliefs and needs are best understood by understanding the older person's life in its entirety. He suggests that life stories are not separate to the person, they are part of them and they help to make sense of the present by using the past. People need to feel understood and it is in trying to make sense of the other person's experience that we begin to develop a relationship with them. Behaviour only provides us with initial information. It is our efforts to try and understand why the person behaves as they do that matters (Morris, 2004).

Case study

Peter was admitted to an older person's ward at the request of his GP. He had been falling almost every day and the doctor could not find out why this was happening. Peter, who was in the early stages of dementia, was a widower who lived alone, however he was visited daily by his daughter who was his main support. Shortly after admission he became angry with the nursing staff and refused to do anything he was asked. He was not sleeping and one night the nurse found him curled up on the floor with his head in his hands.

Lisa, one of the student nurses, had just completed some time learning about person-centred care and decided to try and use this as a way of caring for Peter. She began to spend some time with Peter to get to know him. He loved to listen to classical music and, although Lisa did not like this at all, she sat with him and gradually he began to talk to her. Over the next few days she spent as much time as she could with him; listening to the stories he told her about his life. One evening there was a programme on television about the Second World War and prisoner of war camps. Peter began to get very angry and left the room, she found him again curled up on the floor. This time he was not angry but crying. He finally told her that he had been a prisoner of war in Singapore and that he had been having terrible dreams about what had happened there. These dreams had just got worse after his wife died and he was alone in the house. He had stopped going to bed at night and his daughter did not know. His falls had been caused by exhaustion and lack of sleep.

Activity 1

Choose an older person you are caring for and, with their permission, construct a timeline of their life with them.

Birth   Now

Above the line add all the major events in their life so far, such as going to school, getting married, retirement and so on. Below the line put in all the major events that were going on in the world at that time such as the World Wars, food shortages and the start of the National Health Service.

- What have you learned about the person that you did not know before?
- Do you see them any differently now?

If you wish you can also construct your own timeline of your life so far and compare the experiences you have both had.

- Are there some things that are the same? Or are they different? Were there parts of your life that you found difficult to include? If so, why did you think this was the case?

RELATIONSHIPS

Central to providing holistic, person-centred care are the relationships we build with older people. The nurse needs to see the person as an individual and value their relationship with them, recognising the expectations both have of that relationship. A person-centred approach challenges the view that all older people are the same and values the diversity of older people. Being person-centred is seen as having mutual respect, appreciating the rights of the individual and how these are linked with autonomy. Having positive values that inform our decision making will maximise the person's potential for growth and allow a relationship to develop with them. Fundamental to this approach is the development of a therapeutic relationship between nurse and the older person. Building this relationship needs self awareness on the part of the nurse and an acceptance of the older person as they are.

Central to the development of this relationship is communicating in a person-centred way and not using it simply for the giving and receiving of information. Person-centred communication involves letting others know how you feel, having them recognise these feelings and letting them know you have understood. McCabe (2004) suggests that nurses too often make assumptions about the care needs of their patients, that this type of communication is not person-centred and that this will have a negative effect on the relationship. True person-centred communication is seen as being participative and negotiated (McCabe, 2004).

It is clear that in order to provide person-centred care we need to know the person's care needs. There is no need to be intrusive and we cannot know all about a person as this would be impractical and even unethical (Barker, 2003a). The goal is to have sufficient insight into the person to allow you to modify or tailor care and services to that person.

What you learn about a person may have an impact on how you communicate with them or how you approach their need for assistance (Tuohy, 2003). We need to get closer to understand their needs but, if we get too close, we can get too involved and cannot help; we need boundaries. 'Viewing the person from a distance often feels much safer' (Barker, 2003a: 4). McCabe (2004) suggests that some nurses work in a task-oriented way rather than a person-centred way in order to protect themselves from involvement with their patients. The lack of person-centred communication has also been identified by a number of authors as expressing a need by nurses to protect them from emotional involvement (Barker, 2003a; McCabe, 2004; Kelly *et al.*, 2005).

Case study

Jenny is 86 and lives in her home alone with her little West Highland terrier 'Robbie'. Robbie is getting on too; he is nine years old. Jenny treats Robbie like her child and always puts him first. She has no children and her husband died four years ago. She has no close family and most of her friends are dead too. Jenny's eyesight and mobility are getting poorer and she is not eating well. After a lot of refusals, at last she has agreed to have a carer come in to help her. The carer was to help her eat and gain a little weight. The carer was horrified to learn that Jenny was spending money on the most expensive dog food and treats for Robbie, leaving herself with little money to feed herself. The carer wanted to help and so when she was out shopping she began to buy cheaper meat for the dog and more food for Jenny. Jenny's poor eyesight meant that she did not realise this was happening. Her carer felt she was doing the best thing for Jenny after all. However, after a week or two, Robbie became noticeably thinner and was whimpering a good deal. Jenny was beside herself; to her, Robbie was all she had in the world.

At about this time the carer went on holiday and a relief worker appeared. She listened to Jenny's worries about Robbie and soon worked out what had happened. She was angry at the lack of person-centred care Jenny had received and asked to be placed with Jenny permanently.

Over the next few months she worked with Jenny to balance Robbie's and Jenny's nutritional needs. After a lot of trial and error they all compromised and Robbie and Jenny are now both doing well. Robbie doesn't get the most expensive food and Jenny has been persuaded that if she wants to be well enough to look after Robbie she has to have a good diet. Jenny feels at the centre of her care now and because he is so important to her, so is Robbie.

This case study shows what it is to provide and receive good person-centred care. Jenny feels valued and respected, her circumstances, history and wishes are known and acted upon, she is seen as an individual with rights and choices and, above all, the carer has looked at the world from Jenny's perspective and not her own. She has done this by building a positive relationship based on truthfulness, respect and knowledge about Jenny's past and present concerns.

CHALLENGES

McCormack (2003) in his research found that three factors that enabled person-centred practice are the patient's values, the caregiver's values and the care environment. Each of these factors is discussed in more detail below.

The patient's values

Autonomy is a key issue in the older person's care and choice is the key to autonomy. The threat to autonomy is very real when an older person becomes vulnerable by reason of physical and/or mental health problems. We can often understand the impact that a threat to autonomy can have on the older person but can often find it a dilemma when faced with an older person who has impaired ability to make decisions (Kelly *et al.*, 2005). Having an awareness that this can easily happen to vulnerable older people can help us provide the kind of care that will support older people to have choice and protect their autonomy. Otherwise there is a risk that we begin to make decisions for them when they seem to be finding choices difficult, After all we should not just be caring 'for' the older person but we should also care 'about' them as individuals.

The nurse's values

We need to enhance nursing practice to help us place the older person at the centre of care. All nurses at every level of the organisation can influence the provision of high quality person-centred care. One of the first things nurses need to do is to start to examine the experience of ageing and their own beliefs, attitudes and values related to the older person, as well as considering the older person's experience of care. Our own beliefs and knowledge about old age can shape the way we care for older people. Although McCormack's (2003) study examined specifically the values that it is important for nurses to hold, these could be applied to any person caring for an older adult.

Activity 2

This activity is intended to help you think about being old. It may assist you to explore your own perceptions about what it is to be old. You can do this activity as a reflection by yourself or you can do this as a group exercise and discuss it with your colleagues.

Find a quiet place and sit with your eyes closed. Now imagine you are around 80 years old. Keep your eyes closed and try to examine how you are feeling. There is a mirror on the wall up there and you can see yourself reflected in this. Continue sitting with closed eyes for a few minutes then open your eyes.

- What did you see in the mirror?
- How did you feel?
- Where were you living?

Now reflect on your answers. Why do you think you answered the questions in the way you did? Can you think what could have influenced the way you responded to this exercise? How did the whole exercise make you feel?

We all become old if we live long enough. None of us have any experience of being in that position until we reach it. It is not easy to understand how it feels to be old and this activity can result in some challenging feelings about our own old age. It can also help us to understand and challenge some of our own beliefs about and attitudes to old age and older people.

The care environment

There are a number of factors in a care environment that can have an influence on the implementation of person-centred care. In particular, this approach can be a challenge for those working within a multiprofessional team that is focussed on medical diagnosis as this can have resource constraints and organisational rules. This situation can cause a dilemma for nurses trying to provide person-centred care with all the constraints of modern health care settings.

McCabe (2004) examined the perceptions of nurses' communication patterns by patients who participated in her study. They perceived that the nurses lacked autonomy and were mainly concerned with carrying out orders. Some suggested that the task-oriented way the nurses practised made them feel they were not individuals. This interaction seemed to be influenced by the work and culture of the ward organisation rather than a lack of resources or time; she suggests that it is not more resources that are needed but improved communication and interactions that would move the care to a more person-centred approach (McCabe, 2004).

Involving older people

From the older person's perspective there is an increasing desire for the person to be involved in the decisions about their care. Indeed there is a drive to involve the users of services to help in planning and evaluating the care provided and, more recently, to be involved in research, not just as a participant but also in gathering data and developing the research agenda. Person-centred approaches are being expanded continually in an effort to provide the best service possible to the older person.

Some researchers have attempted to involve older people in the process of their study. Kelly et al. (2005) developed a set of principles for gerontological nursing (they defined gerontological nurses as those who provide nursing care to older people). They presented these principles to a group of older people for comment. However, they felt that this was a rather cursory approach and any further work they did would be more participatory, transparently including the older person throughout the research process. Research that genuinely involves older people is the aim but this has proved difficult to achieve. Dewar (2005) identifies a number of reasons for this, such as the assumption that older people are not capable of becoming involved, are unable to articulate their views and are unfamiliar with the research process. She challenges these ideas and suggests approaches such as programmes of education for the older person to improve their confidence in participation. She also encourages professionals to use language that is easily understood by the older person to increase the opportunity for them to participate (Dewar, 2005).

Implications for joint working

Person-centred care is not exclusive to nursing and has been adopted by both statutory agencies such as social work and non-statutory agencies such as the voluntary sector. Indeed these groups are often in advance of health care in these initiatives. In Scotland, *Joint Futures* is the driving policy on joint working between local authorities and the NHS. The main aim is to provide an approach that will lead to seamless care in the community. There is an expectation that local health and social care partnerships will be able to take person-centred decisions on community care needs (Scottish Executive, 2000). The Single Shared Assessment is one of the key strategies used to implement this person-centred approach. This concept of Single Shared Assessment is that it is person-centred, seamless and effective and is led by a single professional with multidisciplinary support provided as required. The person-centred service is also embedded in policy, such as the National Service Framework for Older People (NSF) (Department of Health, 2001). The NSF set standards for the care of older people. This clearly sets the need to address the needs of the older adult in a person-centred way. Although this framework was developed for English care systems, the standards contained in it are applicable throughout the United Kingdom and also reflect the principles found in the *Joint Futures* agenda in Scotland.

BEYOND PERSON-CENTRED CARE

Person-centred approaches, especially the work of Tom Kitwood in the field of dementia, has given the nursing profession and others a new frame of reference. However, there are continued developments in this area of care. Nolan *et al.* (2006) have developed a more relationship-centred approach called the Senses Framework. It has been suggested that person-centred approaches to care often identify the needs of the older person and their carers separately (Ryan *et al.*, 2008). This is reflected in the Single Shared Assessment where the carer's needs are also addressed. It raises the question of whether person-centred care is enough to provide the best quality of care for older people.

The Senses Framework emphasises the importance of the relationships between older people, their families and carers and those professionals who care for them. It identifies that the needs of each of these groups are equally important and that meeting all these needs can improve quality of care (Nolan *et al.*, 2006). This framework identifies six senses that must be addressed, including a sense of security, continuity, belonging, purpose, achievement and significance (Nolan *et al.*, 2004). Each of these needs are addressed not only from the perspective of the older person, but also for families, carers and professional staff. This is an example of how one of these six senses can be applied.

A sense of security

- For the older person – their needs for fundamental physical and psychological care and safety are sensitively met;
- For family and carers – their needs to be confident in providing care, to have support and help to maintain their own wellbeing and feel able to allow others to help them care;
- For professional carers – their need to feel safe, secure and supported emotionally as they care for others.

(Adapted from Nolan *et al.*, 2006)

CONCLUSION

This chapter has examined the concept of person-centred theories and care frameworks. It is clear from the literature that this central idea of caring for people in a person-centred way is very attractive to us as nurses. It reflects the strong values of care, respect and compassion most caregivers espouse. However, we have also seen that it is not an easy concept to introduce to our practice; it requires self knowledge, good interpersonal skills, and time and resources to implement. It can be challenging to the nurse who may have to work within a culture of care or an organisation that does not value this approach. The individual nurse may be uncomfortable with the concept and may feel challenged by the close working relationship required to facilitate this. Despite this, it is clear that the person-centred approach to care is likely to continue to be developed and refined as we have seen in the work of Nolan *et al.* (2006) in the Senses Framework. The development of relationship-centred care in this framework may simply be the next step to being truly person-centred in our care of the older person, their family and carers and the nurses caring for them. Person-centred care may simply evolve to include everyone involved in the caring process.

FURTHER READING

Baldwin, C. and Capstick, A. (eds) (2007) *Tom Kitwood on Dementia: A Reader.* Maidenhead: Open University Press/McGraw-Hill
A collection of Kitwood's papers with critical and thoughtful commentaries on these.

Brooker, D. (2007) *Person-Centred Dementia Care.* London: Jessica Kingsley Publishers.
This is a guide to implementing person-centred care for the person with dementia.

McCormack, B. (2001) *Negotiating Partnerships with Older People: A Person-Centred Approach.* Aldershot: Ashgate Publishing
This book is a research based approach to person-centred care for the older person.

Nolan, M., Davies, S. and Grant, G. (eds) (2001) *Working with Older People and their Families.* Buckingham: Open University Press
This explores in some depth the relationship-centred and partnership approaches to care of the older person.

Useful websites

www.edenalt.org
The Eden Alternative is a non-profit organisation that aims to improve quality of life for older people in care environments.

www.dementia.stir.ac.uk
The Dementia Services Centre at Stirling University. This is a comprehensive collection of resources for wide ranging materials and information on dementia.

www.cpa.org.uk
The Centre for Policy on Ageing aims to support positive social policy for older people and spread good practice in this field.

www.joycesimard.com/namaste.html
The website for the end of life Namaste care programme. This programme is formulated to help caregivers minister to the spirit and personhood of the person with dementia at the end of their life.

www.un.org/esa/socdev/ageing
This is the United Nations programme on ageing and presents a global view of the needs of the older person.

REFERENCES

Alabaster, E. (2007) 'Involving students in the challenges of caring for older people'. *Nursing Older People*, 19 (6): 23–8

Barker, P. (2003a) 'Assessment – the foundation of practice' in Barker, P. (ed.) *Psychiatric and Mental Health Nursing: The Craft of Caring.* London: Arnold

Barker, P. (2003b) 'Person-centred care: the need for diversity' in Barker, P. (ed.) *Psychiatric and Mental Health Nursing: The Craft of Caring.* London: Arnold

Brooker, D. (2007) *Person-centred Dementia Care.* London: Jessica Kingsley Publishers

Baldwin, C. and Capstick, A. (2007) *Tom Kitwood on Dementia: A Reader.* Maidenhead: Open University Press/McGraw-Hill

Clarke, A., Hanson, E.J. and Ross, H. (2003) 'Seeing the person behind the patient: enhancing the care of older people using a biographical approach'. *Journal of Clinical Nursing,* 12: 697–706

Department of Health (2001) *National Service Framework for Older People.* London: Department of Health

Dewar, B.J. (2005) 'Beyond tokenistic involvement of older people in research – a framework for future development and understanding'. *International Journal of Older People Nursing,* in association with *Journal of Clinical Nursing,* 14 (3a): 48–53

Dewing, J. (2004) 'Concerns related to the application of frameworks to promote person-centredness in nursing with older people'. *International Journal of Older People Nursing,* 13 (3a): 39–44

Ford, P. and McCormack, B. (2000) 'Keeping the person in the centre of nursing'. *Nursing Standard,* 14 (46): 40–4

Kelly, T.B., Tolson, D., Schofield, I. and Booth, J. (2005) 'Describing gerontological nursing: an academic exercise or prerequisite for progress'. *International Journal of Older People Nursing,* 14 (3a): 13–23

Kitwood, T. (1997) *Dementia Reconsidered: The Person Comes First.* Buckingham: Open University Press

McCabe, C. (2004) 'Nurse–patient communication: an exploration of patients' experiences'. *Journal of Clinical Nursing,* 13: 41–9

McCormack, B. (2001) *Negotiating Partnerships with Older People: A Person-Centred Approach.* Aldershot: Ashgate Publishing

McCormack, B. (2003) 'A conceptual framework for person-centred practice with older people'. *International Journal of Nursing Practice,* 9: 202–9

McCormack, B. (2004) 'Person-centredness in gerontological nursing: an overview of the literature'. *International Journal of Older People Nursing,* 13 (3a): 31–8

McCormack, B. and McCance, T. (2006) 'Development of a framework for person-centred nursing'. *Journal of Advanced Nursing,* 56 (5): 472–9

Morris, C. (2004) 'Personal Construct Psychology and person-centred care' in Jones, G.M.M. and Mieson, B.M.L (eds) *Care-Giving in Dementia,* Vol 3. Abingdon: Brunner Routledge

Morton, I. (1999) *Person-Centred Approaches to Dementia Care*. Bicester: Winslow Press

Nolan, M., Davies, S. and Grant, G. (eds) (2001) *Working with Older People and Their Families*. Buckingham: Open University Press

Nolan, M., Brown, J., Davies, S., Nolan, J. and Keady, J. (2006) *The Senses Framework: Improving Care for Older People Through a Relationship-Centred Approach*. Getting Research into Practice Report (GRiP). Sheffield: The University of Sheffield.

Nolan, M.R., Davies, S., Brown, J., Keady, J. and Nolan, J. (2004) 'Beyond person-centred care: a new vision for gerontological nursing'. *International Journal of Older People Nursing*, 13 (3a): 45–53

Price, B. (2006) 'Exploring person-centred care'. *Nursing Standard*, 20 (50): 49–56

Ryan, T., Nolan, M., Reid, D. and Enderby, P. (2008) 'Using the Senses Framework to achieve relationship-centred care services: A case example'. *Dementia*, 7 (71): 71–93.

Scottish Executive (2000) Report of the Joint Future Group at **www.scotland.gov.uk/library3/social/rjfg-00.asp** (Accessed 27 February 2008)

Tuohy, D. (2003) 'Student nurse–older person communication'. *Nurse Education Today*, 23: 19–26

Wilkins, P. (2003) *Person-Centred Therapy in Focus*. London: Sage

Part Two

Chapter 5

Communication and Older People

Susan Royce and F.J. Raymond Duffy

Learning outcomes

Reading this chapter will enable you to:

- explore the complexities of communication both verbal and non-verbal;

- discuss the ways in which verbal and non-verbal communication can be open to different interpretations and the causes and consequences of this;

- consider barriers to communication specifically in relation to older people;

- examine possible strategies to overcome communication difficulties with older people.

INTRODUCTION

This chapter explores the role of communication. It will explore why communication is important and the various influences on and barriers to communication. It will discuss how verbal language is used and what difficulties can arise from its use, the method of its delivery and how this can affect interpretation by others. This interpretation of received verbal language, and the perception through which it is translated, is influenced by culture, age, social class, education and many other factors. The method of speech delivery, speed and volume in which verbal language is delivered (paralanguage) also affects both the meaning intended and the possible interpretations by others. This will be related to how and why older people need to be communicated with effectively, while also considering the problems that older people may have that can affect communication.

WHY DO WE COMMUNICATE?

Hosely and Mollie (2006) suggest that communication is vital to survival. Humans are essentially social animals and their survival is dependent on their ability to socialise with, and be recognised as, part of a group. Communication is an inherent part of this skill and, as such, it is a natural factor in most people's life from birth to death. Communication is an inherent part in the development of attitudes, ideas and emotions and the expression of these. As such, communication plays a large part in our socialisation processes. Communication also assists with maintaining and expressing our individuality and personality. This helps us to adapt and maintain our self-esteem and also how we modify and assert our position within our social groupings.

Activity 1

Write down your answers to the following questions:

- Why is communication important to you?
- What do your answers to the above question say about you?
- Do your answers reflect just your personal life?
- Your social life?
- Your professional life?
- Which of these do you think is most important to you?

Activity 2

Using the answers that you have given in the previous activity, go on and answer these questions:

- In your personal life how would poor communication affect you as an individual?
- What emotional response, if any, would you have to poor communication?
- What could you do about it?
- Would you consider acting on those actions? If yes, why? If not, why not?

Activity 3

Now consider poor communication in your working environment only:

- Have you encountered poor communication in your professional life?
- Was this in relation to you personally or to the client/client group you deal with?
- If it did affect the client/client group you were working with, would you respond differently to it?
- As care workers, do we take on the position of acting as an advocate for our clients more readily than we would advocate for ourselves or our colleagues? Why might this be so?

Within your own professional life reflect on the following questions:

- Have you ever communicated ineffectively with a client/patient?
- What were the causes of this ineffective communication?
- What were the consequences of this ineffective communication?
- What did you learn from the experience?

From these exercises you can see how important communication is to us all, both from a personal and from a professional viewpoint. When communication is ineffective it can cause problems for the individuals concerned and the consequences of this can be far reaching. Social isolation or feelings of being misunderstood, ignored or neglected all have a negative impact on us as individuals. It also inhibits our ability to belong to groups, as ineffective communication makes group cohesiveness difficult. This reflects and impinges on how we feel about ourselves, the social groups that we work and interact with and on other aspects of our lives.

HOW DO WE COMMUNICATE?

There are many definitions of communication as well as numerous attempts to subdivide it into the individual elements that constitute communication. What is generally agreed is that there are two distinct elements, verbal communication and non-verbal communication. However, the rationale for communication is not based on how we communicate, but on why we communicate. Lasswell (1948) was an early guru of visual communication and media. He claimed that an act of communication was adequately explained only when every aspect of his famous questions has been answered: 'Who says what, in which channel, to whom, with what effect?' For communication to be effective we have to satisfy these questions and appreciate why they are important. Communication is more than just telling someone something. It is also about the influence and impact that the information has on the individual (see Figure 1).

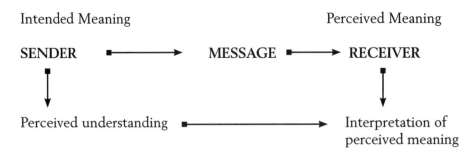

Figure 1 a two-way communication between a sender and a receiver

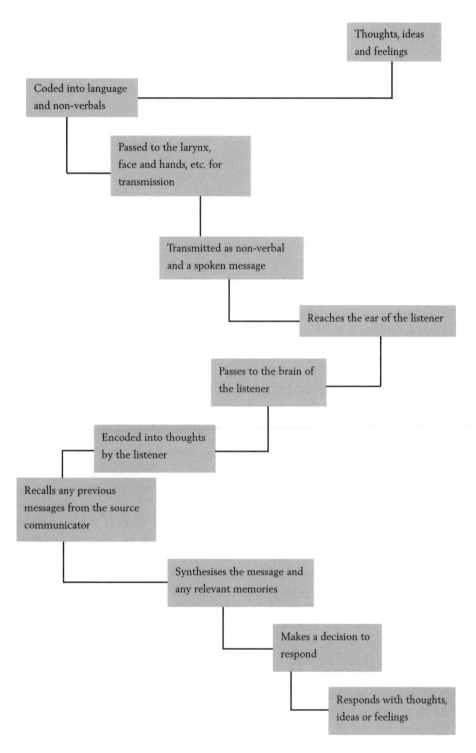

Figure 2 The complexity of apparently simple communication
(adapted from University of Paisley, 2003)

Within this interaction, the verbal language is interpreted and so are the paralinguistics, which include volume, pitch, tone and accent. Non-verbal cues will also be taken into account and utilised. The diagram in Figure 1 shows communication messages being sent and received. It is in the success of encoding and decoding a message where interpretation of any messages occurs. It is failures at this level which cause complications and misunderstandings.

Figure 2 helps to illustrate visually some of the steps involved in the sending and receiving of a communication message. This does not fully show all possible stages, which in itself will help you to realise the complexity of communication. It also helps you to understand how easily problems arise with receiving, encoding and the various complexities that arise that can lead to misunderstandings occurring.

Communication is an extremely complex business because it includes the interchange of ideas, thoughts and emotions, both past and present. Individuals also bring their social, cultural and emotional background to any interaction. Is it surprising then that effective communication is complex?

Verbal and non-verbal communication

The verbal words we choose to use send out a message but this can be influenced by the use of paralanguage, i.e. the way in which these words are delivered. The message that the sender intended may or may not be enhanced by the way in which this paralanguage is used. The visual messages and non-verbal messages that are emitted are extremely important for both the sender and the receiver. It is perhaps no surprise that most analysts of communication agree that during interpersonal relationships verbal language contributes less than 10 per cent of the message, while 50–60 per cent is delivered through body language, with the remainder transmitted via paralanguage (Emap Healthcare, 2000). Perhaps this explains the expressions like 'silence speaks louder than words' or 'we have two ears, two eyes but only one mouth'. Drahota, Costall and Reddy (2008) showed that people can differentiate between at least four different types of smile, clearly showing the variety of interpretations we take from paralanguage and non-verbal cues. Communicating your message clearly and unambiguously involves effort from both the sender of the message and the receiver of the message. It is this process that can be fraught with errors.

There is a Mexican proverb that states that: 'The tongue slow, the eye quick'. This indicates that we interpret visual clues more quickly than we do the spoken word. Even when we use verbal language, we manage to make use of visual signals to emphasise the importance of the verbal language. The receiver responds with non-verbal cues as to how much importance they place on the verbal message. Attentiveness, moving closer, head nodding, etc. all give indications to the sender that they are interested and intent on hearing more. The importance of non-verbal cues both by the sender and the receiver are part of ensuring that the information sent is received and understood. Language has evolved yet we still use the verbal words 'I see' to mean 'I understand', highlighting the importance of our non-verbal cues.

When working with older people it is extremely important to ensure that you are aware of the non-verbal cues that you may be using. Older people are often seen as insatiable users of care services and are often regarded as an unpopular client group to work with (Health Advisory Service, 2000). This makes it even more pressing for care workers to ensure that positive verbal and non-verbal cues are used when working with older people in order not to perpetuate the stigma and discrimination that older people state they experience in healthcare (Roberts, Robinson and Seymour, 2004).

Active communication

For active communication to take place it is important to remember the aim of communication. It is the aim of communication to bring two independent, thinking and feeling human beings with different ideas, concepts, values, upbringing and ages together in order to exchange ideas and attempt to understand each other's perspectives. It is this exchanging of ideas that is the crux of the matter. When working with older people some care workers do not act on or give sufficient importance to older people's ideas and thoughts. It is imperative that care workers see beyond the effects of ageing and disease and respond to the 'real' person who has their own thoughts and ideas and perspective on the situation.

The basis for the need for communication can often be the cause of misunderstanding. For example, care workers often try to persuade or at least get the client to consider some things they may not wish to. Consider the following, what if I wish you to stop smoking, and tell you so? How will this be interpreted? Is this just me asserting my authority over you because I am a health care professional? Do you expect me to say this and so fail to give any attention to my message? By stating my belief, have I failed to give sufficient thought to the complexity of the problem for you? Will you listen to me and will you ask me to tell you why, etc.? To have any idea about what a real person's reaction might be you need to have some idea of their perspectives and views. These problems are intensified by the nature of the relationships between the parties. The older person's previous rivalries and mistrust may prevent this kind of message from ever being offered or accepted at face value. Not only are the language, paralinguistics and verbal and non-verbal components important, we also need to consider the relationship between the two parties involved if successful communication is to take place. It is often the case that we see and hear what we expect, rather than what actually takes place.

Activity 4

Imagine yourself walking into a new health care work environment.

- What is your first action in this new environment?
- How do you adapt to this new environment? Do you use skills from your previous care environment to attempt to fit in?
- Where do you get your cues from as to what is the expected behaviour for this new environment?
- Do you trust the information and cues that you receive? Or are you wary and prefer to double check that information is correct?
- What do you do if you find some of the care practices in this new environment to be unsuitable?
- How do you change these practices or do you adapt to your new environment?

The answers that you give enable you to consider where, when, how and why you survive in a new social environment. They help you to understand how and why social order is achieved and maintained. They may also enable you to understand why some older people need to recheck information regularly. We all, as human beings, have a need to belong to someone or something. We need to belong and fit in to the environment in which we exist; it is part of the socialising process (Warren, Holloway and Smith, 2000).

To put this into a more concrete framework, part of this humanising process is to build and make contact between people. The dynamic process of communication involves continual adaptation and adjustments of a person to each other, whatever and wherever the setting.

Activity 5

Look back on your answers to the previous questions.

- Did you develop as the same person in this new care environment or as someone slightly different?

One of the major factors that encourage us to adapt and fit into a new environment is based around our need to develop and grow as individuals. A healthy interpersonal relationship with those we work with provides for personal growth and development, which in turn is also reflected on those we are caring for in this environment (Wicke, Coppin and Payne, 2004).

Socialisation and its impact on communication

Empathy

As care workers we are aware of the confusion and unnecessary misunderstandings that can occur because of jargon. If you add to this the emotional state of the people being cared for the likelihood of misunderstanding becomes high. For older people in a care setting it is vitally important that the care workers appreciate this. Care workers also need to consider other influences in this situation. One way of achieving this is to consider empathy. Empathy is the ability to see the world as another person does. It is important that we do not let our own personal experiences colour our interactions with our patients/clients. In order to empathise it is necessary to set aside your own perceptions and attempt to consider the way the other person might be thinking. It is impossible to completely enter someone's total frame of reference but it is important that care workers try (Reynolds and Scott, 1992).

For example, as a student nurse I had a placement with a district nurse that was to alter my thinking in relation to how I perceived lack of concordance. During a discussion on this topic after meeting a particularly difficult older lady the district nurse stated that it was her premise that: 'There is no such thing as a non-compliant patient. There are only health care professionals who do not listen enough.' This allowed me to appreciate that most patients would not choose to deliberately not follow medical advice. There are probably other factors, past events or problems, that the nurse is unaware of, that may make the patient choose to disregard the advice/treatment offered. With hindsight, this is a simplistic way to view lack of concordance but it does highlight the need to see and understand the patient's perspective on this issue.

It is difficult not to view situations from a personal perspective, but it is good practice that you are aware of this. Empathy is an important and intrinsic part of a health care worker's required skills. Empathy is also a powerful communication skill that is often misunderstood and underused (Irving and Dickson, 2004). The origin of the word 'empathy' dates back to the 1880s when a German psychologist, Theodore Lipps, used the word 'einfühlung' (in feeling with) to describe the emotional appreciations of another's feelings. Perhaps it can best be described as the capacity to understand another human being's experience from within that person's frame of reference or, to put it more simply, 'to put oneself into another person's shoes'.

BARRIERS TO COMMUNICATION

The need to communicate is an essential need for all of us. However, misinterpretation can and does happen. This makes comprehension, interchange and understanding between people complex. Communication failure occurs for many reasons. It could be that the receiver's language skills may not be sufficient to understand the message because, for example, they may be communicating in a language other than their native tongue. The accent or phonetics used can also make the meaning difficult to understand. The meaning may be altered due to the perception and interpretation of the receiver. People's perceptions and interpretations are also influenced by culture, religion, social class and education. There are whole branches of sociology that deal with perception and interpretation. However, for the sake of clarity, it is best to accept that everyone is different and because of this diversity, they all perceive things differently.

Homonyms

As if communication is not complex enough because of the possibility of misperception and misinterpretation, we need to consider 'homonyms'. Homonyms are words that have more than one meaning. In modern spoken English, many elements of the language have changed over time and developments continue. Each development adds to the list of homonyms. The rise in the use of information technology and increased use of the internet has also had an influence on meanings in current verbal language. In order to illustrate the complexity of homonym uses consider the following:

- **Ball** – a round object that you throw, or a dance that you attended, or a dance that you did whether for joy or not?
- **Pound** – a unit of currency in the United Kingdom, a measure of weight that is becoming redundant, a home where lost dogs are kept, or to hit an object with force.
- **Row** – a line of people, to propel a boat on water, or a noisy argument between people.
- **Sole** – bottom part of the foot, a flat fish, or the only one.

Intergenerational homonyms exist where the homonym has had a different meaning added to the list over the lifetime of an individual. So 'Chip', for example, is a small piece of wood or a fried potato, but had nothing to do with the inner workings of a computer until the 1970s. A few decades ago, 'grass' was mown, but it was never intended to be smoked as a relaxation or recreational drug. 'Coke' was a processed form of coal kept out in the coalshed or an American-based carbonated flavoured drink, but it was never considered to be an illegal drug that could be snorted. 'Aids' was a beauty treatment or help for someone, but it was never thought of as a potentially deadly virus.

Communication and culture

Leininger (1995) and Andrews (2007) have both been advocates of the need for health care professionals to become informed about the cultures of others. They believe in the need to understand how easily offence can be given if you are unaware of cultural difference. In gerontology, it is often stated that the first hazard is the stigma and the discrimination of being old, the second is being both old and female (Letvak, 2002; Duncan and Loretto, 2004) and the third is that of belonging to a different ethnic grouping or cultural background, however this occurs (Cooper, 2002). In this instance 'culture' portrays both those created by belonging to a Black or Minority Ethnic (BME) group and those that arise because of social divisions such as class. There is a need to understand the nuances of other cultures in order not to stigmatise and neglect those from them. The numbers of older people from BME groups within Britain is increasing greatly (Office of National Statistics, 2002). The affect of all the stigmas that these older people face, makes them more likely to need to access health care. It is essential then that care workers understand the need to be aware of cultural and ethnic nuances when communicating, in order to provide required care and avoid causing offence.

Sensory impairments

Hearing loss

Some of the barriers that exist to communication are due to the sensory deficits that accompany age. Of particular relevance are auditory and visual impairments. Presbycusis (the hearing loss expected as you age) can make speech inaudible or distorted particularly with regard to high-pitched sounds. Older people can become self-conscious of this limitation, particularly when interacting in groups and, as a result, they may limit their exposure to group settings, reducing the impact of the problem but also limiting their social contacts. It has also been estimated that approximately 10 per cent of older people have difficulties hearing telephone conversations because of hearing loss (Eliopolous, 2005). There is even growing evidence that older people with hearing loss lose some of their ability to memorise, as subtle effects of hearing loss on memory and cognitive function in older people are being discovered (Wingfield, Tun and McCoy, 2005).

Visual impairment

Visual impairment, which may also accompany ageing, may also affect communication. In 50 per cent of the over 80s there are severe acuity problems, caused by Presbyopia – age-related long sightedness, cataracts, glaucoma, macular degeneration and diabetic retinopathy (Worral and Hickson, 2003). These can all cause communication difficulties, because facial expressions and gestures may be missed or misinterpreted.

Other sensory impairments affecting communication

Some older people may also be affected by trauma, illness or disease that may cause other barriers to communication. For example, during illness the information processing system does not function as well as normal (DeLongis and Holtzman, 2005; Downe-Wamboldt, Butler and Coulter, 2006). Furthermore, some difficulties are illness-specific, for example, touch can be affected by stroke and neuropathic illnesses, thought processing and perception can be affected by dementia-causing illnesses and depression and some older people may have difficulty with speech production such as, for example, in dysphasia or aphasia caused by stroke.

Social barriers to communication

Another range of reported 'barriers' seem to be social in nature. A barrier that is frequently mentioned in health care literature is one that is caused by the generation gap between those who are being cared for and those who are caring. Older people have a different set of values and different expectations from the young. The values and beliefs they have about health care workers mean that they are less likely to challenge their authority. They are also less likely to want to become involved in decision making about their care and may also be less likely to discuss psychological and social issues than their younger counterparts (Davies, Laker and Ellis, 1997). Bethea and Balazs (1997) point out that older adults also appear to seek a higher level of certainty and tend to make more mindful and cautious decisions than younger adults. They may also be slower to adopt technological innovations. Compounding this problem is the fact that medical decisions tend to have a certain level of risk involved and, in recent years, a greater range of choices in health care is available. This failure to understand each other's viewpoint, values and expectations can make effective communication difficult (leMay, 2006).

Barriers resulting from staff attitudes

Of greatest concern perhaps is that a number of barriers to communication related to staff attitudes also exist. Some studies, for example Coupland, Coupland and Giles (1991) and Hummert, Shaner and Gartska (1995), indicate that some health care workers alter the way they speak when addressing older people. They adjust their speech to a type that is simplified, higher in pitch and similar to the manner used to address children; a speech pattern that is quite patronising (see Activity 7 in this chapter). Other signs of underlying ageism in communication can include paternalism (making decisions for the patient rather than with them) and talking over the person or talking to relatives and carers rather than addressing the patient/client directly (Hope, 1994; Lothian and Philp, 2001).

There are also some taboo areas that health care workers rarely discuss with older people. One area is sex and sexual relationships, perhaps because there is a misconception on the part of many professionals that older people are neither interested in nor capable of sex (Kaiser, 1996). There is also a reluctance by practitioners to discuss sex with any age group because most lack experience in the use of sex therapies (Eliopolous, 2005). Another taboo area for many health care professionals involves confrontation and conflict. Again there appears to be a misconception that this should be avoided with older people because they deal less well with the stress of conflict than others (Eliopolous, 2005).

Environmental barriers to communication

A final series of barriers relate to the environment in which communication is occurring or to the circumstances in which communication occurs. For example, in many health care settings the older person is in an area which is shared with others, it is noisy and full of distractions for both the health care professional and the patient/client. There are often few areas available for private conversations (Emap Healthcare, 2000). Older adults and professional carers also have differing agendas because of the circumstances they are in. For example, the patient/client may want social contact and interaction, while the health care professional wants to hurry on to achieve another task (Kralic, Koch and Wotton, 1997). The nurse's role within the ward also affects their agenda, as those with responsibility for the ward are more task-oriented because of the number of interruptions they expect, they have a number of differing priorities to contend with, experience time pressures and other factors that accompany their leadership role (Caris-Verhallen, Kerkstra and Bensing, 1997).

Another environmental issue to note is that ward organisation may also have an impact on communication. Health care staff in wards where primary nursing (nurse-led team care where a named nurse co-ordinates the care of individual patients) was adopted, as opposed to team or functional (task-oriented) nursing, communicated more effectively regardless of their grade. They spent more time offering choice to the people in their care and more time seeking verbal feedback and were also more likely to take into account individual needs (Davies, Laker and Ellis, 1997; Allen and Vatale-Nolen, 2005).

Activity 6

We have all been in situations of stress when someone has tried to give you instructions.

- How well did you receive those instructions?
- Did you follow them?
- Could you recall them when required?

Here you can have empathy with those patients that are receiving information that is going to change their lives. Health care professionals need to be aware that in such situations the information received is likely to be misunderstood. It is necessary to compensate for this by reiterating information in small comprehensive chunks. Feedback from the older person themselves is required in order to ensure that they understand any instructions that are delivered.

It is easy to believe that all health care workers attempt to be effective communicators. However, the research in this area does not readily support this view. Poor communication in clinical settings is the largest source of patient/client dissatisfaction (Calnan, Almond and Smith, 2003). That does not mean that all workers in care settings are ineffective communicators. However, there is a need for greater consideration of how health workers communicate and the difficulties faced by those with whom they are communicating. It is easy to see that the complex nature of the type of communication required does not make this an easy task. The World Health Organisation (2002) considers an ageing population as a triumph of social development and public health and as something that should be viewed as a challenge rather than a crisis. Growing old is neither a disease nor a disability but growing older is associated with an increased likelihood of disease, disability or both. As such, health care workers need to consider all potential impairments to communication in a more positive manner. It is necessary for them to expand their communication skills in order to overcome problems that older people may have. It is by this means that the quality of care to older people will be improved.

Communication is basic to all caring interventions; it is the most important component in the development of all therapeutic relationships. This is one of the most essential aspects of care when working with older people. Stereotyping and ageism (Bytheway, 1995) is just as likely to be seen in the care environment as in any other sphere of life. It is imperative that care workers engage with older people and maintain a positive attitude towards older people. Without this positive attitude the development of a therapeutic relationship will not occur. Without this therapeutic relationship effective care will be difficult to deliver (Kaakinen, Shapiro and Gayle, 2001).

POSSIBLE STRATEGIES FOR OVERCOMING COMMUNICATION DIFFICULTIES

Kruijver *et al.* (2000) suggest that, when carers are communicating with patients/clients, they need to not only inform them about the disease or treatment, but also do this within a therapeutic relationship by assessing the patient's/client's concerns, showing understanding and by providing comfort and support using an empathetic approach.

There are two communicative behaviours that care workers employ. Firstly, there is the instrumental communication, which is informing them about the disease, what's going to happen, etc. and, secondly, there is the affective communication, such as showing respect, sympathy and comforting. It is the non-verbal aspects of communication that are especially important with respect to building rapport with others and conveying empathy and support (Kruijver et al., 2000).

Good communication between health and social care professionals and patients and their families and carers is recognised increasingly as integral to best management (leMay, 2006). Despite this, scant attention is given to communication in the educational process of professionals (Chant et al., 2002). There is also a lack of sound research on how best to teach effective communication. There is no need to explore whether communication skills are necessary for good health care provision, only how best to provide these skills (McCabe and Timmins, 2006). The problem lies with what is the most effective method of transferring these skills from training into daily practice. The adoption of a person-centred approach appears not just to improve communication to older people, but also improves care workers' job satisfaction (Allen and Vatale-Nolen, 2005; McCabe and Timmins, 2006).

It can be argued that dysfunctional or ineffective methods of communication with older people can arise in relation to stereotypical expectations of how older people should behave. This expectation is often influenced by the portrayal of older people through the media (Zhang et al., 2006). As these portrayals tend to be predominantly negative images of older people, it is hardly surprising that this has an effect on the method of communication used by care workers. Hummert et al. (1995) suggest that perceptions of negative decline with ageing are common attitudes among care workers and they believe that these negative attitudes affect how health care workers interact with older people. This is personified by patronising behaviour, speaking slowly and loudly, the use of diminutives such as 'honey' and 'love', almost to the degree, as Simpson (2002) suggests, of what is called 'elderspeak' or secondary baby talk. In 'elderspeak', care workers tend to use a singsong voice, changing pitch and exaggerating tones, use a limited vocabulary and repeat and paraphrase what has just been said during conversation.

Activity 7

- Have you ever noticed someone talking to an older person in 'elderspeak'?
- Have you ever found yourself doing this?
- Were you just mimicking what everyone else did?
- Were you aware of doing this?
- Are there any circumstances that you can think of that appear to encourage this manner of conversation?
- What impact do you think it has on the older person and the likelihood of them conversing further with those who do this?

Among other things that 'elderspeak' conveys, it includes an implication that the older person is not competent. It indicates that miscommunication is occurring and that this is the fault of the older person. It may reinforce stereotypes about ageing and erode the self-esteem of the older person. The older person may also see it as a method for indicating who is superior in the relationship and may view it as a distant and cold way to communicate. Most aspects of 'elderspeak' actually decrease comprehension. It is confusing if a word is exaggerated. It is also hard to understand a statement that sounds like a question and talking too slowly may make it difficult for some older people to focus on the main point of the communication (Kemper and Harden, 1999).

Unfortunately, it is perhaps worth noting that the environments where elderspeak is encountered are the environments where it may do the most damage. Older people in long-term institutions have fewer opportunities for social interaction than most. It is in these environments where you, the health care professional, will meet the neediest group of older people. It is these health care professionals that require the highest levels of communication skills in order not to miss any opportunities as they arise to engage in communication with older people in this setting. It is in these settings where effective and respectful communication is most needed (Carpiac-Claver and Levy-Storm, 2007).

CONCLUSION

Although this chapter does not examine this in any depth, the importance of taking into account the views of service users has been a recurrent theme of recent gerontological practice and government policy (see Chapter 1). Despite this, care workers working with older people still do little to take account of the views of service users (Calnan, Almond and Smith, 2003). Older people themselves often feel that their encounters with care workers are based on the care worker's need to be seen as powerful. By acting in this manner the care worker makes the older person feel demeaned (Lothian and Philp, 2001; Nordgren and Fridlund, 2001). Respect for older people's dignity is inherent in good gerontological practice. Woolhead *et al.* (2004) suggest that older people find it easier to talk about the lack of dignity than how to maintain it. Therefore, it is necessary for the care workers to ensure that respect for older people's dignity is uppermost and this is dependent on effective communication.

Effective communication with older people requires the emotional engagement of the professional with their client. In fact, older people are usually very aware of whether communication is patient-focussed or nurse-focussed and whether responses may be spontaneous or learned. They do not, after all, lack experience of good communication.

Essentially, contemporary communication research and writing suggests that health care professional–patient communication ought to be patient-centred and that the professional needs to work with sincerity, warmth and empathy to maintain a patient focus during all communication (McCabe and Timmins, 2006). It is also worth noting that advances in communication and information technology will certainly have an impact on what will be considered effective communication in the future. Many of these changes will be positive and will enhance both the number and the nature of communication contacts that the health care professional has with older people. However, the ways in which new technologies will enhance communication with older people are still being explored. There is a positive interest among health care professionals and older people to engage with and utilise new technologies to enhance communication, but currently only a few examples of what might be achievable exist – see Philipson and Roberts (2007) and Gilleard, Hyde and Higgs (2007).

FURTHER READING

Balzer-Riley, J. (2000) *Communication in Nursing* (4th edn). Edinburgh: Elsevier/Mosby

A clear and concise and well organised book looking at the skills required by nurses in order to improve their communication skills. It looks at wider issues affecting communication than the previous book.

Harwood, J. (2007) *Understanding Communication and Ageing: Developing Knowledge and Awareness*. Thousand Oaks, CA: Sage
A new book looking at communication and ageing and attempting to overcome the stereotyping of older people. However it is from the USA.

Suly, P. and Dallas, J. (2005) *Essential Communication Skills for Nursing*. Edinburgh: Elsevier/Mosby
A clear, concise book that looks at useful communication skills for nurses. Useful as a reference guide although does not look specifically at problems with older people.

Worral, I. and Hickson, L.M. (2003) *Communication Disability: From Prevention to Intervention*. Florence, KY: Thomson Delmar
An interesting and informative book that explores how the ageing process may affect communication. It also explores possible methods and tools that may be used to overcome these problems.

Useful websites

www.communicationmatters.org.uk
Communication Matters is the UK Chapter of the International Society for Augmentative and Alternative Communications (ISAAC) which focusses on the needs of people with complex communication needs who may benefit from AAC systems to maximise their opportunities and enhance their life. Augmentative and alternative communication (AAC) systems include eye pointing, gesture, signing, using symbol/word boards, and electronic speech devices. Worldwide, there are 11 National Chapters of ISAAC, co-ordinated by a Secretariat based in Canada.

www.library.nhs.uk/laterlife
The NHS Library for Health have a Later Life Specialist Collection that aims to meet the information needs of health care professionals who work with older adults. It is also freely available to the general public unlike some other areas of the library. It holds many resources that older people's health care professionals will find useful including access to the best practice statement on maximising communication with older people who have hearing disability.

www.aphasianow.org
Aphasia Now is a website created by and for aphasic people of working age. It came about with the help of the Tavistock Trust for Aphasia, a leading UK charity which works in this field.

www.rnid.org.uk
The Royal National Institute for the Deaf is the largest charity working to assist the UK's 9 million deaf and hard-of-hearing people. They campaign and

lobby on relevant issues as well as raising awareness of deafness and hearing loss. They also provide services to deaf people and conduct social, medical and technical research. The site has extensive information and resource pages.

www.rnib.org.uk
The Royal National Institute for the Blind is a leading UK charity offering information, support and advice to over two million people with sight loss. Like RNID they campaign, lobby, provide services and conduct and commission research on issues relevant to those who have partial sight or sight loss, as well as attempting to raise awareness of sight loss and how this might be prevented. Again this website has extensive information and resource pages.

REFERENCES

Allen, D.E. and Vatale-Nolen, R.A. (2005) 'Patient care delivery model improves nurse job satisfaction'. *The Journal of Continuing Education in Nursing.* 36 (6): 277–83

Andrews, M.M. (2007) *Transcultural Concepts in Nursing Care* (5th edn). Philadelphia, PA: Lippincott, Williams and Wilkins

Bethea, L.S. and Balazs, A.L. (1997) 'Improving intergenerational health care communication'. *Journal of Health Communication*, 2, 129–37

Bytheway, B. (1995) *Ageism.* Buckingham: Open University Press

Calnan, M., Almond, S. and Smith, N. (2003) 'Ageing and Public Satisfaction with the Health Service: An Analysis of Recent Trends'. *Social Science and Medicine*, 57, 757–62

Caris-Verhallen, W.M.C.M., Kerkstra, A. and Bensing, J.M. (1997) 'The Role of Communication in Nursing Care for Elderly People: A Review of The Literature'. *Journal of Advanced Nursing*, 25, 915–33

Carpiac-Claver, M.L. and Levy-Storm, L. (2007) 'In a Manner of Speaking: Communication between Nurse Aides and Older Adults in Long-Term Care Settings'. *Health Communication*, 22 (1): 59–67

Chant, S., Jenkinson T., Randle, J. and Russell, G. (2002) 'Communication Skills: Some Problems in Nursing Education and Practice'. *Journal of Clinical Nursing*, 11 (1): 12–21

Cooper, H. (2002) 'Investigating socio-economic explanations for gender and ethnic inequalities in health'. *Social Science & Medicine*, 54 (5): 693–706

Coupland, N., Coupland, J. and Giles, H. (1991) *Language, Society and the Elderly.* Cambridge: Blackwell

Davies, S., Laker, S. and Ellis, L. (1997) 'Promoting autonomy and independence for older people within nursing practice: a literature review'. *Journal of Advanced Nursing*, 26: 408–17

DeLongis, A. and Holtzman, S. (2005) 'Coping in context: The role of stress, social support, and personality in coping'. *Journal of Personality*, 73 (6): 1633–56

Downe-Wamboldt, B., Butler L. and Coulter, L. (2006) 'The relationship between meaning of illness, social support, coping strategies, and quality of life for lung cancer patients and their family members'. *Cancer Nursing*, 29 (2): 111–19

Drahota, A., Costall A. and Reddy, V. (2008) 'The vocal communication of different kinds of smiles'. *Speech Communication*, 50 (4): 278–87

Duncan, C. and Loretto, W. (2004) 'Never the right age? Gender- and age-based discrimination in employment'. *Gender, Work & Organization*, 11 (1): 95–115

Eliopoulos, C. (2005) *Gerontological Nursing* (6th edn). Philadelphia, PA: Lippincott, Williams and Wilkins

Ellis, R. B., Gale, B. and Kenworthy, N. (1995) *Interpersonal Communication in Nursing: Theory and Practice* (2nd edn). Edinburgh: Churchill Livingstone

Emap Healthcare (2000) *Professional Perspectives in the Care of the Older Person*. London: Emap Healthcare Ltd

Gilleard, C., Hyde, M. and Higgs, P. (2007) 'Community and communication in the third age: The impact of internet and cell phone use on attachment to place in later life in England'. *Journal of Gerontology: Series B: Psychological Sciences Social Sciences*, 62: S276–S283

Health Advisory Service (2000) *Not Because They are Old: An Independent Enquiry into the Care of Older People in General Hospitals*. London: Health Advisory Service

Hope, K. (1996) 'Nurses' attitudes towards older people: a comparison between nurses working in acute medical and acute care of the elderly settings'. *Journal of Advanced Nursing*, 20: 605–12

Hosely, J. and Mollie, C. (2006) *A Practical Guide to Therapeutic Communication for Health Professionals*. New York: Elsevier

Hummert, M.L., Shaner, J.L. and Gartska, T.A. (1995) 'Cognitive processes affecting communication with older adults: the case for stereotypes, attitudes and beliefs about communication' in Nussbaum, J.F. and Coupland, J. (eds) *Handbook of Communication and Ageing Research*. Hillsdale, NJ: Erlbaum

Irving P. and Dickson, D. (2004) 'Empathy: towards a conceptual framework for health professionals'. *International Journal of Health Care Quality Assurance*, 17 (4): 212–20

Kaakinen, J., Shapiro, E. and Gayle, B.M. (2001) 'Strategies for working with clients: a qualitative analysis of elderly client/nurse practitioner communication'. *Journal of the American Academy of Nurse Practitioners*, 13 (7): 325–30

Kaiser, F.E. (1996) 'Sexuality in the elderly'. *Urologic Clinics of North America*, 23: 99–109

Kemper, S. and Harden, T. (1999) 'Experimentally disentangling what's beneficial about elderspeak from what's not'. *Psychology and Aging*, 14: 656–70

Kralic, D., Koch, T. and Woton, K. (1997) 'Engagement and detachment: Understanding patients' experiences with nursing'. *Journal of Advanced Nursing*, 26: 399–407

Kruijver, I.P.M., Kerkstra, A., Francke, A.L., Bensing, J.M. and Van de Weil, H.B.M. (2000) 'Evaluation of communication training programs in nursing care: a review of the literature'. *Patient Education and Counseling* 39: 129–45

Lasswell, H.D. (1948) *Power and Personality*. Kansas, OH: Norton Library

leMay, A. (2006) 'Communication challenges and skills' in S.J. Redfern and F.M. Ross (eds) *Nursing Older People* (4th edn). Edinburgh: Elsevier Churchill Livingstone

Letvak, S. (2002) 'The myths and realities of ageism and nursing'. *Association of Operating Room Nurses (AORN) Journal*, 75 (6): 1101–7

Leininger, M. (1995) *Transcultural Nursing: Concept, Theories, Research and Practices* (2nd edn). New York: McGraw

Lothian, K. and Philp, I. (2001) 'Maintaining the dignity and autonomy of older people in the healthcare setting'. *British Medical Journal*, 322 (7287): 668–70

McCabe, C. and Timmins, F. (2006) *Communication Skills for Nursing Practice*. Basingstoke: Palgrave Macmillan

Mackenzie, C. (2000) 'Adult spoken discourse: the influences of age and education'. *International Journal of Language & Communication Disorders*, 35: 269–85

Nordgren, S. and Fridlund, B. (2001) 'Patients' perceptions of self determination as expressed in the context of care'. *Journal of Advanced Nursing*, 35 (1): 117–25

Office of National Statistics (2002) *Census 2001: National Report for England and Wales*. London: The Stationery Office

Philipson, G. and Roberts, J. (2007) 'Caring for the future: the impact of technology on aged and assisted living'. *Electronic Journal of Health Informatics*, 2 (2): 1-9

Reynolds, W.J. and Scott, B. (2000) 'Do nurses and other professional helpers normally display much empathy?'. *Journal of Advanced Nursing*, 31 (1): 226–34

Roberts, E., Robinson, J. and Seymour, l. (2004) *Old Habits Die Hard: Tackling Age Discrimination in Health and Social Care*. London: King's Fund

Simpson, J. (2002) *Elderspeak – Is It Helpful or Just Baby Talk?* The University of Kansas, OH: Merrell Advanced Study Center. **www.merrill.ku.edu/IntheKnow/sciencearticles/elderspeak.html** (Accessed 24 May 2008)

University of Paisley (2005) On-line Learning Support Material: Ageing Matters – Meeting Healthcare Needs of Older Adults. Paisley: University of Paisley

Warren, J., Holloway, I. and Smith, P. (2000) 'Fitting in: maintaining a sense of self during hospitalisation'. *International Journal of Nursing Studies*, 37: 229–35

Wingfield, A., Tun, P.A. and McCoy, S.L. (2005) 'Hearing loss in older adulthood: what it is and how it interacts with cognitive performance'. *Journal of the American Psychological Society*, 14 (3): 143–248

Wicke, D., Coppin, R. and Payne, S. (2004) 'Team working in nursing homes'. *Journal of Advanced Nursing*, 45 (2): 197–204

Woolhead, G., Calnan, M., Dieppe P. and Tadd, W. (2004) 'Dignity in older age: what do older people in the United Kingdom think?' *Age and Ageing*, 33 (2): 165

World Health Organisation (2002) *Active Ageing: A Policy Framework*. Copenhagen: World Health Organisation Noncommunicable Diseases and

Mental Health Cluster; Noncommunicable Disease Prevention and Health Promotion Department; Ageing and Life Course

Worral, L.E. and Hickson, L.M. (2003) *Communication Disability in Ageing: From Prevention to Intervention.* Australia: Thomson/Delmar Learning

Zhang, Y.B., Harwood, J., Williams, A., Ylanne-McEwan, V., Wadleigh, P.M. and Thim, C. (2006) 'The portrayal of older adults in advertising: a cross-national review'. *Journal of Language and Social Psychology.* 25: 264–82

Chapter 6

Promoting Dignity Through 'Compassionate Care' for the Older Adult in Hospital

Michelle Walters

Learning outcomes

Reading this chapter will enable you to:

- understand the importance of delivering nursing care which is compassionate and promotes dignity to the older adult in hospital;

- recognise and reflect on your own competence in delivering nursing care which is compassionate and promotes dignity.

INTRODUCTION

In today's modern world people are living longer and enjoying better health, when compared with the past, as a result of improved medical advances and scientific research (Tadd, 2005). It has been estimated that, within the next 20 years, the number of people over the age of 85 years residing in the United Kingdom (UK) will increase by two thirds (Royal College of Nursing, 2007). The largest group of hospital service users are older adults who often have complex needs and evidence shows that older adults over the age of 75 years tend to have longer episodes in hospital than those aged between 16 and 45 years (Higgs, 2006). This has implications for the delivery of health care for older adults which requires specialist care, skills and knowledge.

Older adults are one of the most vulnerable groups within society and are often viewed in a stereotypical way as being dependent or having a poor quality of life. Moreover, as cited by Tadd (2005), old age is seen as inevitable decline, which fails to consider the diversity of older people, denying older adults their individual dignity as human beings. This chapter will discuss the importance of delivering nursing care within a hospital environment that is compassionate and promotes patient's rights and maintains their dignity. As a student nurse you are required to be competent in delivering care that is compassionate in approach and maintains the patient's dignity. To enable you to reflect upon your ability to put this into practice there are four case studies for you to read, followed by activities that will help your reflections.

COMPASSION AND DIGNITY

It is generally acknowledged within the nursing profession and general population that an essential component of nursing practice is providing care that is 'compassionate' and 'promotes dignity'. It has been argued in the nursing literature that the concepts of 'compassion' and 'dignity' are too complex to define, and vary according to the context in which they are applied (Dietze and Orb, 2000; Anderberg, *et al.*, 2007; Jacobson, 2007). However, this should not deter nurses from understanding how to deliver 'dignified' care as argued by Walsh and Kowanko (2002).

Compassionate care

Modern nursing literature continues to emphasise the significance of 'compassionate care' within nursing practice (Dietze and Orb, 2000). The term 'compassion' is to do with emotions and feelings and the *Cambridge Dictionary* defines compassion as 'a strong feeling of sympathy and sadness for the suffering or bad luck of others and a desire to help them' (*Cambridge Dictionary*, 2008). The word compassion originates from the Latin – *com* (together with) and *pali* (to suffer), which literally means 'to suffer with' (Dietze and Orb, 2000). Debates about the meaning of compassion as a human experience have been discussed for decades within disciplines such as religion, philosophy and sociology but the essence of compassion is to do with what it means to be human (Kanov *et al.*, 2004).

Compassion within nursing has tended to be viewed as an essential component of nursing practice with the common assumption that nurses, through their professional knowledge and competence, develop the ability to deliver 'compassionate care' (Dietze and Orb, 2000). However, as suggested by Dietze and Orb (2000), within nursing practice compassionate care is more than just a natural reaction to suffering; it takes on wider aspects such as nurses making moral choices. Contemporary nursing literature highlights the difficulties of defining 'compassion' or 'compassionate care' because of the terms being used synonymously with expressions such as empathy and sympathy (Schantz, 2007). According to Schantz compassion in nursing practice is more than being empathetic or sympathetic. It is, as described by Dietze and Orb, about 'entering into that person's experiences so as to share their burden in solidarity with them, hence enabling them to retain their independence and dignity' (Dietze and Orb, 2000: 169). Furthermore, Rinpoche (1992) argues that compassion is about being actively determined to do what is necessary to help alleviate an individual's suffering, which involves being more than just empathetic or sympathetic. The active process of delivering nursing care within a compassionate approach is being sensitive to the needs of others and fundamental to this is being there for patients, not just doing things for them (Kitson, 2004). Showing such compassion by using interpersonal skills when carrying out tasks for patients illustrates the way the moral virtue is applied to the situation. Compassionate caring has the ability to help with healing (Dietze and Orb, 2000) and is an intrinsic part of maintaining and restoring dignity in care (Finfgeld-Connett, 2008).

Dignity in caring

Defining the term 'dignity' has proved difficult due to the complexity of the various meanings and characteristics that can be related to its meaning (Tadd et al., 2002). The word 'dignity' originates from the Latin word dignus, which means 'worthy of esteem and honour' (Borowski, 2007). As stated by Borowski 'human dignity means that we are to respect and behave towards others in ways that increase their gravitas, their importance or worthiness' (Borowski, 2007: 724). Ensuring human dignity within all aspects of life is the cornerstone of the United Nations Declaration that can be traced back to 1948 in the General Assembly of the United Nations Declaration, which highlights dignity as being a basic right of everyone which should always be maintained (Matiti and Trorey, 2004). However, it was not until the enactment of the 1998 Human Rights Act that public bodies in the UK were obligated to comply with the European Convention on Human Rights, which draws attention to various rights such as rights to life, civil rights and social rights (Glasby, 2007). Furthermore, as cited by Glasby (2007), since the introduction of the 1998 Human Rights Act there has been a growing number of legal challenges that have had the effect of changing areas within health and social care services.

Health and social care policies nationally and internationally have increasingly highlighted the right of and need for older people to be treated with dignity but the evidence continues to show that older people are often treated with disrespect and experience undignified care. Providing nursing care for the older adult in a dignified manner needs careful consideration and understanding as providing undignified care impacts negatively on older adults' experiences of health care provision and may lead to poorer health outcomes for some patients (Walsh and Kowanko, 2002).

Over recent years care for older adults in hospital has become a government priority with set standards being introduced to improve service delivery. The publication in March 2001 of the National Service Framework (NSF) for Older People identified itself as a ten-year programme that would address the needs of older people by ending age discrimination, ensuring older people were being treated with respect and dignity and encouraging services to support independence and promote good health (Squires, 2002). Moreover, as Squires states:

> Although a lot of effective work is known to exist within services for older people, the many reported variations in service provision and quality have caused public and professional concern. The NSF aims to develop higher quality services for older people, specialised services for key conditions, and a culture change that will ensure that all older people and their carers are always treated with respect, dignity and fairness. A key strategy for successful implementation will be active engagement of primary, secondary and tertiary care.
>
> (Squires, 2002: 88)

Five years after the introduction of the NSF, Professor Ian Philp, National Director for Older People, highlighted in his report *A New Ambition for Old Age* the continued concerns by some service users of receiving care that was undignified and lacked respect (Department of Health, 2006a). In response, the government put a greater emphasis on the need for services to put dignity at the heart of caring for older people (Agnew, 2007) with greater focus on human rights. In November 2007 the *Dignity in Care* campaign was launched, detailing for service users what they should expect from a service that respects dignity. Taylor (2007) highlights the elements in the campaign:

- The ten areas include zero tolerance of all forms of abuse and respect of people's right to privacy. Service providers, commissioners and the public have been challenged to ensure services are up to scratch.
- A Dignity in Care Champions network is being set up to raise the profile of dignity in care locally. The volunteer network has access to an online resource with examples of best practice and information on events.
- An online practice guide has been developed to help frontline workers, managers, commissioners, older people and their carers to take up the dignity challenge.
- Local authorities will be given £67 million to improve the physical environment of care homes.

(Taylor, 2007)

Dignity model and preserving dignity

Woolhead *et al.* (2006) from their study *Dignity and Older Europeans* devised a model that highlights four types of dignity that should be considered when working with older adults. This incorporates the aspects of respect, either self-respect or respect for others. This model of dignity includes:

- **Dignity of merit** – giving respect to older adults and acknowledging their social status, for example, 'an office holder such as a mayor or bishop has a certain status, which is recognised by other people and for which they are given respect'.
- **Dignity of moral status** – allowing individuals to make choices for themselves within their own moral values, for instance, 'if an individual is able to live according to his or her own moral principles then that person will experience a sense of dignity'.
- **Dignity of personal identity** – allowing an individual to have their own identity, which must be respected and, as cited by Woolhead *et al.*, 'this dignity can be violated by physical interference as well as by emotional or psychological insults such as humiliation'.
- *Menschenwürdig* – ensuring human rights are maintained. 'It is this aspect of dignity that provides a justification of the moral requirement to respect all human beings, regardless of their social, mental or physical properties'.

(Woolhead *et al.*, 2006: 365)

While identifying the importance of dignity Anderberg *et al.*, (2007) discuss the importance of preserving dignity within caring.

Ways of preserving dignity within nursing practice

- **Individualised care** – caring for the individual in a holistic way and recognising the person's wishes and needs at spiritual, social, physical and psychological levels. Taking the time to get to know individuals and valuing them as people by listening and understanding their needs, choices and hopes and aspirations.
- **Control restored** – supporting the older adult to remain in control through transitional changes caused by health problems until they have adjusted and accepted their adapted level of capacity. The older adult should be encouraged to preserve and develop new capabilities.
- **Respect** – this is a fundamental value that many older adults hold dear and they often link dignity and respect. Self-respect for the older adult is preserved if those around them treat and speak to them in a dignified and respectful manner. That is, allowing the older adult to continue with their own habits and allowing them their own space with time to think and reflect on thoughts.
- **Advocacy** – nurses often act as advocates but can become over protective in this role, which can create greater levels of dependency in the older adult. It is important that the nurse is aware of how much support to give to ensure the person's dignity is not lost.
- **Sensitive listening** – being sensitive when communicating with the older adult is important in preserving their dignity and this has been related to the way in which the older adult is addressed. They are often treated in a patronising way and are spoken to as though they are a child.

The list above highlights aspects of holistic care, which means getting involved with the whole person rather than isolating the disease process. Compassionate care is embedded in such holistic care and this happens when you, as a student, learn to go beyond the daily routine of care and treat patients and family members as partners in care (Kelly, 2005; Finfgeld-Connett, 2008).

Compassionate care and your competence as a student

To ensure you as a student are competent to undertake care that is compassionate, promotes dignity and is respectful, the Nursing and Midwifery Council (2007) has introduced 'Essential Skills Clusters' to complement existing proficiencies (Nursing and Midwifery Council, 2007). One of the Essential Skills Clusters that student nurses are required to demonstrate competence in is 'Care, compassion and communication' whereby patients/clients can be reassured that you as a newly qualified registered nurse will have these skills. This cluster states that 'As a newly qualified nurse you should be able to:

Concern has highlighted that although the majority of inpatients within the NHS are older adults the service is not organised to meet their needs. These charities have campaigned for the rights of older adults using health and social services to be treated with respect and dignity wherever that care is being undertaken. There are various charities within the UK which are working in collaboration with the NHS to support older adults in the community and to promote wellbeing through their daily care (Help the Aged, 1999; Age Concern, 2006; British Geriatrics Society, 2007).

Critics have highlighted the way in which health and social care policy and practice has hindered the delivery of consistent and holistic support for older people due to their separation (Glasby and Littlechild, 2004; Tanner and Harris, 2008). In response, the government, under the leadership of the then Prime Minister Tony Blair, placed at its heart the need for improved services for older people through better co-ordinated strategies and services (Tanner and Harris, 2008). Moreover, as cited by Tanner and Harris:

> A central theme within New Labour's health and social care policy is the need for co-ordinated and joined up strategy between all key agencies, not just health and social services.
>
> (Tanner and Harris, 2008: 61)

The implications for greater joint working for health and social services can be seen in the government's White Paper *Our Health, Our Care, Our Say* (Department of Health, 2006b). This document places greater emphasis on a model of service provision that is person-centred, promoting more individual choice and ensuring services overcome any barriers to inclusion and treating people with respect and dignity (Brotherton, 2008).

CASE STUDIES

Consider the following case studies and relate these to what you have learned about dignity and compassionate care so far. Then undertake the related activities.

Going into hospital for the first time can be a very traumatic time for everyone, especially for older adults who are from a different generation with different traditions. Examine the following case study.

Case study 1

Ward story – admission to hospital

Mrs Harris, an 82-year-old lady, is admitted to your medical ward for assessment and is accompanied by her son and daughter. She has not been managing very well at home and her daughter is finding it difficult to cope. As a first year student nurse, part of your learning programme is about ward admission protocols and you have been asked by your mentor to start taking the admission details, which you are keen to do as you want to make a good impression. As you approach Mrs Harris she seems a little agitated and begins to stand up and proceeds to urinate on the floor. Her son and daughter become very upset and embarrassed by this and demand to know where the nearest toilet is, saying that they will manage to clean her. Mrs Harris seems confused and unaware of what is happening.

Activity 1

1. How would you deal with this situation?
2. How would you support Mrs Harris, her son and her daughter in a caring and compassionate way?
3. In what ways could you maintain Mrs Harris's dignity?
4. Can you relate these circumstances to other incidents in your nursing training to date? Think about how you felt and coped in these types of situations.
5. On reflection what could you have done differently?

Once a patient has been in hospital for several days, an assessment profile of them will have been recorded. This profile often changes as the patient progresses and sometimes the unexpected can occur, which will lead you to re-evaluate the patient's care. Consider the following case study.

Case study 2

Ward story – assessment in hospital
You are a second-year student on duty in a busy medical rehabilitation ward. It is lunchtime and you are part-way through your shift. While the lunches are being given out, you are called to the duty desk to answer a telephone enquiry. While you are on the phone, you glance across the ward and notice that Mr Brown, an elderly gentleman with expressive dysphasia, appears to be choking on his food. The carer helping to feed him continues to place food in his mouth, occasionally slapping him on the back. You finish your telephone conversation before going over to check on this patient.

Activity 2

1. Is the carer acting in a compassionate way towards the patient?
2. Do you think the manner in which Mr Brown is being fed is dignified?
3. How would you deal with this situation?
4. What is the protocol within your clinical placement when caring for patients with any feeding difficulties?
5. Can you relate this type of situation to other incidents in your nursing training to date? Think about how you felt and coped in these circumstances.
6. On reflection what could you have done differently?

The majority of elderly patients make good progress in hospital and, when following through the patient's journey, it is always satisfying to help the patient plan for discharge home. A nurse once said that one of the most satisfying aspects of her job in nursing the elderly was 'to follow through a patient who on admission was considered to be too ill to make any progress and over the weeks that followed made excellent progress, [and that] it made her feel that she had achieved something very special'.

Sometimes when a patient is physically better, there may be other issues that you will need to consider when helping a patient plan for discharge home. Consider the following case study.

Case study 3

Ward story – planning for home
Mrs Patel, a 60-year-old Asian woman who understands English but can only speak a few words, is making very good progress following a stroke. The ward team are now considering planning her discharge home and you are a senior third-year student nurse and have been asked by your mentor to start to discuss with Mrs Patel the plan for her discharge.

Activity 3

1. How do you think you will communicate with Mrs Patel in a caring and compassionate manner in order to establish her needs?
2. How will you plan to preserve Mrs Patel's dignity once she has a date to be discharged – what community care teams could be involved with her continuing care?
3. How do you feel about being involved in patient discharge planning?
4. Reflect on your experiences, thinking about your strengths and limitations in discharge planning.

Compassionate care is about being there for patients, not just doing things for them. Sometimes this can be difficult for junior student nurses as they tend to concentrate on getting ward procedures right in the allocated time and forget that patients are real people, who need time to be listened to and supported in the decision-making process about their care. Examine the following case study.

Case study 4

Ward story – the ward routine
As a third-year student nurse you are asked to be a 'buddy' to a first-year nurse student as this is her very first practice placement. The ward is a busy stroke rehabilitation unit and you allocate the student to a bay of six male patients and tell her to ascertain the needs of each patient for their personal hygiene that morning. You observe the student pass along the row of patients with a piece of paper on which she ticks off patients' needs against a list of bath, shower or assisted wash. There is limited conversation with each patient as to what exactly they would prefer and you doubt if the student has given herself the time to get to know the patients' names as she is too anxious to get her workload completed. When you ask how the student is getting on she tells you that she has almost finished her bay of patients, which is the task completed, and asks you what needs to be done next.

Activity 4

1. Has the first-year student acted in a compassionate way towards the patients she has been allocated?
2. Reflecting on this scenario, what feedback would you give to the first-year student for formative learning focussing on the aspects of compassionate and dignified care?

CONCLUSION

This chapter has provided an overview of the difficulties in defining the concepts of 'compassion' and 'dignity'. However, while the concepts are not easy to define it is crucial that, as nurses, we understand how the two terms relate to each other. More importantly, providing care that is compassionate should lead to dignified care being given. Caring for older adults requires a holistic approach but, from the evidence provided, this is not always the case in health and social care policy or practice. The Labour Party since coming into government have made a commitment to ensuring service provision is person-centred, promotes individual choice, respect and dignity. Caring for older adults can be challenging but it is also very rewarding.

Summary points

- Through compassionate care dignity can be maintained or restored.
- Caring for older adults needs to be undertaken with a holistic approach.
- Health and social care services working in partnership can help to ensure older people are placed at the forefront, respecting their dignity as service users.

FURTHER READING

Barry, A. and Yuill, C. (2008) *Understanding the Sociology of Health: An Introduction*. (2nd edn). London: Sage
An interesting chapter on ethnicity, race and health.

Brotherton, G. and Parker, S. (2008) *Your Foundation in Health and Social Care: A Guide for Foundation Degree Students*. London: Sage
This is a comprehensive and readable book with chapters that will provide further support when answering the questions on the case studies.

Tanner, D. and Harris, J. (2008) *Working with Older People*. Abingdon: Routledge
This book has been written for social work students and qualified social workers but for students working within health care it provides a comprehensive account of the importance of partnership working and how social policy has evolved in trying to meet the needs of older adults.

Useful websites

www.dh.gov.uk
Department of Health

www.healthcarecommission.org.uk/_db/_documents/Caring_for_dignity.pdf
The Healthcare Commission

www.rcn.org.uk
Royal College of Nursing

www.scotland.gov.uk
Scottish Executive Health Department

www.nmck.org/aArticle.aspx?ArticleID=1815&Keyword=skills%20and%20clusters
NMC *Proposals Arising from a Review for Practice at the Point of Registration*

www.york.ac.uk/healthsciences/mentors/escsapril07.pdf
NMC *Essential Skills Clusters*

www.cf.ac.uk/medic/subsites/dignity/resources/Educating_for_Dignity.pdf
Educating for dignity *The Dignity Europeans Project: A Multi-disciplinary workbook – Dignity and Older Europeans.*

REFERENCES

Anderberg, P., Lepp, M., Berglund, A. and Segesten, K. (2007) 'Preserving dignity in caring for older adults: a concept analysis'. *Journal of Advanced Nursing,* 59 (6): 635–43

Agnew, T. (2007) 'Dignity in care: a genuine commitment?'. *Nursing Older People,* 18 (12): 7-8

Age Concern (2006) *Hungry to be Heard: The Scandal of Malnourished Older People in Hospital.* London: Age Concern

Borowski, A. (2007) 'Guest editorial: On human dignity and social work'. *International Social Work,* 50, 9 (6): 723–6

Brotherton, G. (2008) 'Planning and managing care' in Brotherton, G. and Parker, S. (2008) *Your Foundation in Health and Social Care: A Guide for Foundation Degree Students.* London: Sage

British Geriatrics Society (2007) *Dignity Behind Closed Doors.* London: British Geriatrics Society

Cambridge Dictionary (2008). 'Compassion' **http://dictionary.cambridge.org/define.asp?dict=CALD&key=15573&ph=on** (Accessed 20 February 2008)

Commission for Healthcare Audit and Inspection (2007) *Caring for Dignity: A National Report on Dignity in Care for Older People While in Hospital.* London: Commission for Healthcare Audit and Inspection

Dearnley, B. (2007) 'Dignity in hospital'. *Nursing Older People,* 19 (4): 19

Department of Health (2006a) *A New Ambition for Old Age: Next Steps in Implementing the National Service Framework for Older People. A Report From Professor Ian Philp, National Director for Older People.* London: Department of Health

Department of Health (2006b) *Our Health, Our Care, Our Say: A New Direction for Community Services* (White Paper). London: Department of Health

Dietze, E. and Orb, A. (2000) 'Compassionate care: a moral dimension of nursing'. *Nursing Inquiry,* 7: 166–74

Finfgeld-Connett, D. (2008) 'Meta-synthesis of caring in nursing'. *Journal of Clinical Nursing,* 17 (2): 196–204

Glasby, J. (2007) *Understanding Health and Social Care.* Bristol: Policy Press

Glasby, J. and Littlechild, R. (2004) *The Health and Social Care Divide: The Experiences of Older People.* Bristol: Policy Press

Hayes, N., Dearnley, B. and Robson, B. (2007) 'Involving older people in improving general hospital care'. *Nursing Older People,* 19 (4): 27–31

Help the Aged (1999) *Dignity on the Ward: Promoting Excellence in Care in Acute Settings.* London: Help the Aged

Higgs, P. (2006) 'Older people, health care and society' in Scambler, G. (ed.) *Sociology as Applied to Medicine* (5th edn). Edinburgh: Saunders

Jacobson, N. (2007) 'Dignity and health: a review'. *Social Science and Medicine,* 64: 292–302

Kanov, J., Maitlis, S., Worline, C., Dutton, E., Frost, J. and Jacoba, M. (2004) 'Compassion in organizational life'. *American Behavioural Scientist,* 47 (6): 808–27

Kelly, T. (2005) 'Describing gerontological nursing: an academic exercise or pre-requisite for progress?'. *International Journal of Nursing Older People,* 14 (3a): 1–11

Kitson, A. (2004) 'The whole person'. *Nursing Standard,* 19 (12): 14–15

Lothian, K. and Philp, I. (2001) 'Care of older people: Maintaining the dignity and autonomy of older people in the healthcare setting'. *British Medical Journal,* 322: 668–70

Matiti, M. R. and Trorey, G. (2004) 'Perceptual adjustment levels: patients' perceptions of their dignity in the hospital setting'. *International Journal of Nursing Studies,* 41: 735–44

Nursing and Midwifery Council (2004) *'The NMC Code of Professional Conduct: Standards for Conduct; Performance and Ethics'.* London: NMC

Nursing and Midwifery Council (2007) Circular 07/2007 Annex 2, *Essential Skills Clusters (ESCs) for Pre-registration Nursing Programmes.* London: NMC

Rinpoche, S. (1992) *The Tibetan Book of Living and Dying.* London: Rider Books

Royal College of Nursing (RCN) (2007) *Three Years On: Caring in Partnership: Older People and Nursing Staff Working Towards the Future.* An RCN Nursing Older People Strategy process and evaluation report. London: Royal College of Nursing

Schantz, M. (2007) 'Compassion: A concept analysis'. *Nursing Forum,* 42 (2): April–June

Squires, A.J. (2002) 'The National Service Framework For Older People: Timely and challenging' in Squires, A.J. and Hastings, M.B. (eds) *Rehabilitation of the Older Person: A Handbook for the Interdisciplinary Team* (3rd edn). Cheltenham: Nelson Thornes Ltd

Tanner, D. and Harris, J. (2008) *Working with Older People.* Abingdon: Routledge

Taylor, J. (2007) 'Has dignity gone out of care?' *Nursing Times,* 103 (4)

Tadd, W. (2005) 'Editorial: Dignity and Older Europeans'. *Quality in Ageing,* 6 (1)

Tadd, W., Bayer, T. and Dieppe, P. (2002) 'Dignity in health care: reality or rhetoric?'. *Clinical Gerontology*, 12: 1–4

Woolhead, G., Tadd, W., Boix-Ferrer, J. A., Krajcik, S., Schmid-Pfahler, B., Spjuth, B., Stratton, D., Dieppe, P. and on behalf of the Dignity and Older Europeans Project (2006) '"Tu" or "vous" A European qualitative study of dignity and communication with older people in health and social care settings'. *Patient Education and Counseling*, 61 (3): 363–71

Walsh, K. and Kowanko, I. (2002) 'Nurses' and patients' perceptions of dignity'. *International Journal of Nursing Practice*, 8: 143–51

Chapter 7

Assessment and Care Planning

Austyn Snowden

INTRODUCTION

Learning outcomes

Reading this chapter will enable you to:

- demonstrate the link between collaboration and effective care;
- critically analyse the process of planning care;
- apply the principles of care planning outlined in this chapter.

Planning care is difficult. Condensing somebody's strengths and problems into three or four statements of need is impossible. This can lead to disengagement with the process. The purpose of this chapter is to provide a discussion of some of the more challenging care planning decisions by considering a complex case study. You may agree with some of the decisions here or you may disagree, but you will at least understand the rationale behind them and therefore be able to counter with your own rationale.

A more mundane reason for disengagement with care planning is that nurses have often considered that when they are planning care they are primarily recording the needs of organisational administration and not the care of the patients (Lee *et al.*, 2002). Some nurses feel that care plans are of no use in their everyday work, nor do they use the language and terminology of care plans in their oral reports (Griffiths, 1998). This implies that care planning is futile and that there is a lack of connection between the process of caring and the recording of it. However, this may not necessarily be the fault of the care plan process *per se*. For example, consider an 'ideal' care plan. What should it contain? How could the process be more meaningful to everybody?

The 'ideal' care plan

I would suggest that an ideal care plan should accurately reflect an 'agreement on action'. Note therefore that negotiation and communication are at the heart of this process. For example, studies have shown that when the care plan was made together with the patient, and when its main purpose was to report the patient's state of health, the attitude to recording was positive and the subsequent care plan quality improved (Kirrane, 2001; Kärkkäinen, 2005). This should be no real surprise as it acknowledges the benefit of genuine partnership or an attempt to really engage with someone. Real engagement need not necessarily be complex either. In fact it is often quite the opposite. Atkinson (2000) makes a powerful case for considering the simple action of recording a person's details as therapeutic in itself. In other words, if the care planning process is genuinely meaningful to all concerned the likelihood is that the plan will be both more relevant and more likely to succeed. The trick is therefore in making and keeping the process meaningful to all.

Gega (2004) defines a care plan as a:

- legal document;
- means of communication;
- practice guide;
- progress record;
- teaching tool;
- means of user involvement.

(Gega, 2004)

I would argue that Gega's last point is the most important. If the person with whom the care is planned is genuinely involved, it is easy to see that the plan will function as a better means of communication, a relevant practice guide, an accurate progress record and a functional teaching tool. How is this collaboration translated into a written care plan?

The answer is: systematically. That is, care should be taken to ensure that the negotiated plan is grounded in accurate and relevant assessment, and prioritised according to agreed need. It should be easily measurable and clearly evaluated over a particular timescale. A period of reflection on action will then underpin the rationale for specific changes as necessary (see Figure 1). This sounds straightforward, but it isn't. This is because agreement isn't always possible however much you try. Communication is never straightforward even when you think you couldn't possibly be misunderstood and measurement is easier said than done. This is before consideration of some of the more difficult issues which may arise like, for example, the capacity of the individual to understand, consent and fully participate in this process.

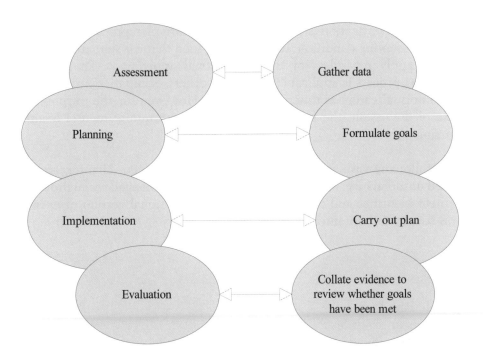

Figure 1 The nursing process in the UK

THE CASE STUDY

In order to discuss these issues in a practical manner this chapter focusses on the systematic construction of a care plan with an older adult. It cannot cover every potential problem and so, for the purpose of describing the process, it focusses on one of the major health problems in older adult care: depression. In the case that follows the process could just as easily have focussed on arthritis or lack of sleep, for example. Some would argue that these factors cause depression, as inferred in the Case study on page 120 (Smith, 2006), and many others look at care as a hierarchy that should naturally address physical problems first (Maslow, 1943). These issues will be returned to throughout the chapter and discussed in particular in the evaluation. However, as a starting point, depression is why the GP referred Bob to you in the first place, following significant attempts to address his physical issues.

A single case is particularly useful in emphasising the individuality of the care planning process. I would strongly argue against the notion of 'generic' care plans, which require little thought and offer a **mechanistic approach** to care. That said, it should be noted that a systematic approach to clinical investigation is transferable to the care plan process regardless of the presenting condition. It is further argued that a systematic process should apply regardless of the professional applying it. That is, the following process is applicable to social workers, occupational therapists and informal carers as much as to nurses. However, for the purpose of ease of discussion, the focus here is on the community mental health nursing input.

The following case study is developed throughout the chapter, and is based on a real case. Names and details have been changed throughout to protect identities and consent to publish this fictional version of events was sought and obtained from the original family.

Case study

Bob: Part 1

Bob is an 85-year-old retired accountant who lives with his wife Jane. They have two children and six grandchildren who live away. Bob is normally active in the local church and keeps an interest in village life. This has lapsed in the last two months. Recently he has become anxious about impending building work at home to the point where he can't sleep well. His arthritis appears to be troubling him and he is finding it increasingly difficult to get dressed and to shave in the morning. Jane tells you that he doesn't appear to have any energy any more or any interest in anything, other than the impending building work. You have been asked to see Bob by his GP, who is concerned that Bob may be depressed. His GP has known Bob for 30 years and fears his current presentation may be exacerbated by his propensity to low mood. He has a long history of bipolar depression.

Part 2

You say to Bob that you think he may be depressed. You explain that this is because his GP thinks so and that he reports himself to be lacking in energy, not sleeping well and ruminating excessively on matters others consider less concerning, particularly his wife. He gives this some thought. He then responds that he doesn't consider the building work to be trivial because the last time any work was done on the house it went on longer than was initially planned and the family ended up in dispute with the builders. His main problem is his arthritis as far as he's concerned.

Part 3

You ask Bob to be more specific about how his arthritis is affecting his quality of life. He tells you that the pain and lack of power in his hands prevents him from shaving efficiently, and the trauma of having to shave first thing in the morning is the first thing on his mind. This is what he wakes up thinking about at 3 a.m. most mornings. He lies awake worrying about not being able to do it. He eventually gets up to shave at 7 a.m. He is often so exhausted when he has finished that he feels the need to go back to bed. Instead he gets himself dressed, which takes over an hour. While conveying this information, the look of distress on his face and the frustration in his body language is unmistakable. As he appears to be communicating a desperate state of affairs you ask him if he has ever felt like harming himself. He goes silent for a long time and looks down. 'Not really,' he eventually says. 'What do you mean by "not really"?' you ask. 'I sometimes wish I was dead,' he says.

Part 4

On further discussion with Bob and Jane you explore the functional side of Bob's problems. You discover that he has always wet shaved and worn a shirt and tie. He feels improperly dressed without these. However, Jane seems pleased that the subject has been brought up and suggests buying an electric razor and some smart casual shirts. Although Bob feels this to be a drop in standards he acknowledges the logic that his current difficulties may be addressed by doing this. He agrees to this temporary arrangement and the plan in general.

Part 5: one week later

Bob has new shirts and trousers that are easier to manage. He says he is pleased with them. He has followed the diet as agreed in the plan and had his medication reviewed. He now rates his arthritic pain at 7, which is a reduction. However, this information is skipped over quickly. As he was feeling better Jane managed to persuade him to go to church for the first time in months. Bob thinks this was a grave mistake as one of the parishioners looked at him 'in a funny way', as if he knew exactly what he was thinking. Bob remembered a disagreement he had with this man's wife 35 years ago. He can't remember if he ever apologised for this and fears he and his family may be banned from the church. He has been unable to get these thoughts out of his mind ever since. Jane's version of events is that the man in question shook Bob's hand and said it was good to see him again.

Initial assessment

Reflection

Read Part 1 of the Case study.

On meeting Bob for the first time you find him to be a very welcoming but clearly a very serious and preoccupied man. His speech is slow and ponderous and appears to be an effort. He looks very tired but is immaculately dressed in shirt and tie. He lives in a traditional detached house in a popular village. The house has a beautiful garden that Bob and his wife manage themselves. However, instead of being able to enjoy this achievement Bob begins to tell you how difficult it is to maintain, especially because the arthritis in his hands makes work difficult for him. This leads into discussion of other worries, such as the impending building work, which turns out to be relatively minor cosmetic work according to his wife. His wife assures you they are financially secure and the work is in hand.

> ## Reflection
>
> Take a moment to consider your initial thoughts. What is going on here? What other information have you noticed?

One of the first things you may notice is Bob's presentation. His appearance is clearly important to him. Surely if he was depressed he wouldn't care so much about this? His speech is slow, however, and he appears to be having difficulty in thinking. You may then have noticed the apparently exaggerated worry Bob seems to feel towards jobs his wife considers minor. That is, his wife doesn't share these worries. Could this be a source of comfort or tension? You may also notice he doesn't appear to be sad in any obvious way. This doesn't seem to fit with a typical depression does it? Yet this is why his GP referred him.

> ## Reflection
>
> Read Part 2 of the case study again. This seems a rational response doesn't it? Would you accept this reasoning at face value? Is arthritis Bob's main problem? He says it is so surely it is, isn't it?

An open mind is always important, but particularly at this initial assessment stage. Consider in more detail other factors that could be significant here. A structured approach helps elicit pertinent information. Two of the more popular mnemonics to help at this stage are SWIPE and TROCARSS. These are:

- When did it Start?
- What makes it Worse?
- What causes Improvement?
- Is there a Pattern?
- What is the Evaluation (what is currently being done to make it better?).

TROCARSS is along the same lines but more detailed – Time, Rapidity, Occurrence, Characteristics, Associations, Relief, Site and spread, Severity. These are both useful in any consultation. These methods of systematic enquiry will therefore help explore his arthritis in purposeful detail, as it would any presenting complaint.

Arguably consultation in mental health assessment is more detailed still (Harrison, 2004), with more focus on subtle communication such as nuance, tone and cognition for example. History is often taken in greater depth, possibly an artefact of its psychodynamic roots, but the approach remains systematic. For example, the following issues are suggested as having direct correlation with concordance in mental health treatment (Nolan *et al.*, 2004: 2). Nolan *et al.* suggest these issues should be established on first contact:

- how the person presents – their general demeanour;
- how they talk about their problems;
- what the condition means to them;
- why they think their illness has occurred at this time;
- whether they have felt this way before;
- what they think the appropriate treatments should be;
- what they think about other treatments;
- what their family and friends think about (e.g. depression) and its treatment;
- whether they intend to comply with whatever treatments are prescribed;
- what important things they are currently not able to do;
- what important things they would most like to do;
- how long they think it will take before they are well again.

Reflection

Read Part 3 of the case study again. Do you still think arthritis is Bob's major problem? Could he be depressed as well? What could be causing this?

Defining depression

If you suspect a particular problem exists it is very important to understand it. For example, if you assess someone as having high blood pressure then you would be expected to have detailed knowledge of hypertension: its cause, diagnosis, manifestation, presenting symptoms, its likely outcome, risk factors and its treatment. Therefore, it is important in this case to have a working knowledge of equivalent factors of depression. Consider the evidence. In short, depression is categorised as mild, moderate or severe according to the following criteria.

- Persistent sadness, anhedonia (loss of pleasure), fatigue AND one or more associate symptoms:
    - sleep disturbance, appetite disturbance, poor concentration, agitation/opposite, decreased libido, low self-confidence, suicidal thoughts/acts, and guilt;
        - 4 = mild depression (for example, sadness, anhedonia, fatigue AND suicidal thoughts/acts);
        - 5–6 = moderate depression (for example, sadness, anhedonia, fatigue AND poor concentration, sleep disturbance and suicidal thoughts/acts);
        - 7+ = severe depression (for example ALL the symptoms).

(World Health Organisation, 2007)

Depression was the third most common of all diseases in the year 2002, and it is expected to continue as a rising trend during the coming 20 years (Imperidore *et al.*, 2007). More sceptical authors such as Barondes (2003) and Healy (2004) interpret this trend as an indication that the drug companies have successfully medicalised unhappiness for profit. However, alternative viewpoints point to the historical under-diagnosis of depression. For example, Isacsson (2000) found that a fivefold increase in the use of antidepressants was followed by a 25 per cent decrease in the Swedish suicide rate.

One of the major complications for Bob is that older adults don't always fit the typical picture of depression (Segal *et al.*, 2007). Many depressed older adults don't claim to feel sad at all, which is a primary symptom of typical depression. They may complain instead of a lack of energy or physical problems. Physical complaints, such as arthritis pain, are often the predominant symptom. Older adults with depression are also more likely to show symptoms of anxiety or irritability. They may constantly wring their hands, pace around the room, or fret obsessively about money, their health, or the state of the world. In other words, Bob's apparently atypical presentation is actually typical for his age group.

The reported prevalence of depression in the over 65s varies greatly depending on the source of the information, assessment tools used and variables studied. However, the range seems to suggest between 10–20 per cent of the population suffer with some level of depression, indicating a significant health problem. As regards variables involved in depression, studies point to a massive range of factors, from the smallest biological

Metabolic disturbances
Acid-base disturbance
Azotemia, uremia
Dehydration
Hypo- and hypercalcemia
Hypo- and hyperglycemia
Hypo- and hyperkalcemia
Hypo- and hypermatremia
Hypoxia

Endocrine
Addison's disease
Cushing's disease
Diabetes mellitus
Hyper- or hypoparathyroidism
Hypo- and hyperthyroid

Neurological disease
Aneurysms
Brain tumours
Cerebral arteriosclerosis
Cerebral infarct
Cerebrovascular disease (stroke; transient ischemic attacks)
Dementia: all types
Intracranial tumours (malignant or benign)
Meningitis
Neurosyphilis
Normal pressure hydrocephalus
Parkinson's disease
Subarachnoid haemorrhage
Temporal lobe epilepsy

Respiratory infections
Brucellosis
Hepatitis
Influenza
Pneumonia

Tuberculosis

Cancer
Occult carcinomas
Pancreatic

Cardiovascular disorders
Congestive heart failure
Endocarditis
Myocardial infarction

Pulmonary disorders
Chronic obstructive lung disease
Malignancy

Gastrointestinal disorders
Hepatitis
Irritable bowel
Malignancy
Other organic causes of chronic abdominal pain, ulcer, diverticulosis

Genitourinary
Urinary incontinence
Urinary tract infections

Musculoskeletal disorders
Degenerative arthritis
Osteoporosis with vertebral compression or hip fracture
Paget's Disease
Polymalgia rheumatica
Rheumatoid arthritis

Collagen vascular disease
Systemic Lupus Erythmatosis

Anemias
Folate and iron deficiencies
Megaloblastic anemia
Pernicious anemia

Metal intoxications
Thallium
Mercury

(Smith, 2006)

Box 1 Physical illnesses that are associated with depression nuance to social contentions that the roots lie in relative deprivation. Box 1 illustrates some of the more common physical illnesses that have been correlated with depression. Arthritis is one of them.

Effective clinical decision making and care planning therefore rests with the practitioner being able to make sense of this web of causality.

Further assessment

Reflection

You are likely at this point to suspect some sort of depressive episode, possibly secondary to Bob's physical problems. Do you suspect anything else? What about his cognitive function? Could anything else be responsible for his apparent low mood? How would you confirm this? What would be the purpose of further testing? What is the most important information you need?

There is a need to objectively assess Bob's suspected depression both to confirm the suspicion and to provide a baseline for the effectiveness of future interventions. In this case it would also be worthwhile assessing his cognitive abilities as he appears to be struggling with his thinking. The quickest and therefore best way to take a snapshot of these is to use the Geriatric Depression Scale (GDS) (Sheikh *et al.*, 1986) and the Mini Mental State Examination (MMSE) (Folstein and Folstein, 1975). The reason you would use these very brief tests is that somebody who is apparently struggling to think would not appreciate a lengthy and potentially pointless cognitive assessment. The most important consideration at this early assessment stage is to gather enough information to ensure your client is safe. If this is assured then other information can be gathered at a pace suitable to the client. This shows respect and empathy which, in turn, will be more likely to generate a mutually beneficial therapeutic relationship (Peplau, 1952; Reynolds, 2000).

Is your client safe?

The ultimate harm in Bob's case is death, as the major risk is suicide. In identifying someone with depression you have also identified a person who is at far greater risk than the norm of taking their own life, especially in older age (see Box 2). This is a desperate place to be and quite impossible to generalise from. However, the attempt to do so is

- The suicide rate is higher among older adults than any other age group.
- Older adults are less likely to *attempt* suicide, but are more likely to use more lethal methods that result in death (compared to younger adults).
- People over the age of 65 make up 13 per cent of the population but commit 20 per cent of all reported suicides.
- White men aged 80 years and over, are at highest risk of suicide.

(Smith, 2006)

Box 2 Suicide correlations in older adults

necessary in order to potentially save a life. From the literature there appear to be two ways of significantly reducing risk:

1. Understand the level of risk in order to take appropriate action;
2. Ensure the tools are not available for the person to harm themselves.

The second measure is effective only to the extent that the individual is unmotivated or unable to seek another method. The first measure involves a deeper and more sophisticated engagement with the person in order to individualise risk. For example, individual belief in whether a particular suicide method would work or not is far more indicative of suicidal intent than the apparent severity of a suggested method. Rihmer *et al.* (2002) provide a useful hierarchical classification of risk in Box 3. Eliciting and acting on this information requires great skill based on a rich therapeutic relationship (Kroll, 2007). However, there is a lot to be said for just asking if a person has considered harming themselves if you feel that there is a risk. Bob is clearly at risk and should be asked. In 22 years I had only one person take exception to the question. The lady was deeply religious and offended by the insinuation, even though she was deeply depressed at the time and exhibited all the risk factors except suicidal ideation identified by the World Health Organisation (2007). The fact that I asked the question appeared to do no lasting damage to our therapeutic relationship, a finding supported by ASIST training which supports asking someone directly in order to validate their feelings.

1. Primary (psychiatric–medical) suicide risk factors

(a) Major psychiatric illness (depression, schizophrenia, substance use disorders)
± Co-morbid anxiety or personality disorder, serious medical illness
± Feeling of hopelessness and insomnia, concomitant anxiety
(b) Previous suicide attempt(s)
(c) Communication of wish to die/suicide intent (direct or indirect)
(d) Suicide among family members (biological or social 'inheritance')
(e) Disregulated serotonergic system, low total serum cholesterol, abnormal dexamethasone suppression test during depression

2. Secondary (psychosocial) risk factors

(a) Childhood negative life-events (separation, parental loss, etc.)
(b) Isolation, living alone (divorce, separation, widowhood, etc.)
(c) Loss of job, unemployment
(d) Severe acute negative life-events
(e) Smoking

3. Tertiary (demographic) suicide risk factors

(a) Male sex
(b) Adolescent and young men, old age (both sexes)
(c) Vulnerable intervals (spring/early summer, pre-menstrual period, etc.)
(d) Minority groups (relatives of suicide victims, victims of disasters, bisexuality, same-sex orientation, etc.)

Box 3 Hierarchical classification of suicide risk factors (Rihmer *et al.*, 2002)

Reflection

How would you feel about asking somebody if they wanted to kill themselves? How else could you find out? How can you be sure anybody is safe?

Less immediately deadly but also potentially very risky are other issues of personal safety. For example, can the person look after their own needs? If not why not and what would they need to do so? Do they need other forms of support? Are they at risk of falling? How about polypharmacy? Could his lack of sleep be affecting his cognitive ability? These issues are nicely summarised but less pleasantly named as the 'giants of geriatrics' according to Cape (1978) and illustrated in Figure 2. They are: falling, iatrogenic disorders, impaired homeostasis, incontinence, confusion against a backdrop of psychosocial factors. This model has been used more recently to discuss systematic nursing intervention, Olenek *et al.* (2003), and remains a useful baseline despite its outdated terminology.

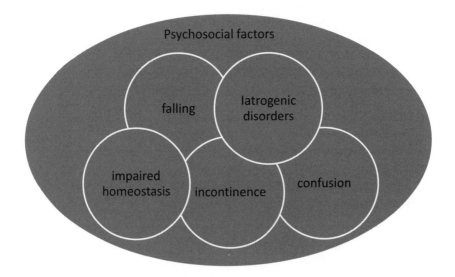

Figure 2 'Geriatric giants' (Cape, 1978)

You may be thinking at this point that there is an overwhelming amount of background information to know. Not only that but this information needs to be combined with unique comprehensive individual history, in order to establish an effective and agreeable plan. How can this be achieved?

Care planning

Defining and prioritising problems is the first step. Goals can then be set. Formulating goals is a collaborative process based upon all the information you have collated so far. Most importantly, what may seem a problem to you may not be so to your client and vice versa. For example, in the case of Bob the actual work that needs doing on the house is not really a problem according to his wife. His major problem is his arthritis. You may feel his major problem is his suicidal ideation. However, the problem just might be a history of very poor building work.

Reflection

What then is his problem? Is it the actual work? If so, does he have a problem communicating with his wife? What do you think is the problem? How will you find out?

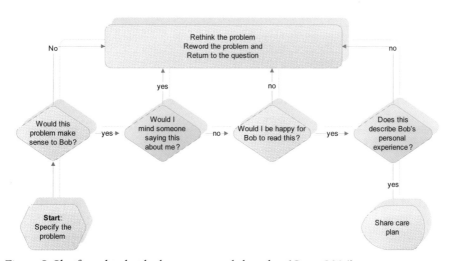

Figure 3 Clarify and individualise your initial thoughts (Gega, 2004)

A good way of testing whether or not you are close to clarity and partnership is to ask the following questions of your initial thoughts (Gega, 2004) (see Figure 3).

For example, instead of saying that the problem is, 'Bob appears to be depressed', which will certainly be one of your thoughts, define it in his terms. For example, 'Bob has problems sleeping', 'Bob feels as if he has no energy', 'Bob feels stressed about the impending building work'. The correct terminology requires negotiation.

Go back to Smith's (2006) summary of physical illnesses that are correlated with depression (Box 1). Arthritis is one of them. Perhaps this needs to be addressed first? As far as Bob is concerned this is his major problem. Yet in Part 3 of the case study the conversation moved from the building work to his arthritis, and then from his arthritis to his desperate exhaustion. Your concern for his safety was justified with his admission that he sometimes wished he was dead. You therefore have enough information to discuss a preliminary list of mutually agreeable problems:

- Bob sometimes wishes he was dead;
- Bob's arthritis is his major concern;
- Bob is tired of being tired;
- Bob worries all the time.

Bob agrees with this summary of his current problems.

Reflection

Do you agree with these problems? What is wrong with them for the purpose of care planning?

The problem with these problems is that they are not specific or prioritised. Words like 'sometimes' are meaningless in a care plan. Being tired of being tired likewise means nothing for the purpose of setting goals. That is, how would you know if Bob is not quite as tired of being tired after intervention? In a way, this is a semantic issue but it is the area of care planning that many nurses struggle with. Agreeing a broad statement of problems is essential as a first step towards collaborative care planning. It is subsequently important to ensure the problems, and hence the goals or objectives, are sensible to everybody. This means clarity. To use a very popular and enduring acronym, the objectives that follow should be SMART (Doran, 1981):

- Specific.
- Measurable.
- Achievable.
- Relevant.
- Time-bound.

Specific

'Specific' in the context of objectives refers to a definable and observable action. It can be any quantifiable event. For example, it can be a frequency, rate, number or ratio. In the case of Bob then it would be non-specific to state that his arthritis will improve. This is not quantifiable. The plan would have to state by how much. This depends on how it is measured.

Measurable

A measurable objective is specific. This doesn't have to be a validated assessment tool, just genuinely meaningful. For example, Bob could self-rate his arthritic pain on a personal scale of zero to ten in order to be specific about it. He could measure it by rating how easy it is to get dressed. These rating scales would then provide a measurement by which to assess change.

Achievable

The concept of 'achievable' makes the care planners focus on what are meaningful and realistic aims for the person. Undoubtedly Bob would like to feel better immediately. However, he will probably view this as unlikely. Consequently he is less likely to engage with any plan promising immediate eradication of his symptoms. An achievable goal requires a reasonable amount of effort. Not too much and not too little. This requires skilful negotiation.

Relevant

'Relevant' goals are goals the individual can actually impact upon. That is, change in this regard is both desirable and appropriate to the situation. In practical terms a relevant goal is one identified by the individual. Again then, this requires skilful negotiation. This would be the case even with the most apparently rudimentary medical measurement. For example, lowering blood pressure is an obvious objective in addressing hypertension. However, this will still have to be relevant to the individual concerned or the plan won't work.

Time-bound

Finally the goals need to be reviewed in order to see if the objectives have been met. This is why they need to be 'time-bound'. In other words, clarify exactly when this care planning cycle finishes. Then start again if necessary.

Reflection

How would you apply SMART objectives to Bob's problems?

Let's start with his arthritis as this remains Bob's explicit major concern, even though you may be more worried about his overall presentation. Arthritis refers to a group of conditions that cause damage to the joints of the body. So, from a SMART perspective, arthritis itself is not specific. History reveals that Bob has 'gouty' arthritis, which is a result of accumulation of uric acid in the joints. The cause of gouty arthritis is a high serum level of uric acid, which accumulates through a combination of high input (diet) and poor output (excretion) of uric acid. Risk factors in diet appear to include beef and seafood (Choi et al., 2004), suggesting avoidance of these foods may be helpful in reducing intake. On the output side taking 500 mg vitamin C every day has been shown to increase serum uric acid excretion. A small dose of lithium may also be useful and has been associated with the treatment of 'gouty mania' since 1850 (Cade, 1949). However, the evidence for these interventions is unclear. For example, larger doses of vitamin C have been harmful in some patients with gout and lithium can be a very toxic drug, increasingly so in older adults.

From a nursing perspective then the most sensible next move would be to investigate his diet further (Saag and Choi, 2006) and also the functional problems his arthritis presents. Suggesting a reduction in his beef and seafood intake may possibly have further benefit without risk. There is also some evidence that ice therapy may provide relief (Schlesinger et al., 2002) for affected joints. This is also risk free. Bob's major complaint, along with his shaving, is the difficulty he has fastening the smaller buttons of his shirt and trousers. Home help may be appropriate here. Discussing these issues specifically with Bob and Jane leads Jane to suggest temporary alternatives to buttoned clothes and wet razors.

General problem area	Specific statement of problem	Goal	Intervention	Evaluation
Bob sometimes wishes he was dead because of how bad his arthritis makes him feel. He worries excessively about everything.	1. Bob has stated that he wishes he was dead. Geriatric Depression Scale (GDS) score seven out of 15, indicative of a moderate depression.	1. Bob will remain safe. He will not wish he was dead at any time. He will score less than 7/15 on GDS after one month.	Nurse will build and maintain a therapeutic alliance in order to discuss Bob's and Jane's views of the presenting problems and suggest options.	See page 136.
	2. Bob's arthritis causes him pain and distress which he rates as scoring ten on a personal pain scale of one to ten.	2. Bob's arthritic pain will be less than ten in one week.	Bob will initiate sleep hygiene measures as discussed with nurse.	
	3. Bob wakes at 3 a.m. every morning and worries about his inability to dress and shave. He rates this worry as scoring ten on a personal worry scale of one to ten.	3. Bob will wake later than 3 a.m. His worry will be less than ten after one week.	Bob will use an electric razor instead of a wet razor and go 'button free' with his clothing.	
			Bob will eliminate beef and seafood from his diet for one week.	
			Nurse will contact GP to review medication for arthritis.	

Figure 4 Bob's care plan

135

> ### Reflection
>
> Are these discussions likely to lead to SMART objectives? How do you turn this into a care plan? Does a change of shirt address your concerns about his potential suicidal ideation?

Implementation

The implementation phase is one of action. That is, the care plan is put into practice. The care plan is shown in Figure 4 on page 135.

Evaluation

It is very difficult to isolate any aspect of care, yet that is what is required to a degree in care planning. Bob has so many potentially interconnected factors impinging on one another. No matter how specific your objectives are, real life is likely to complicate them in unplanned ways. However, the principle of evaluation is the same as it has been throughout the process: Involve the person. That is, the best possible evaluation will centre on Bob's and Jane's perspective of how the care plan worked.

> ### Reflection
>
> Please read Part 5 of the Case study on page 122. This is one week after the implementation of the suggested care plan. What has succeeded? What hasn't been successful? What do you think has gone wrong?

According to Part 5 Bob is complaining of enduring (and apparently worsening) rumination to the point of **psychosis**. He believes he has caused his family great distress through seemingly innocuous comments made years ago. He is grinding his teeth, has a dread of socialising ever again, continues with early wakening despite following the care plan and now also exhibits a lowering of appetite. His concentration is noticeably worse than on the last visit, and he struggles to complete the GDS, in which he scores nine, a two-point increase on last time, indicative of a worsening depression. He continues to make vague allusions but non-specific threats of self-harm, although he now denies this on direct questioning.

Reflection

The plan doesn't seem to have worked. What do you do now?
Has all of it failed? Why has it gone so wrong?

Bob's overall presentation is undoubtedly worse. This may often happen in older adult care. However, the plan hasn't completely failed as the interventions to address his functional problems with arthritis appear to be working. This is very important as these were the areas of distress Bob was most keen to focus on last week. As a consequence of this Bob is more likely to be open to negotiation this week. That is, the review of this week's problems takes place within an established therapeutic relationship where Bob knows he will be listened to and heard.

IMPLICATIONS FOR JOINT WORKING

The concept of collaborative working in the assessment and co-ordination of care for individuals is not new, and is certainly as old as the NHS (McTavish and Mackie, 2003). The latest attempt to systematically formalise a partnership approach to older adult care in Scotland has been driven through the *Joint Future* agenda (Scottish Executive, 2000). The UK approach as a whole mirrors this drive towards formalising existing partnerships and extending them to include other agencies where possible (Department of Health, 2007).

The main ideas were to have agencies working in partnership with better operational and strategic planning through joint budgeting (Scottish Office, 1998). One operational consequence of these ideas was the emergence of jointly funded and jointly managed community teams. The day-to-day impact on front line health and social work staff was the application of single shared assessment within these teams (Box 4).

In practice this means that the care plan process discussed here would have taken place within a jointly-managed community mental health team. This effectively means that should further social support be necessary for Bob then this can be organised efficiently by the 'lead professional' or care manager, thus reducing the need to duplicate any part of this plan as has been historically the case. For example, home support could have been offered if Bob continued to struggle to get dressed. Respite can be organised much more easily if needed.

Single, Shared **Assessment:**
- is person-centred and needs-led;
- relates to level of need; and
- is a process, and not an event.

Single, Shared Assessment
- seeks information once;
- has a lead professional who co-ordinates documents and shares appropriate information;
- co-ordinates all contributions; and
- produces a single summary assessment of need.

Single, **Shared** Assessment
- actively involves people who use services and their carers;
- is a shared process that supports joint working; and
- provides results acceptable to all agencies.

Box 4 The fundamentals of single shared assessment (Scottish Executive, 2001: 10)

The most relevant aspect from the point of care planning is that the process should be the same regardless of the professional undertaking the care management role. Although it could be argued that the purpose of the care plan is different in different professions, the process of arriving at that care pan should be similarly systematic.

CONCLUSION

This case study didn't appear to have a happy ending. It was complicated and difficult to know what to do. Even after deciding what to do it didn't seem to be the right thing to do, otherwise surely the outcome would have been better? However, this is why the care planning process is cyclic, reflective and person-centred. All parties should now review the situation and start the process again. The key points are:

- care planning is a collaborative process;
- care planning is a systematic process;
- care planning is a reflective process;
- care planning is a hierarchical process;

- care planning is a goal-directed process;
- care planning is a specific process and therefore,
- care planning is a measurable process;
- care planning is a cyclical process.

FURTHER READING

There are many textbooks on the art of care planning. If you are going to buy one make sure it has a UK focus. A lot of international books include diagnosis as part of the process, which, although interesting and increasingly relevant, is rarely a specific aspect of the process in the UK. Roper, Logan and Tierney are widely credited with introducing the nursing process. In the UK their four-stage model is generally preferred, and this is what was discussed in this chapter. In the USA, the five-stage model is the most popular. Both versions of this model are effectively the same. Roper, Logan and Tierney remain essential reading and their final publication together on the topic was:

Roper, N., Logan, W. and Tierney, A.J. (2000) *The Roper, Logan, Tierney Model of Nursing; Based on Activities of Daily Living.* London: Churchill Livingstone
Holland *et al.*'s (2003) application of this process is very popular with students:
Holland, K., Jenkins, J., Solomon J. and Whittam, S. (2003) *Applying the Roper-Logan-Tierney Model in Practice: Elements of Nursing.* London: Elsevier/ Churchill Livingstone

There is less literature devoted specifically to care planning with older adults because the process itself is transferable. Information on what is different about older adult care does not therefore necessarily focus on the planning process. Most undergraduate textbooks have a dedicated section on the nursing process, and therefore any modern text on older adult nursing care will reinforce the information given here. A good modern text from the USA focussed on practical rather than theoretical perspectives is:

Wallace, M. (2007) *Essentials of Gerontological Nursing.* New York: Springer Publishing Company Inc.

Useful websites

www.nimh.nih.gov/health/topics/older-adults-and-mental-health/index.shtml
This is a good web resource about depression in older adults written by the National Institute for Mental Health. Further links to ongoing research projects on depression:

www.rcpsych.ac.uk
Very simple to understand and navigate. Excellent section on older adult mental health. Links to more complex information.

http://en.wikipedia.org/wiki/Nursing_process
Wikipedia offers a good summary of the nursing process, linked to Maslow's hierarchy of needs. It includes diagnosis as the focus is American, but the logic and further reading advice is excellent.

www.nursesnetwork.co.uk
Nursesnetwork runs a forum and a blog. This is a good way of taking part in practical discussion on nursing topics. The academic accuracy of content cannot be guaranteed however. There are already threads on the nursing process.

http://nursingcrib.com
This is one of many sites posting generic care plans as examples. While I do not support this method of problem solving the practical examples here are useful as exemplars.

REFERENCES

Atkinson, J. (2000) *Nursing Homeless Men: A Study of Proactive Intervention.* London: Whurr Publishing

Barondes, S.H. (2003) *Better than Prozac.* Oxford: Oxford University Press

Barraclough, B., Bunch, J., Nelson, B. and Sainsbury, P. (1974) 'A hundred cases of suicide: clinical aspects'. *British Journal of Psychiatry* 125: 355–73

Cade, J. (1949) 'Lithium salts in the treatment of psychotic excitement'. *Medical Journal of Australia* 36: 349

Cape, R. (1978) *Aging, Its Complex Management.* Hagerstown, MD: Harper & Row

Choi, H., Atkinson, K., Karlson, E., Willett, W. and Curhan, G. (2004). 'Purine-rich foods, dairy and protein intake, and the risk of gout in men'. *New England Journal of Med* 350 (11): 1093–103

Department of Health (2007) *Making Partnerships Work: Examples of Good Practice.* http://www.dh.gov.uk/en/Publicationsandstatistics/Publications/PublicationsPolicyAndGuidance/DH_072998 (Accessed 9 September 2008)

Doran, G. (1981) 'There's a S.M.A.R.T Way to Write Management Goals and Objectives'. *Management Review,* November, pp. 35–6, in Weiss, J.W. and Wysocki, R.K. (1992) *5-Phase Project Management: A Practical Planning and Implementation Guide.* Sydney: Addison Wesley, p.13

Folstein, M.F. and Folstein, S. (1975) *Mini Mental State Examination.* www.minimental.com (Accessed 20 February 2008)

Gega, L. (2004) 'Problems, goals and care planning' in Norman, I. and Ryrie, I. (eds) *The Art and Science of Mental Health Nursing.* Maidenhead: Open University Press/McGraw-Hill

Griffiths, P. (1998) 'An investigation into the description of patients' problems by nurses using two different need-based nursing models'. *Journal of Advanced Nursing*, 28 (5): 969–77

Harrison, T.C. (2004) *Consultation for Contemporary Helping Professionals.* Auckland: Pearson Education

Healy, D. (2004) *Let them eat Prozac.* New York and London: New York University Press

Imperadore, G., Cipriani, A., Signoretti, A., Furukawa, T.A., Watanabe, N., Churchill, R., McGuire, H.F. and Barbui, C. for the Meta-Analysis of New Generation Antidepressants (MANGA) Study Group. (2007) 'Citalopram versus other anti-depressive agents for depression.' (Protocol) *Cochrane Database of Systematic Reviews*, Issue 2. Art. No.: CD006534. DOI: 10.1002/14651858.CD006534

Isacsson, G. (2000) 'Suicide prevention – a medical breakthrough?' *Acta Psychiatrica Scandinavica*, 102:113–17

Kärkkäinen, O. (2005) 'Recording the content of the care process'. *Journal of Nursing Management*, 13 (3): 202–8

Kirrane, C. (2001) An audit of care planning on a neurology unit. *Nursing Standard*, 15 (19): 36–9

Kroll, J. (2007) 'No-Suicide Contracts as a Suicide Prevention Strategy'. *Psychiatric Times*, 24 (8): 1–2. **www.psychiatrictimes.com/showArticle. jhtml?articleId=200001448** (Accessed 27 August 2007)

Lee, T., Yen, C.-H. and Ho, L.-H. (2002) 'Application of a computerized nursing care plan system in one hospital: experience of ICU nurses in Taiwan'. *Journal of Advanced Nursing*, 39 (1): 61–7

Maslow, A. H. (1943) 'Theory of Human Motivation'. *Psychological Review*, 50: 370–96

McTavish, D. and Mackie, R. (2003) 'The Joint Future Initiative in Scotland: The Development and Early Implementation Experience of an Integrated Care Policy'. *Public Policy and Administration*, 18 (3): 39

Nolan, P., Bradley, E. and Carr, N. (2004) 'Nurse Prescribing and the Enhancement of Mental Health Services'. *Nurse Prescriber*, 1 (11): 1–9

Olenek, K., Skowronski, T. and Schmaltz, D. (2003). 'Geriatric nursing assessment: A holistic approach to patient care incorporating the "giants of geriatric nursing" and patient psychosocial issues can improve nursing assessment'. *Journal of Gerontological Nursing*, 29 (8): 5–9

Peplau, H. E. (1952). *Interpersonal Relations in Nursing.* New York: G.P. Putnam & Sons

Reynolds, W. (2000) *The Measurement and Development of Empathy in Nursing.* Aldershot: Ashgate Publishing

Rihmer, N., Belso, N. and Kiss, K. (2002) 'Strategies for suicide prevention'. *Current Opinion in Psychiatry* 15: 83–7

Saag, K.G. and Choi, H. (2006) 'Epidemiology, risk factors, and lifestyle modifications for gout'. *Arthritis Research and Therapy*, 8 (1): S2

Schlesinger, N., Detry, M.A. and Holland, B.K .(2002) 'Local ice therapy during bouts of acute gouty arthritis'. *Journal of Rheumatology*, 29 (2): 331–4

Scottish Executive (2002) *Report of the Joint Future Integrated Human Resource Working Group.* Edinburgh: HMSO

Scottish Executive (2000) *Community Care: A Joint Future*. Report of the Joint Future Group. Edinburgh: HMSO

Scottish Executive (2001) *Guidance on Single Shared Assessment of Community Needs*. Edinburgh: HMSO

Scottish Office (1998) *Modernising Community Care – An Action Plan*. Edinburgh: HMSO

Segal, J., Jaffe, J., Davies, P. and Smith, M. (2007) *Depression in Older Adults and the Elderly: Recognising Symptoms and Getting Help*. **www.helpguide. org/mental/depression_elderly.htm** (Accessed 14 November 2007)

Sheikh, J.I, Yesavage, J.A., Brooks, J.O. III, Friedman, L., Gratzinger, P., Hill, R.D., Zadeik, A. and Crook, T. (1986) 'Proposed factor structure of the Geriatric Depression Scale'. *International Psychogeriatrics*, 3 (1): 23–8

Smith, M. (2006) Revised from Buckwalter, K.C. and Smith, M. (1993) 'When you are more than "down in the dumps": Depression in the elderly'. *The Geriatric Mental Health Training Series*, for the Hartford Center of Geriatric Nursing Excellence, College of Nursing, University of Iowa

WHO (2007) *ICD-10 Chapter V. Mental and Behavioural Disorders (F00-F99)* **www.who.int/classifications/apps/icd/icd10online** (Accessed 15 August 2007)

Chapter 8

Involving Relatives and Carers

F.J. Raymond Duffy

Learning outcomes

Reading this chapter will enable you to:

- understand why the number of informal carers, and the average age of informal carers, is rising;

- recognise the importance of informal carers to our society;

- show an awareness of the emotional, psychological, physical, social and financial cost of informal caring;

- appreciate that informal caring has rewards;

- be aware of the nature and type of support that carers may benefit from;

- discuss the impact on healthcare professionals of adopting a 'caring for carers' approach.

INTRODUCTION

The aim of this chapter is to highlight the importance of informal caring, some of the difficulties **informal carers** may face and how they can be assisted by health care professionals. Informal caring (often also called lay caring in other literature) is unpaid care by family, friends and neighbours, as distinct from the care offered by statutory services, professional carers or organised volunteers (Mackenzie and Lee, 2005). The great bulk of care worldwide is provided by informal carers, who play a vital role in looking after those who are sick, disabled, vulnerable or frail. It is highly likely that we will all need to provide or arrange care for a friend, a family member, a child or a loved one at some point. Most informal carers, as a result, are making a conscious choice to care, for reasons of love, loyalty, friendship or support, for others that they know well. In the initial stages of the process of becoming an informal carer many do not realise that, in the help they are offering, they are becoming informal carers. Once they are carers though, their main aim is to ensure that the person they care for is safe and is getting the best help and support possible. The person or persons being 'cared for' also usually value the help and support received. They also usually want that caring relationship to continue.

Informal caring can – as you may know from your own experience – bring sleepless nights, involves physical effort and sometimes feelings of being an intruder in someone else's business. At the same time however, most people who are, or have been carers, recognise how close and rewarding a caring relationship can be.

WHAT DOES THE LITERATURE SAY?

To get some idea of the extent of informal caring and what it involves, it is worth considering some statistics related to this issue. Taking the UK as an example of a Westernised economy, the UK population in April 2004 was 59.8 million people (National Statistics Online, 2006). The Office of National Statistics in 2002 reported that, in the UK, 6.8 million adults care for a sick, disabled or older person. Of that total almost 2 million devote at least 20 hours a week to caring. Over a million provide care in excess of 50 hours per week. People who share a household with the person they are caring for tend to spend more of their time caring. For that reason, spouses are most likely to be in-house carers. They are also the oldest group of carers and are the most likely to be carrying sole responsibility for care. They are also more likely to be involved in providing personal or physical care or both (Mackenzie and Lee, 2005). A similar pattern is seen across Europe, with most older people being cared for by their spouses or close family. In some instances, less common in the UK than elsewhere, caring may be devolved further when there is an extended family, but no immediate relatives (Mesthenos and Triantafillou, 2005).

The Office of National Statistics Census (2002) reports that the majority of carers look after someone who is over 65 years of age. Nearly a quarter of carers have been looking after the person for whom they were caring for at least ten years, and a further quarter had looked after the person for whom they were caring for between five and nine years (Department of Health, 1999).

Who does the caring?

If we examine who does this informal caring, a significant number are very young. There were 114 000 children in the UK aged five to 15 years providing care in 2001 (about 1 per cent of the total number of informal carers), with 9 000 of them caring for 50 or more hours a week (National Statistics Online, 2006). Most informal carers (about 45 per cent) are aged between 45 and 64. However, it is worth noting that, as well as receiving informal care, older people are also major providers of informal care. In 2001, 2.8 million people aged 50 and over in England and Wales were providing unpaid care. This is about 17 per cent of all people aged 50 and over. Around a quarter of older informal carers are providing 50 hours or more of unpaid care per week.

The number of hours of care given also seems to be related to age, with a higher percentage of older carers providing 50 or more hours' caring a week. The proportion of carers providing this level of care rises sharply from age 65 (National Statistics Online, 2006). As an illustration of this effect, around 44 000 people aged 85 and over provide care, with around half of these (51 per cent) spending 50 or more hours a week caring (National Statistics Online, 2006).The majority of informal carers are women by a ratio of about three women to two men (National Statistics Online, 2006). Yet, where care is provided by older people to each other, then there is a greater gender balance. For example, Poland and Switzerland reported equal proportions of male family carers in the 50+ age groups while the UK reported no gender differences in family care for co-resident carers (Mesthenos and Triantafillou, 2005). From the statistics it becomes clear that older people are increasingly more likely to become carers for other old people. There are several sociological reasons that help explain this. Life expectancy is increasing, so the number of the older population is increasing. The age at which people become frail and may require care is also increasing, so family carers overall are often older before beginning a carer's role. Other social factors such as women being in employment, lower birth rates, the migration of family members away from older relatives, result in fewer adult children actually being available to be caregivers. Therefore, care from within the family network has to be given by an older person and, generally, that person is the spouse of the dependent person. The high demand for formal care has also led to limited availability of many health care services, which further limits the personnel and agency support available to older dependents, leaving many older people little choice but to take over caring responsibilities.

There is also a need to recognise that factors such as race and culture affect the way that carers respond to the experience of caring. In the UK, little is known of the patterns of caring among Black and other minority ethnic groups (BME groups). An assumption is made that because of the strong kinship networks and large extended families that exist in these communities, they will contribute willingly to caring for their older relatives. However, Blakemore (2000) reports that families are not as supportive to older people as they once were, due to changes in family structures and residence patterns. As the number of older people within minority ethnic communities increases, the support that can be offered from within their own community will become diluted. Merrell *et al.* (2006) indicate that language barriers led to a lack of awareness of what was available and how to access those services. BME carers also believed that there was a lack of understanding of their culture by service providers and services would be unable to meet cultural and religious needs. These issues all significantly impede the accessibility of services for BME carers. These problems are added to, by the limited information that is available to service providers concerning family obligations and community care for minority ethnic groups and the lack of research in this whole field (Merrell *et al.*, 2006).

THE BURDEN AND COST OF CARING

Before looking at this issue it is worth considering the differences between the roles of formal and informal carers. The following activity is based in part on a small study carried out by Pickard and Glendinning in 2002. They compared and contrasted the work of carers and nurses in the domestic setting and, from this, tried to outline some of the differences between the role of formal carers and the role of the informal carers.

In Activity 1 the formal care role is listed. Using the description of that role as guidance, complete the informal carer's role side of the table given below (see Table 1).

Activity 1

Formal Care Role	Informal Care Role
Specific care is delivered, for example, wound dressing, medication giving, bathing, etc.	
There is a concentration on performing or supervising technical care, e.g. Colostomy care, monitoring blood sugar levels, injection giving, dialysis, etc.	
An organisational role that involves liaising with other services.	
Limited involvement with social aspects of care.	
Education of the carer and the cared for.	
Contact is time limited.	
Formal carers are entitled to frequent breaks and time off.	
If care becomes continuous a team will be involved in delivering care and it won't be an individual responsibility.	
Should a formal carer become sick or injured replacement is possible.	
It is possible to maintain professional detachment from the emotional aspects of caring.	

Table 1 Comparing and contrasting informal and formal carers' roles (adapted from Pickard and Glendenning, 2002; and University of Paisley, 2005).

On completing the table you should be aware that informal carers may have to deliver a wide variety of care that may consist of social, personal and technical care. They may choose to liaise with other professionals or may rely on those professionals they already have contact with. They are highly involved in the social aspects of care, may be involved in educating themselves and the person they are caring for, even if the care professional considers that as part of their role. Their contact time with the 'cared for' may be unlimited, they may get few breaks from caring, may be responsible for all aspects of care outside that given by formal caregivers, may have to liaise with their family as a member of a caring team, may not be replaced when they are sick and cannot distance themselves from the emotional aspects of care giving. As Pickard and Glendinning (2002) put it, family carers' care giving, particularly if given in what the older person considers to be their 'home', is boundless.

Informal caring requires a great investment of time, as well as physical and emotional energy. Caregivers, as a result, may feel that at times caring is challenging and difficult, especially the primary care giver who bears the brunt of responsibility for the older person (Greenberger and Litwin, 2003). The stress caused by taking on this role comes at a cost to both the physical and mental health of carers. It can increase psychological and stress-related disorders; it can cause personal strain and social isolation. Depression in the carer is always a possibility as a result (Runciman, 2003). Carers themselves often describe caring as 'burdensome' and the burdens of caring can be emotional, psychological, physical, financial and social.

The emotional and psychological cost

For most carers this is the most important stress that they experience and the burden most likely to lead to burnout and ill-health (Hirst, 2004). Caring for another person is emotionally stressful for a number of reasons. The first consideration though, has to be the relationship that exists between the carer and the 'cared for'. Love for, and commitment to, the person that you are caring for is an important basis for most caring relationships. The very fact that there is love and commitment there may mean that people underestimate or deny the emotional strain or burden that they are under (Mackenzie and Lee, 2005).

Feelings of love and affection for the recipient can also make it easier for the person to provide care but, paradoxically, can also prevent people from caring, as it can make the task of caring emotionally difficult. Carers may suffer pain and feel less able to cope when they witness deterioration or growing debilitation and handicap in their loved ones (Greenberger and Litwin, 2003).

Another consideration is the dependency level of the person being cared for. Reductions in the autonomy of the person being cared for can induce emotional stress in the carer, as the carer has to make more and more stressful decisions on behalf of the person in their care. The more areas of decision making that the carer has responsibility for, the greater this stress is likely to be. This may be exacerbated by the changes in social role that may accompany the adoption of the carer's role, for example sons and daughters become carers of, rather than being cared for, by their parents. Carers may also need to adopt unfamiliar roles, for example a wife may find she has to take over financial control of the family from her husband, a husband may have to assume responsibility for domestic tasks. Such changes and the difficulties that they can produce, may lead to complex feelings of guilt, frustration, embarrassment, anger, fear, hate and resentment in both parties and can lead to wider family conflict (Neufeld and Harrison, 2003).

Not surprisingly, satisfaction in the caring role reduces as the emotional stress caring creates increases. Behaviours that are too demanding, upsetting, or difficult to deal with, like verbal or physical aggression or abuse, or the 'cared' for becoming incontinent, can make the carer's burden seem more pronounced and helplessness and depression may result, if the emotional feelings accompanying these factors are not addressed (Mackenzie and Lee, 2005).

The emotional and psychological stress that carers experience may also be linked to the uncertainty of the outcome of their care and an inability to visualise a future (Nolan, Grant and Keady, 1996). Perhaps this can best be imagined by considering two questions carers may have to ask themselves at some point in their caring journey:

- What traumas lie ahead before caring ends?
- How will this relationship end?

The physical cost

For many carers there are physically demanding activities associated with their role. The most physically demanding activities and the most problematic for older carers, are lifting, bathing and dressing. Older carers are also likely to have chronic illness themselves, which may limit their ability to perform some of the caring tasks they would like to tackle. These physical demands often require older carers to seek assistance from outside agencies. The physical demands of caring may threaten carers' physical health further and causes tiredness, which is known to be a very common complaint among carers (Mackenzie and Lee, 2005).

Carers themselves also report an increasing vulnerability to physical illness. This includes increasing vulnerability to back problems, strains, sprains, colds and chest infections, as well as chronic fatigue (De Frias, Tuokko and Rosenberg, 2005). Although it is likely that carers experience a level of physical exertion in their lives perhaps greater than the norm, the relationship between that caring and ill-health is not clear. This is partly because most carers accept their role when they are older and begin caring with already existent chronic health problems (Mackenzie and Lee, 2005). Caring may not cause physical ill-health, but if you are already unwell or have a chronic disease it may exacerbate your condition and delay your recovery from illness (Carers UK, 2004).

Social cost

For most carers the demands of caring lead to a reduction in their opportunities for social contact. The opportunities to interact with others, usually provided by employment and by involvement in social activities outside the home, are the most likely to be restricted. For carers who remain in employment, caring duties tend to restrict social activities and reduce the time available for, and the opportunity to have, holidays (Mackenzie and Lee, 2005).

The social circle that carers come into contact with may also shrink. Caring can reduce the carer's contact with friends, can cause reduced entertainment opportunities and cause an increasing feeling of isolation. The demands of caring can also lead informal carers to neglect their own needs, an inability to remain in employment and decreasing family contact. As a result, carers can commonly feel that they have no private time, are lost or trapped and are missing life's opportunities (Neufeld and Harrison, 2003). The cost of this burden can be increased by a lack of family support, or if conflict and other negative interactions exist in the relationship the carer has when in contact with their family. In order for this burden to be overcome, many carers when asked, express a need for companionship and a feeling that they have some support from outside the caring relationship. They particularly need someone to talk to, when family and other immediate forms of social support are lacking (Stoltz, Uden and Willman, 2004).

Financial cost

Caring also has financial cost implications for the carer. The extra expenditure involved can include the cost of heating, laundry, the need to buy foodstuffs required to meet special dietary requirements and increased travel costs. Carers may also find themselves required to cover medical treatment fees and the cost of aids and home adaptation for the person. They may also have to meet the cost of paying for assistance or additional care. Many carers are also faced with the prospect of giving up paid work, or going to part-time, to take on a caring role, both of which seriously restrict the financial resources available to them (Mackenzie and Lee, 2005).

Many older carers also live on fixed incomes (basically their pensions) and the financial burden of caring can squeeze their financial resources to a point where the monetary burden alone further increases their poverty and increases their stress. This has a detrimental effect on their health status and their ability to continue caring (Hirst, 2004).

Carers UK (2007) reported that one in five UK carers has to cut back on food, one in four has cut back on heating and, worryingly, nearly half have no savings at all. They also report that six out of ten carers worry about their finances a lot, or all of the time and over half believe this has an effect on their health (Carers UK, 2007). Many Westernised governments, including the UK Government, do provide financial support in the form of a variety of carers' allowances aimed at replacing lost earnings, but these rarely compensate adequately for the lost savings, loss of earnings and time spent on caring (Mesthenos and Triantafillou, 2005).

There are other reported burdens of caring over and above those discussed here. For example, the cost to the family unit because of the increased tensions that caring places on it. The cost and strains, when combined, can eventually stress and burnout the carer if they are not dealt with appropriately. As a consequence of all these cumulative burdens, anxiety and depression can result, both for the carer and in the 'cared for' (Greenberger and Litwin, 2003). However, most carers want to continue to care for as long as is possible, feasible or practical and that is because caring also has important rewards associated with it.

THE REWARDS OF CARING

Although we appear to know quite a lot about the burdens of caring, few studies have focussed on the rewards of care giving. Care giving relationships provide opportunities for those involved to learn more about each other. They also provide a spouse or younger person with an opportunity to give something back to the person who has made sacrifices for them, a repayment for past care and kindness. In many societies caring is also seen as a cultural duty or an obligation which lends a carer status (Eliopoulos, 2005).

Many carers view caring as a worthwhile challenge. As it involves the act of giving, which is in itself viewed as rewarding, caring can improve the perceived life quality of the carer. This sense of reward can be increased when the person receiving care shows appreciation for what is being done for them. Appreciating that the person being cared for is stable in health or improving during care, also acts as a reward and increases carers' satisfaction (Mackenzie and Lee, 2005).

Care givers also take satisfaction in recognising their own achievements and ability to care. Care giving can provide a sense of pride and satisfaction at being able to cope with crises and difficulties. As a result, caring can lead to personal growth and a deepening sense of self-awareness. Carers state that they become stronger, more tolerant, less judgemental, more sensitive and empathetic toward others and were more assertive in their demands on welfare services (Grant et al., 2001). A sense of achievement can also be gained from helping the older person avoid institutional care. Care at home, which is generally the preference of the older person being 'cared for', is viewed as a much better alternative to institutional care. The common perception being that institutional care is poor, undesirable or both (Mackenzie and Lee, 2005).

SUPPORT FOR CARERS

Meeting the care needs of older people can be seen as a balance between informal and formal care. There has however been a tremendous growth in informal care over the past two decades for various economic and social reasons. Carers UK's research has suggested that the number of carers is likely to increase in the future. Carers UK (2002) demonstrates that demographic change, coupled with the direction of community care policy, will see a 60 per cent rise in the number of carers needed in the UK by 2037 – an extra 3.4 million carers.

Informal care has been considered more economic and, given the numbers to be involved in the future, will remain so. It is also considered to be socially desirable because it accords with the wishes of older people for closeness with family and friends, while at the same time maintaining autonomy and independence within the community. If there are many carers coping in the community, then the research evidence would suggest that they need support to continue to cope. Clearly, with more carers emerging within the population, support of carers is an area of care that health care professionals need to address. Supporting carers is a multi-dimensional task and requires multi-disciplinary input. Support of carers then is a key role for all health care professionals and this needs to be recognised (Pickard and Glendinning, 2002).

Since carers are so important to the UK's wealth and social stability, the National Strategy for Carers (Department of Health, 1999) acknowledges that carers play a vital societal role and notes three key approaches to supporting people who choose to be carers. Carers must be given:

- information on the means to provide care and about available help and services;
- support from communities in planning and the provision of services;
- care that promotes choice, maintains health and recognises their role.

For health care professionals then, there is a need to address each of the suggested areas within the strategy. There is also a requirement to assess and address the needs of individual carers. Nolan and Grant (1989) highlighted that there is remarkable consensus among carers as to what services they feel are important. Five areas identified by carers that they feel there is a need for services in are:

1. information;
2. skills training;
3. emotional support;
4. respite;
5. social support.

Carers' information needs

Health care professionals, particularly community-based nurses, are the main group who provide information to carers and are key to meeting this need, particularly for older carers (Mackenzie and Lee, 2005). It is believed that the provision of information can reduce carers' levels of anxiety, improves outcomes by encouraging adherence to treatment and rehabilitation programmes, contributes to the patients' and carers' sense of control, improves patients' and carers' satisfaction and can improve the relationship between health professionals, patients and carers (Wiles *et al.*, 1998).

Meeting carers' needs for information is not a simple task, however, as they need information from a wide range of areas, such as the person's condition, treatment, physical and psychosocial aspects of caring, sources of financial aid, sources of legal assistance, availability of community services and resources, and information regarding their own coping and adjustment strategies. Given the extent of their needs for information, carers express concern that the information that they are given by health care professionals is not always appropriate, or given at the right time, or in the right form. In fact, Morris and Thomas (2002) indicate that the key area of unmet need for carers is the need for information. They suggest that the perception of carers is that health care professionals seem to give too little, too late, often give too much information and much that is irrelevant. Most carers in fact seek additional information outside that given by the professionals that they are in contact with, and outside the health care system, suggesting that health care professionals probably can't meet all their needs (Morris and Thomas, 2002). Improving information giving is helped by using a variety of methods (for example, video, audio discs and tapes) and using more written information, particularly in conjunction with oral information. The satisfaction with, and success of, information giving can be improved, if the provided information can be tailored or customised to meet the needs of a wide range of individuals. In fact, as a general principle, the more individualised the information becomes the more successful it is likely to be (Wiles *et al.*, 1998). Perhaps the key to successful information giving is to remember that carers do need to know things to succeed. As health care professionals perhaps our role is to try to determine what that information is, and when they need to know it (Morris and Thomas, 2002).

Skills training

As informal carers are untrained, they will certainly benefit from education and training in tasks such as lifting, moving, use of disability aids, medication effects and side-effects, and dealing with continence issues. However, although skills training may help to improve their confidence and competence in carrying out caring tasks, it is dealing with the emotional aspects of caring that create the most turmoil for informal carers (Pickard, Jacobs and Kirk, 2003).

Emotional support

There is abundant evidence that emotional support is perceived by carers to be the most important. Carers must be listened to. Being recognised and valued for their work is fundamental to supporting them. Health care workers need to give them more explicit recognition. They should be praised for their efforts, and both they and the care recipients and other significant people should be involved in the development of the plans for care. Carers have to be helped to deal with a number of emotions arising from caring and helped to find meaning in their situation. Life review, pet therapy, group interactions, hobbies and music therapy can all aid this. At times referral to more intensive counselling may be needed. If necessary, referral to formal services like, for example, mental health services, may greatly assist the older person in a care-giving situation (Mackenzie and Lee, 2005).

Respite

Informal carers need to address their own needs and regular respite should be made available to them. Offering chances for carers to retain normality allows them opportunities to reduce their negative feelings towards their dependents and helps them to maintain their caring relationships. Most carers, older carers especially, support the idea of home-based respite care because this is the least distressing to the care recipient. Often, though, home respite is limited in availability, inflexible in the way that it is delivered and is rarely available outside office hours This leads to respite services being rejected quite quickly by many carers (Innes *et al.*, 2005). Respite care has to match the needs of informal carers and the people they care for, not conflict with their needs and create more disharmony. Informal carers also need to realise the importance of respite to their own health and need to understand the variety of forms that it can take. Unless they have this information, they are unlikely to make best use of respite services when they are offered.

Other forms of respite care, which tend to be offered in institutional settings, are also often inflexible and there is often a lack of choice regarding the type of respite service on offer. Everyone involved in caring needs to be aware of the importance of a break for a carer. Short-term breaks should be of an acceptable quality and be individually tailored, so the main provision is not always within an institution. Additionally, a partnership approach between all relevant services has to be developed so that respite is not seen as the responsibility of just one agency or profession. Greater involvement of the carer and the 'cared for' in the design and delivery of respite services is also required (Jarvis, Worth and Porter, 2006).

Activity 2

- If you were asked by an informal carer in your own area or in the area in which you currently work about what respite services were available locally, could you answer them?
- How would you suggest they find out about what is available to them?
- How difficult do you think it would be for them to access appropriate information about locally available services?

Consider that the respite they require may vary from a few hours to allow them to do some necessary shopping regularly, to a few weeks to allow them to go on holiday. They may also wish for overnight respite to allow them to catch up on much needed sleep or to allow them to attend an important family occasion.

Social support

The desire for carers' (peer) support groups is one that is often expressed by carers themselves. Social support, via a support group, can meet the carers' esteem needs, and may help them feel valued and cared for. Support within the group can come from both the formal and informal carers who are participants. Support groups are valuable as an opportunity for carers to share experiences with people in a similar situation and to exchange information and emotional support (Pickard, 2003). The reported gains of joining a support group include:

- Significant increases in morale and feelings of wellbeing because of the increased emotional support that comes with group involvement.
- Increased knowledge. The supportive environment of the group allowed assimilation of knowledge that was already known and allowed acceptance of the real nature and course of long-term illness and this helped carers to cope with their situation.
- The development of a more positive outlook to their caring role.
- A high satisfaction level with the support received and a feeling that participation in the support group is worthwhile.

(Arksey *et al.*, 2002)

Work with support groups indicates that their needs change over time. When first established the focus is on information sharing, friendship and social contact. For a longer-established group (perhaps two years plus), members become concerned with lobbying for change and trying to raise awareness of the problems of carers. Involving carers in self-help groups early in the caring experience helps reduce the frequency of crises and the subsequent emotional burnout that these stresses cause. Not all carers will want to join a support group or will find it helpful, but research suggests that carers who have links with a support group are better able to continue to provide care. For this reason, local carers' support groups should be seen as an integral part of service delivery (Carers UK, 2005). In fact, Greenberger and Litwin (2003) commenting on the fact that a care giver's ability to cope can be bolstered by health professionals, believe that efforts to strengthen a care giver's self-esteem, social support and confidence by involving them in support groups may be more effective in guaranteeing quality care than attempts to relieve their sense of burden. Pickard (2003), however, does point out that although support groups are valued by those who attend, there is no conclusive evidence regarding the effectiveness of support groups. She goes on to state that, despite the reports, there is no evidence that support groups produce direct improvements in the wellbeing of carers or in their ability to continue caring. It should also be noted that no research has been carried out in the UK into the cost-effectiveness of support groups (Pickard, 2003).

INVOLVING CARERS

Health care professionals who work in the community in particular have the privilege of entry into the private lives of the people that they care for, and can see at first hand the difficulties that exist for carers. They can make a major contribution, particularly with the help of other professionals and care providers in assessing, planning and supporting carers. Carers often praise the help that they receive from the caring professions, but they may also complain of being taken for granted or not being understood. The views that carers and professionals hold of each other can affect the relationship that they have. Carers are often intimidated by professionals and hold them in awe. This may be because they cannot perceive the professional as an individual, but hold a collective and generalised view of all the professionals they come into contact with (Mackenzie and Lee, 2005). Professionals, on the other hand, can often be unrealistic regarding carers, viewing them as selfless and morally sound characters, when the caring relationship may be far more turbulent than they suspect and may, at times, even be abusive. Such perceptions can make it difficult for professionals and informal carers to be open with each other (O'Keeffe *et al.*, 2007).

Another factor to consider is that professional training, particularly prior to professional registration for many health care professionals, does not or has not included any in-depth education on how to recognise a carer's needs. This can make it very difficult for some professionals to accurately assess informal carers' needs. Professionals may also ignore carers' needs, for fear that, in identifying them, they may be unable to do anything to meet them. If this is the case, it may be the professional who ends up feeling helpless and guilty (Twigg and Atkin, 1994).

In 1994, Twigg and Atkin drafted a framework in an attempt to provide some understanding for the ambiguity that exists in the relationship between formal and informal carers. They stated that, on examining interactions between formal carers and informal carers, formal carers viewed the informal carers in at least four ways. They viewed the carer's role as shown in Table 2:

Role	Description
A resource	Carers seen as a community resource and a cheap source of labour. Services are provided to keep the carer capable but at minimal cost.
A co-worker	Service providers recognise the importance of the carers' role and work to maintain their morale and the support that they offer to their patient.
A co-client	Carers seen as having needs in their own right in a similar manner to the patient.
A superseded carer	The aim is to move the client from this family care regime to independent living in a different environment (including hospitalisation and care home).

Table 2 Formal carers' views of the role of the informal carer (adapted from Twigg and Atkin, 1994)

Consider these roles from the informal carer's perspective. If you, the informal carer, believe that you are a 'resource' only, then you will not be happy about how you are being treated and may feel that you are being taken advantage of. You may also feel poorly supported. Those informal carers who experience 'co-workers' or 'co-client' status are more likely to be positive about their experiences and may express a view that they felt supported and felt they were partners in formal care giving. Those viewed as 'superseded carers' may have accepted that their caring role has altered and be positive that formal carers have 'taken over', but perhaps they are more likely to feel that their experience in caring was undervalued and may feel left out of decision making once formal care started. If this is the case, they are unlikely to be happy with the experience. If health care workers are aware of these perceptions and the restrictions that they may impose, then perhaps they can act to offer carers more supportive attitudes and choices.

It would also appear that, in order for health care professionals to offer carers effective support and to make them feel more valued, they need to understand what carers really want. Carers UK (2004) state that ultimately carers want a good quality of life for the person that they care for. Besides this key aim they also want to:

- be fully informed;
- be recognised and have their own health and wellbeing considered;
- use high quality services that they can depend on;
- have some time off and breaks from caring;
- have some emotional support which can offer some relief from their sense of isolation;
- training, advice and support on how to care;
- financial security;
- their voice to be heard both in their own individual situations and in the development of local services.

(Carers UK, 2005)

IMPLICATIONS FOR JOINT WORKING

The importance of informal carers as part of the UK and European political agenda has grown over the last 20 years, with the realisation that carers form the bedrock of community care. There is a growing belief that the role of public authorities is to sustain and develop where necessary this form of support and care (Forbat, 2008). This has been labelled a 'caring for carers' approach and has been recognised in UK legislation since the Carers (Recognition and Services) Act 1995 (Department of Health, 1995), which gave all informal carers the right to have a separate and independent assessment of their needs. The Carers National Strategy (Department of Health, 1999), which is called *Caring About Carers*, enshrines this approach, which has been the basis for further policy development in this field. Another attribute of the 'caring for carers' approach is that informal carers are now being recognised as a group of citizens with special rights – see Table 3 overleaf.

Policy document and/or Legislation name and citation

Department of Health (1995) *The Carers (Recognition and Services) Act 1995.* London: HMSO.

Department of Health (1997) *The New NHS, Modern Dependable.* London: Stationery Office.

Department of Health (1999) *National Strategy for Carers: Caring About Carers.* London: Stationery Office.

Department of Health (2000) *The Carers and Disabled Children Act 2000.* London: Stationery Office.

Department of Health (1999) *The National Service Framework for Mental Health.* London: Stationery Office.

Department of Health (2001) *Valuing People.* London: Stationery Office.

Department of Health (2001) *The National Service Framework for Older People.* London: Stationery Office.

Department of Health (2001) *The Carers (Equal Opportunities) Act 2004.* London: Stationery Office.

Department of Health (2005) *Everybody's Business.* London: Stationery Office.

HM Government (2008) *Carers at the Heart of 21st Century Families and Communities: a Caring System on Your Side, a Life of Your Own. (The New Carers Strategy for England).* London: Department of Health.

Scottish Executive (1999) *Strategy for Carers in Scotland.* Edinburgh: Stationery Office.

Scottish Executive (2002) *Community Care and Health (Scotland) Act 2002.* Edinburgh: Stationery Office.

Scottish Executive (2003) *Partnership for Care.* Edinburgh: Stationery Office.

Scottish Executive (2003) *National Care Standards – Short Breaks and Respite Care Services for Adults.* Edinburgh: Stationery Office

Scottish Executive (2005) *Delivering for Health.* Edinburgh: Stationery Office

Department of Health, Social Services and Public Safety (2002) *Caring for Carers: Recognising, Valuing and Supporting the Caring Role.* Belfast: DHSSPSNI.

Department of Health, Social Services and Public Safety (2002) *Carers and Direct Payments Act (Northern Ireland) 2002.* Belfast: DHSSPSNI.

Department for Employment and Learning (2006) *The Work and Families (Northern Ireland) Order 2006.* Belfast: DELNI

Table 3 UK Government documents that enshrine a 'Caring for Carers' approach.

However, carers' awareness of their rights, particularly their right to independent assessment, is low and social services often do not consider this usual practice and may fail to offer it. In fact, in the UK, present health and social service infrastructures mean that countrywide there are no consistent methods of support for informal carers. There is also an absence of a strategic service delivery. Such an irregular response to a known need seems very inadequate (Carers UK, 2002). Carers in the UK and elsewhere need to be made more aware of their rights, particularly their entitlement to have their needs assessed. As a result, health professionals need to become allies and effective advocates for carers' rights, as well as for the rights of their own clients. There is also a need for local health care workers and local health and social services to evaluate the quality of the care they provide to their carers. Part of this evaluation has to involve how they can identify those in the community not receiving services, as these carers may be ones experiencing or feeling the greatest burden, since they are often relying on the support of families and friends alone (Pickard, 2004).

However, changing social patterns, particularly in Northern Europe where there is an increase in 'partner' relationships without the legal ties of marriage and an increase in divorce and re-marriage, mean that new family networks are being created where a lack of clarity exists regarding obligations and willingness to care. As a result, the situation developing in the UK and some other European countries is one where there are low social expectations of the family providing all the care and increasing political and legal recognition of the role of informal carers (Mesthenos and Triantafillou, 2005).

Recently there has been a growing move in several countries to develop a 'Carers' Charter' or 'Carers' Bill of Rights' (Carers UK, 2005; Scottish Executive, 2006). Among the rights being debated are the following:

- That the payment system for carers needs to change from one based loosely on income replacement, to one which properly recognises their contribution to society.
- That national and local government organisations and the health care system should make considerable efforts to look after the health and wellbeing of carers.
- That carers should have increased access to counselling and emotional support services and occupational health provision, that matches that provided to formal carers.
- That there should be national standards regarding addressing carers' needs.

- That local organisations offering carer support should be strengthened.
- That carers are given a statutory entitlement to respite breaks from caring.
- That carers should be involved in the development of all policies that may impact upon them.

In the UK, the government recently created the Standing Commission on Carers with a view to putting carers at the heart of policy-making in order to explore new ways of maximising independence and developing services fit for the twenty-first century. The standing Commission is working with Ministers on overseeing the revision of the UK's Strategy on Carers which is called *Carers at the Heart of 21st-century Families and Communities*. (Department of Health, 2008).

As our current health and social care systems would collapse under the cost of replacing even a small proportion of the care that informal carers provide, perhaps it is the duty of government and all health care professionals to recognise the important role played by informal carers and support any moves that would improve their lives and improve their status in society. Professionals need to be more responsive to the needs of informal carers, and should recognise them as key stakeholders and partners in providing the most appropriate care to meet their clients' needs (Department of Health, 2001; Scottish Executive, 2003). After all, the likelihood is that many of us will become informal carers to our parents, spouses, siblings or other people that we know.

The health professional's ability to provide support will be enhanced by knowing what carers find difficult, how they manage these difficulties and what they find satisfying. By having an understanding of the often invisible difficulties and, equally, individual ways of managing and finding satisfaction, they may better appreciate why some carers appear to manage the stresses of caring and others struggle with less demanding loads (Jarvis, Worth and Porter, 2006).

CONCLUSION

There is no doubt that, both socially and politically, the role of the informal carer providing health and social care to older people is vitally important. There is increasing political and professional awareness that informal carers are so key that they require to be supported in their efforts to care with information, training, financial and where required peer and professionally-led support services.

As the number of older people in societies rises worldwide, there is an increasing need for the professional training of all health care staff to include a substantial input that relates to their role in supporting informal carers as partners in patient care in all health care settings. They also need to be well prepared to assess carers' real needs and work co-operatively across the health, social care and voluntary sectors to ensure that identified carers' needs are met. Health care professionals also need to be able to take account of the diversity of informal carers in order to ensure that they meet the needs of the whole caring community, taking account of carers with specialised needs and the specific cultural and language needs of the minority ethnic groups they encounter.

Government also has a role to play by recognising the rights of informal carers, reducing the financial difficulties that becoming a carer can bring and ensuring that the health and social care system is receptive when carers require support.

FURTHER READING

Carers UK (2002) *Without Us . . . ? Calculating the Value of Carers' Support*. London: Carers UK
Carers UK (2004) *In Poor Health: The Impact of Caring on Health*. London: Carers UK
Both are available to download from the Carers UK website: **www.carersuk. org**

Mesthenos, E. and Triantafillou, J. (2005) *EUROFAMCARE Group: Supporting Family Carers of Older People in Europe – the Pan-European Background*. Hamburg: EUROFAMCARE-Consortium
This is a very informative report on many aspects of informal caring for older people in 23 countries of the European Union. It is available to download from: **www.uke.uni-hamburg.de/extern/eurofamcare**

Scottish Executive (2005) *Care 21: The Future of Unpaid Care in Scotland: Headline Report and Recommendations*. Edinburgh: Scottish Executive
This is more than just a government report, it is also an important piece of research that attempts to provide a comprehensive picture of the issues currently facing informal carers and how they might be tackled now and into the future. The report and a number of responses and associated documents can all be downloaded from:
www.carerscotland.org/Policyandpractice/Keylegislationandpolicy/ Care21-reports

Useful websites

www.direct.gov.uk/en/CaringForSomeone/index.htm
This is part of the UK Government's Directgov website called 'Caring for Someone'. The page provides details of the services and benefits affecting carers that are available throughout England and Wales.

www.carersuk.org
Carers UK (formerly the 'Carers National Association') is a charity and campaigning organisation that states that it is the voice of carers and is the only UK carer-led organisation working for all carers.

www.princessroyaltrust.org.uk
The Princess Royal Trust for Carers is the largest provider of comprehensive carers' support services in the UK.

www.ukcarers.net
UK Carers is a campaigning group that collects the views of carers through a series of message boards and 'blogs' by UK carers and then campaigns on their behalf.

www.crossroads.org.uk/index.php?mid=1&pgid=1
Crossroads is a service aimed at improving the lives of carers by giving them time to be themselves and have a break from their caring responsibilities. Its aim is to provide a reliable service, tailored to meet the individual needs of each carer and the person they are caring for. The main organisation serves England and Wales.

www.crossroads-scotland.co.uk
In Scotland the organisation is called Crossroads Caring Scotland.

REFERENCES

Adams, T. (ed.) (2008) *Dementia Care Nursing: Promoting Well-being in People with Dementia and their Families.* Basingstoke: Palgrave, Macmillan

Arksey, H., O'Malley, L., Baldwin, S., Harris, J., Mason, A. and Golder, S. (2002) *Services to Support Carers of People with Mental Health Problems. Literature Review Report for the National Co-ordinating Centre for NHS Service Delivery and Organisation R&D (NCCSDO).* University of York: Social Policy Research Unit

Blakemore, K. (2000) 'Health and social care needs in minority communities: an over-problematized issue?' *Health and Social Care in the Community*, 8 (1): 22–30

Braithwaite, V.A. (2000) 'Contextual or general stress outcomes: Making choices through caregiving'. *Gerontologist*, 40: 706–17

Carers UK (2002) *Without Us . . . ? Calculating the Value of Carers' Support.* London: Carers UK

Carers UK (2004) *In Poor Health: The Impact of Caring on Health.* London: Carers UK

Carers UK (2005) *A Manifesto for Carers*. London: Carers UK

Carers UK (2007) *Real Change Not Short Change*. London: Carers UK

De Frias, C.M., Tuokko, H. and Rosenberg, T. (2005) 'Caregiver physical and mental health predicts reactions to caregiving'. *Aging & Mental Health*, 9, (4): 331–6

Department of Health (1995) *The Carers (Recognition and Services) Act 1995*. London: Stationery Office

Department of Health (1999) *Caring About Carers: A National Strategy*. London: Stationery Office

Department of Health (2001) *Valuing People*. London: Stationery Office

Department of Health (2008) *Advisory Bodies: Standing Commission on Carers (SCOC)*. Available at: **www.advisorybodies.doh.gov.uk/scoc/index.htm** (Accessed 20 April 08)

Eliopoulos, C. (2005) *Gerontological Nursing* (6th edn) Philadelphia, PA: Lippincott, Williams & Wilkins

Forbat, L. (2007) 'Social Policy and Relationship-centred Dementia Care Nursing' in Adams, T. (ed.) *Dementia Care Nursing: Promoting Well-being in People with Dementia and their Families*. Basingstoke: Palgrave Macmillan

Gaugler, J.E., Zarit, S.H. and Pearlin, L.I. (1999) 'Caregiving and Institutionalisation: Perceptions of family conflict and socio-emotional support'. *International Journal of Aging and Human Development*, 49: 1–25

Grant, G., Ramcharan, P., Mc.Grath, M., Nolan, M. and Keady, J. (2001) 'Rewards and gratifications among family caregivers: Towards a refined model of caring and coping'. *Journal of Intellectual Disability Research*, 42 (1): 58–71

Greenberger, H. and Litwin, H. (2003) 'Can burdened caregivers be effective facilitators of elder care-recipient health care?' *Journal of Advanced Nursing*, 41 (4): 332–41

Hall, J. (2002) 'Assessing the health promotion needs of informal carers'. *Nursing Older People*,14 (3): 14–18

Hirst, M. (2004) *Hearts and Minds: The Health Effects of Caring*. London: Social Policy Research Unit and Carers UK

Innes, A., Blackstock, K., Mason, A., Smith, A. and Cox, S. (2005) 'Dementia care provision in rural Scotland: Service users' and carers' experiences'. *Health and Social Care in the Community*, 13 (4): 354–65

Jarvis, A., Worth, A. and Porter, M. (2006) 'The experience of caring for someone over 75 years of age: Results from a Scottish general practice population'. *Journal of Clinical Nursing*, 15: 1450–9

Mackenzie, A. and Lee, D.T.F. (2005) 'Carers and lay caring' in Redfern, S.J. and Ross, F.M. (eds) *Nursing Older People* (4th edn). Edinburgh: Elsevier/ Churchill Livingstone

McGarry, J. and Arthur, A. (2001) 'Informal caring in later life: a qualitative study of the experiences of older carers'. *Journal of Advanced Nursing*, 33 (2): 182–9

Merrell, J., Kinsella, F., Murphy, F., Philpin, S. and Ali, A. (2006) 'Accessibility and equity of health and social care services: Exploring the views and experiences of Bangladeshi carers in South Wales, UK'. *Health and Social Care in the Community*, 14 (3):197–205

Mesthenos, E. and Triantafillou, J. (2005) *EUROFAMCARE Group: Supporting Family Carers of Older People in Europe – the Pan-European Background.* Hamburg: EUROFAMCARE-Consortium

Morris, S.M. and Thomas, C. (2002) 'The need to know: Informal carers and Information'. *European Journal of Cancer Care,* 11: 183–7

National Statistics Online (2006) *Focus on Health: Caring & Carers: 6 million Unpaid Carers in the UK.* **www.statistics.gov.uk/CCI/nugget.asp?ID=1336 &Pos=3&ColRank=1&Rank=208** (Accessed 1 March 2008)

Neufeld, A. and Harrison, M.J. (2003) 'Unfulfilled expectations and negative interactions: Non-support in the relationships of women caregivers'. *Journal of Advanced Nursing,* 41 (4): 323–31

Nolan, M. and Grant, G. (1989) 'Addressing the needs of informal carers: A neglected area of nursing practice'. *Journal of Advanced Nursing,* 14 (11): 950–61

Nolan, M., Grant, G. and Keady, J. (1996) *Understanding Family Care: A Multi-dimensional Model of Caring and Coping.* Buckingham: Open University Press

O'Keeffe, M., Hills, A., Doyle, M., McCreadie, C., Scholes, S., Constantine, R., Tinker, A., Manthorpe, J., Biggs, S. and Erens, B. (2007) *UK Study of Abuse and Neglect of Older People: Prevalence Survey Report.* London: National Centre for Social Research

Office of National Statistics (2002) *Census 2001.* London: National Statistics

Pickard, S. (2004) *The Effectiveness and Cost Effectiveness of Support and Services to Informal Carers of Older People – A Review of the Literature Prepared for the Audit Commission.* Wetherby: Audit Commission Publications

Pickard, S. and Glendenning, C. (2002) 'Comparing and contrasting the role of family carers and nurses in the domestic health care of frail older people'. *Health and Social Care in the Community,* 10 (3): 144–50

Pickard, S., Jacob, S. and Kirk, S. (2003) 'Challenging professionals' roles: lay carers' involvement in health care in the community'. *Social Policy and Administration,* 37 (1): 82–96

Runciman, P. (2003) 'Family carers' experiences: Reflections on partnership'. *Nursing Older People,* 15 (3):14-16

Scottish Executive (2003) *Partnership for Care.* Edinburgh: The Stationery Office

Scottish Executive (2006) *Scottish Executive Response to Care 21 Report: The Future of Unpaid Care in Scotland.* Edinburgh: Scottish Executive

Stoltz, P., Uden, G. and Willman, A. (2004) 'Support for family carers who care for an elderly person at home – A systematic literature review'. *Scandanavian Journal of Caring Science,* 18: 111–19

Twigg, J. and Atkin, K. (1994) *Carers Perceived.* Buckingham: Open University Press

University of Paisley (2005) *Online Learning Support Materials: Ageing Matters Meeting the Healthcare Needs of Older People.* Paisley: University of Paisley

Wiles R., Pain H., Buckland S. and Mc.Lellan, L. (1998) 'Providing information to patients and carers following a stroke'. *Journal of Advanced Nursing,* 28 (4): 794–801

Chapter 9

Older People and Advocacy

Rick Henderson

Learning outcomes

Reading this chapter will enable you to:

- gain an overview of current advocacy services and issues for older people in the UK;

- explore the policy context for current advocacy provision and practice;

- explore the skills required for effective advocacy with older people, and key dilemmas in acquiring and maintaining those skills;

- through the use of case studies, illustrate the impact that advocacy can have on the lives of older people;

- understand the difference between advocating as part of a wider role and the specific provision of independent advocacy services.

INTRODUCTION

This chapter aims to introduce the reader to the current situation regarding advocacy and related services for older people in the United Kingdom (UK). There has been a significant increase in awareness of the need for and benefits of advocacy in recent years. Advocates and advocacy schemes can make a real difference in the lives of older people through the provision of independent support and representation. This is slowly being recognised by government and a number of recent policy initiatives have championed the cause of older people's advocacy, notably the Adults with Incapacity (Scotland) 2000 Act and the Mental Capacity Act 2005. However, this recognition has not necessarily been accompanied by a corresponding increase in funding. This poses problems for a sector that has been traditionally under-funded. While some attempts have been made to inform and educate funders and commissioners of advocacy, there is still some way to go. As a result, advocacy schemes have sought pragmatic solutions to the dilemmas caused by increasing demand, notably through the use of volunteers.

The UK advocacy sector is diverse and a number of advocacy 'models' have developed, which will be explored in greater detail later in this chapter. There has also been a growing focus on the advocacy needs of older people with dementia and those from Black and minority ethnic (BME) communities. Another significant development has been the increasing role of independent advocates in adult protection and elder abuse situations. But a distinction needs to be made here between 'independent advocacy' as a service model, provided by independent (mainly voluntary) organisations, and the kinds of 'everyday advocacy' practised by health and social care staff, informal carers and others. This chapter focusses primarily on issues for independent advocacy practitioners, although, of course, many of the issues and skills are transferable.

A REVIEW OF THE CURRENT LITERATURE

The first independent advocacy scheme in the UK was established as recently as 1983. The first few schemes were established in response to concerns about the neglect and ill-treatment of people living in long-stay institutional environments (Henderson and Pochin, 2001). Advocacy was seen as a way of providing some form of safeguard to very vulnerable people, as well as an empowering process that focussed on rights as well as needs. For older people, advocacy has an even more recent history, and it is only in the past few years that older people's advocacy has become more commonplace, alongside information and advice services (Dunning, 2005).

Definitions of advocacy

It has been a feature of the advocacy sector that agreement on a common definition of advocacy has been difficult to achieve. This is in part due to the fact that most advocacy schemes have developed from the grassroots up and, therefore, have sought their own definitions of what they do.

In its most basic form, advocacy can be defined as supporting a person to speak for themselves or, where necessary, speaking up for them. A more comprehensive definition, taken from the Advocacy Charter (Action for Advocacy 2002: 2), is as follows:

> Advocacy is taking action to help people say what they want, secure their rights, represent their interests and obtain services they need. Advocates and advocacy schemes work in partnership with the people they support and take their side. Advocacy promotes social inclusion, equality and social justice.

What is advocacy?

In theory, anybody can act as an advocate, either for themselves (self-advocacy) or for another person (third party advocacy). Individual acts of advocacy are commonplace in our everyday lives. Consider the following examples:

- Peggy remonstrates with the man who pushed in front of her in the queue.
- John sends back his wife's meal in the restaurant because it is cold.
- Edna speaks to the doctor's receptionist on behalf of her older neighbour who needs a home visit.
- Geevan tells the teacher that his best friend is being bullied at playtime by some other children.
- Julian accompanies his partner to the medical appointment for moral support.

In all these cases there is a sense that people are acting, either on their own behalf or on behalf of another, to challenge a perceived injustice, or stand up for a right or entitlement. However, it is important to make the distinction between 'formal' and 'informal' approaches to advocacy. Not everyone has a friend or relative who can advocate for them in the ways mentioned above. Additionally, many people are unable to speak for themselves with the confidence or articulacy that certain situations require. This could be because of frailty or illness, fear, lack of confidence or information. For many older people, especially those with dementia, effective self-advocacy is extremely difficult. In these circumstances, and without access to family or friends, an independent advocate can have a huge impact. The advocate forms a relationship with the older person and supports them to access and understand information, know their rights and options and, ultimately, have a say in decisions that affect them. Dunning (2005) describes a dual advocacy role which is both expressive (providing emotional support) and instrumental (providing practical support). A skilled advocate will know when and how to combine these twin roles to best effect.

Advocacy skills

The skills of effective advocacy are many and varied. At the core of advocacy is an empathy with the position of the older person. Often, older people seek advocacy support at the point at which things have already gone wrong for them. The older person may feel that they have exhausted all available avenues in seeking redress for themselves. Many older people report that they value the advocate's independence from 'the system' as well as their ability to 'get things done'. Key skills of effective advocacy include:

- listening skills – taking time to listen to the person in a confidential and safe environment;
- empathy – showing a genuine interest in the older person's point of view; being non-judgemental and open-minded to the person's perspective;
- knowing the system – understanding what rights and entitlements people have, having knowledge of local service systems and procedures;
- negotiation skills – being assertive without being aggressive, having excellent communication skills across a range of audiences;
- tenacity – being persistent, not taking no for an answer, trying all available options;
- independence – being free from conflicts of interest, having support from an established advocacy organisation.

MODELS OF ADVOCACY

A number of advocacy forms or models have emerged during the past 25 years, each with its own strengths and weaknesses. All share a common desire to ensure that the vulnerable person's voice is heard and understood. These models have been summarised as follows (Henderson and Pochin, 2001):

- **Citizen advocacy**: a long-term, one-to-one relationship between a vulnerable person and an unpaid volunteer advocate.
- **Self-advocacy**: people speaking up for themselves, often with the support of friends, family or support staff.

- **Peer advocacy**: where the advocate shares a common experience with their advocacy 'partner', for example where they are also an older person or disabled person.
- **Professional advocacy**: advocacy provided by paid advocates who have a 'caseload' of people they support.
- **Collective advocacy**: groups of individuals coming together to take action on issues of common concern.

It is important to note the distinction between advocacy and other supportive services such as advice, mediation and befriending. The advocacy relationship is unique in that it has no agenda other than the active representation of the older person's own views and concerns. Advocates will often signpost people to these other services if they are more appropriate and if the older person is happy for this to happen. Generally speaking, the advocate will not give advice or undertake any activities without the express permission (referred to as 'instruction') of the older person. However, Dunning (2005: 14) suggests that:

> . . . the link between information, advice and advocacy resembles inter-related circles, in which each links to the other. In such situations, rather than being different points along the same continuum, information, advice and advocacy may best be described as circles of support.

Here the suggestion is that older people may be most effectively served, not by one sector working in isolation, but rather by a spectrum of support services that includes advocacy, information and advice, as well as more practical 'hands on' support. However, the reality of advocacy provision is that it is often unavailable as a result of 'patchy' funding. Many advocacy schemes are reluctant to publicise their services for fear of being overwhelmed with referrals that they are inadequately funded to deal with. Hence, it may be the case that many older people are unaware of the availability of advocacy locally even if it does exist. Older people may find out about advocacy via social workers or medical staff such as GPs or a nurse, via publicity materials or, often, by word of mouth from other older people. A full list of advocacy schemes for older people can also be found at **www.actionforadvocacy.org.uk**

THE POLICY CONTEXT

The policy framework within which older people's advocacy schemes operate has changed dramatically over the past decade. Central to the government's current public service reform agenda are the twin themes of choice and control. The agenda is driven by the belief that 'people power' can be a major driver for improving the delivery of public services, to ensure that the needs of individuals and their communities are met. Government policy stresses the importance of people being able to have a say in how services are run and for services to be more user- or consumer-led (for example, Health and Social Care Act 2001, *Our Health, Our Care, Our Say*, 2006). Citizenship highlights people's rights as well as their responsibilities. In this context, older people are perceived, not as a burden that needs to be managed and 'cared for', but as active, empowered citizens capable of contributing to society. The link between advocacy and active participation of older people has been made in the literature as well as in practice. Atkinson (1999) states that:

> Not only is advocacy seen to be a 'good thing' in its own right, as a means of enabling people's voices to be heard, it becomes more of a necessity where legislation assumes the involvement of the users of services in their design and delivery.
>
> (Atkinson, 1999: 5)

This level of active participation requires older people to have a voice and not to be afraid to use it.

For those older people who do need the support of services, there is some recognition that those services are often inappropriate. In relation to advocacy, *A Sure Start to Later Life* concludes that:

> Advocacy services for older people can be the only way to ensure that excluded older people receive their entitlements and get the best support from unresponsive services.
>
> (Social Exclusion Unit, 2006: 50)

As a result of this general shift towards recognition of the value of advocacy, many local authorities and, to a lesser extent, Primary Care Trusts (PCTs) have sought to commission advocacy services from local voluntary organisations such as Age Concern or local independent advocacy providers. However, the issue of value for money is never far away, whichever funding body is involved. Jones (2004) in a study of an older people's advocacy service working in the London Borough of Westminster concludes that:

Based on an analysis of the current caseload . . . the equivalent of about one and a half full-time posts, costing about £50,000 a year, would be needed by statutory service providers to work on cases, had advocacy provided by the voluntary sector not been available to them.

(Jones, 2004: 5)

In particular, the study identifies support for people wishing to make complaints and support to prevent people from 'falling through the net' as key benefits of local advocacy provision. She goes on to argue that the statutory sector, in this case the Local Authority, should consider increasing their grant to the advocacy service proportionately. This is a good example of advocacy providers demonstrating their worth in monetary as well as moral terms. However, as Jones subsequently warns: Few funders will provide longer term funding, and everyone associated with (the advocacy scheme) lives with the possibility that sufficient ongoing funding will not be found.

This reinforces a view held by Harding that:

Information, advice and advocacy services tend to be seen as luxuries by funders such as local authorities – as not a real service and therefore less important when cuts are having to be made.

(Harding, 1997: 37–8)

More recently a survey of Welsh advocacy schemes for older people carried out by Age Concern Cymru, found that seven of the 45 respondents had funding that was either ending or being reduced in the following 12 months. This was despite predictions of a substantial increase in the number of people aged 60 or over in the general population (Age Concern Cymru, 2007). The Welsh data suggests that advocacy is still not perceived by commissioners as an 'essential' service for older people. This view is supported by a recent study of commissioning arrangements for older people's advocacy schemes conducted by Get Heard on behalf of the Older People's Advocacy Alliance (OPAAL). The authors conclude that:

Commissioners, however, did not always appreciate that the role of the advocate was to represent the voice of the client and sometimes viewed advocacy as something that had been paid for by them and should therefore be arranged primarily for their benefit.

(Get Heard consultancy, 2006: 9)

NON-INSTRUCTED ADVOCACY

A significant group of older people accessing advocacy services are those with dementia-causing illnesses. There is a growing body of expertise in the field of dementia advocacy, as illustrated by the recent formation of the National Dementia Advocacy Network (DAN) and several publications on the subject (Kileen, 1996; Wells, 2006). Older people with dementia represent an especially vulnerable group and advocacy can help to ensure that people are supported to have a voice in key decisions. One of the challenges of dementia advocacy is that it is often 'non-instructed' (Henderson, 2006), meaning that the older person with dementia is unable to give the advocate a clear indication of what their wishes or views might be in a given situation. Wells (2006) proposes that dementia advocacy should focus on the three inter-related issues of Communication, Capacity and Consent:

- What level of **communication** does the client have?
- Does s/he have the **capacity** to reason and make sense of the issue and any relevant information?
- Does the client have the **capacity** to make a decision about a specific issue?
- Is she able to **consent** to the advocate working with them?

Another approach to non-instructed advocacy, known as the 'Watching Brief', has been developed by the Asist advocacy project in Staffordshire (Asist, 2007). 'Watching Brief' is based on a number of 'quality of life domains' and empowers the advocate to pose questions to the relevant decision maker about proposed courses of action and consequences for the older person.

Case study – John

Non-instructed Advocacy
An advocate visits John who is 87 and has a dementia-causing illness. He currently lives in a residential home. While sitting with John in the dining room, the advocate notices that he is not given a pudding although all the other residents get one. When the advocate asks staff about this, she is told that John is a slow eater and takes longer to eat his main course. Hence, there isn't time for John to eat his pudding before the dining room is cleared. The advocate takes this up with the catering manager and requests that John be given a) extra time in the dining room, b) support to eat more quickly or, c)

the option to take his pudding to his room. The advocate argues that John is being treated less favourably than his peers are as a result of his disability. The catering manager agrees to try the various options put forward by the advocate and adopts the most successful one.

The above Case study clearly illustrates the potential benefits of the advocacy role. By intervening on John's behalf, the advocate ensures a 'level playing field' in which John is not unfairly disadvantaged because of his situation. The catering manager agrees to change his position towards John and try other options. However, the intervention required little of the advocate by way of forming a relationship with John. She simply observed an injustice and acted accordingly. No effort was made to seek instruction from John or to check that he actually liked or wanted pudding.

One of the key features of non-instructed advocacy with older people is the need for the advocate to spend a greater amount of time getting to know the person and developing a relationship with them. In this way, the advocate is able to build up a picture of how the older person lives, their likes and dislikes and preferred ways of communicating. However, this significant investment in time and resources is often difficult to achieve within hard-pressed services (Wells, 2006).

ADVOCACY CASE STUDIES

Case study – Ivy

Ivy Hall is 79 years old and has lived alone since her mother died eight years ago. She has gradually lost her independence and is now housebound. She has home carers that visit twice a day. Six months ago Ivy had a serious fall in her bathroom and lay undiscovered for more than 24 hours because the carers failed to turn up twice in a row. Ivy has now recovered and wants to make a complaint against the home care agency. However, she is worried that the agency will withdraw her service if she makes a fuss. She was told about the advocacy service by her Care Manager, who suggested she refer herself to get support in making a complaint.

Case study – Stanley

Stanley is in hospital awaiting discharge following a stroke that has left him confused and unable to speak. There is disagreement between his daughters and his ex-wife as to where Stanley should live when he leaves hospital. His ex-wife, whom he divorced two years ago, wants him to move in with her, but his daughters would prefer him to be transferred to a care home close to where they live, some 60 miles away from the town where he has lived all his life. The consultant refers Stanley to the Independent Mental Capacity Advocacy (IMCA) service and an advocate is appointed to try to ascertain what Stanley's wishes are.

Note: the IMCA service was created by the Mental Capacity Act 2005. IMCAs can be appointed where people lack capacity to make certain key decisions (of which long-term care moves is one) and where there are no family or friends appropriate to consult.

Case study – Mr Khan

Mr Khan has recently moved to a residential home as he could no longer look after himself. However, he is the only Asian person in the home and has very poor spoken English. He has lost touch with his relatives and has few friends. The home staff are finding it difficult to engage with Mr Khan, who seems down and has taken to spending all his time alone in his room. One of Mr Khan's few friends has contacted the local advocacy scheme because he had asked (on Mr Khan's behalf) for Asian food to be served at the home and they had refused. The friend had previously used the advocacy service himself for a housing issue.

Case study – Jean

Jean is 64 and has cared for her disabled mother all her life. Jean had lived with her mother in a council flat but was not officially a tenant. When Jean's mother died, the council insisted that Jean move out of the flat as quickly as possible and claimed that she had no tenancy rights as Jean could not prove that she had lived there permanently. Jean has poor reading and writing skills. She contacts the advocacy scheme in a distressed state, having seen a poster advertising the service in the housing office. She explains that she has received an eviction notice. She says she knows it must be bad news because 'it's written in red ink and that always means trouble'.

Activity 1

Using the case studies above, think about what you would do if you were the advocate. Try to work out:

- What are the advocacy issues?
- What does the service user hope to achieve?
- What would your action plan consist of?
- What skills and knowledge would you need to have?
- What would constitute a successful outcome?

THE SERVICE USER PERSPECTIVE

A consultation exercise with older people undertaken by the Older People's Advocacy Alliance (OPAAL) concluded that older people were generally unfamiliar with the term advocacy. The motivation or need for advocacy was broadly related to protection from abuse, combating discrimination, obtaining and changing services, securing and exercising rights – as well as being involved in decision making and being heard (OPAAL, 2006). Hence there is no one reason why older people might seek advocacy support nor is there a sense of what constitutes the 'ideal' advocate. In a study of the views of people from Black and minority ethnic service users, Kapasi and Silvera (2002) noted the following characteristics of an effective advocate:

- listens to and respects their views and opinions;
- is not judgemental (about their culture, religion, accent, dialect, political affiliation or the situation of their home country), condescending or discriminatory;
- is sensitive to their cultural and religious needs;
- is dependable and punctual;
- is honest and trustworthy;

- has high standards of personal integrity and can maintain confidentiality;
- can represent them confidently;
- has good bilingual skills;
- will give them the confidence to do things for themselves.

Solle (2006) in his survey of the views of mental health service users on advocacy presents the following vignettes:

'Advocacy is my safety net – in fact when I'm unwell it's my only safety net.'

'An independent voice helps to ease the strain, particularly when matters you are dealing with drag you down and so your voice is stifled.'

'I have felt more able to handle meetings with the professional deciding my fate when I have had an advocate with me.'

Dunning (2005) also notes that the issue of independence is crucial in the eyes of older people. He offers this quote from an older service user:

The professionals will say it is good for older people to have services to help them to make informed choices, offer good advice [and] represent their views. But, if people are not getting out of hospitals quickly enough or not being happy with what they are given, they come down like a ton of bricks. That's where there is strength in independence.

IMPLICATIONS FOR JOINT WORKING

Independent advocacy presents significant challenges to joint working. The advocacy role is unlike any other, in that the advocate's loyalty is exclusively to the service user. Anything that compromises this loyalty is deemed to be a 'conflict of interest' that should be minimised. In this way, the advocate is not subject to any of the constraints and pressures that face other professionals. For service users, knowing that there is someone on their side who is not directly employed by the statutory sector (although they may be funded by them) is reassuring. This is especially true in situations where a complaint is being made against health or social services. In this sense, the advocate is not impartial; rather they are 'partial' to the views, wishes and interests of the older person. This is not to say that the advocate will necessarily agree with the service user's perspective, but the advocacy role is to ensure that that perspective is heard. The following quote from the *Elder Abuse Advocacy Toolkit* illustrates the point:

> The relationship that an advocate has with an older person is . . . unique within the health and social care field. Unlike a social worker it is not a relationship that is defined by legislation such as the Community Care Act. Unlike a social care worker in a residential or domiciliary care setting it is not a relationship designed to meet a particular physical need.
>
> (Action on Elder Abuse, 2006: 10)

However, the potential for confusion and conflict with other professionals is clear. In supporting and representing the older person, the advocate can find themselves positioned in opposition to other professionals working with that person. As a result, advocates are often perceived as troublemakers or as being 'difficult' to work with. This problem can be compounded by a lack of awareness about the advocacy role and a lack of clear engagement protocols for working alongside advocacy schemes. Advocates often need to have good relationships with other agencies in order to 'get good results' for service users, but these relationships should not be at the expense of independence.

Case study – Eleanor

Eleanor lives in a residential home for older people. She likes to spend her personal allowance on alcohol and cigarettes, but tends to spend it all in one go, meaning that she has nothing left for later in the week. This often leads to Eleanor becoming distressed and angry, and she often begs for money or cigarettes from other residents, staff and visitors. The staff in the home have taken to rationing her money, allowing her a certain amount each day. However, Eleanor states that she is 'not a child' and wants all her allowance in one instalment. Eleanor contacts the advocacy scheme and Jean, the advocate, presents this view to the staff in the home. The staff state that they are acting in Eleanor's 'best interests' and are frustrated that Jean has 'taken sides' with Eleanor.

In this example the advocate is simply 'doing her job', that is, ensuring that Eleanor's views, wishes and interests are central to the decision-making process. But, in doing so, she is at risk of being perceived by other staff as naïve or even troublesome. But it is Jean's independence that makes her such a useful asset to Eleanor. Consider the following, more serious example.

Case study – Mr Roberts

Mr Roberts is a voluntary patient on a psychiatric ward. He contacts the advocate and claims that another patient has threatened to strangle him in his sleep. As a result, he has become extremely anxious and is having great difficulty sleeping. Mr Roberts tells the advocate that he has told ward staff and even his psychiatrist about his fears, but they have told him that he is 'delusional' and have offered him medication to aid his sleep. What Mr Roberts really wants is to be moved to a different ward away from his tormentor.

In this scenario the advocate is presenting an opposing view to the doctor and ward staff, and one that is likely to prove unpopular. Staff may feel that the advocate is interfering with the therapeutic process by colluding with what they perceive as Mr Roberts's delusional thoughts. However, it may well be that Mr Roberts is telling the truth, and is indeed living in fear of some form of assault. The advocate in this case does not have decision-making power, but is obliged to ensure that Mr Roberts's concerns are taken seriously.

Activity 2

Look at the case studies above. How do the actions of the advocates in these cases differ from those of other professionals? What conflicts of interest might have occurred if the advocates were not independent?

The Action for Advocacy *Code of Practice for Advocates* (Action for Advocacy, 2006) offers a useful guide, for both advocates and other professionals, to reach a better understanding of the advocacy role. Where such an investment has been made in raising awareness, a positive relationship can flourish and grow.

CONCLUSION

There is growing recognition among government departments, health and social care commissioners and providers, voluntary organisations and service users that advocacy plays a vital and empowering role in society. This is true for all disadvantaged groups and for anyone who struggles to make their voice heard. For older people, the reasons why people seek advocacy support are many and varied. They include lack of information on choices, rights and entitlements, fear or lack of confidence, social isolation, ageism and discrimination, and cognitive impairments such as dementia. For all these reasons and more, an older person may find themselves in a position of needing support to make their views known and access the services they need to live full and active lives. Advocacy is a means to an end – that end being the full participation of older people in everyday life. Advocacy serves to ensure that the older person is at the centre of the decision-making process and is in control of their own life. Advocacy is not by nature confrontational, although there are times when the worst excesses of poor service delivery or misguided government policy need to be challenged vigorously. In these instances, collective forms of advocacy (such as the pensioners' movement) can have a major impact on both legislation and in individuals.

Advocacy works best where there is a degree of discretion available to the decision maker or service provider. It is, in essence, the art of persuasion, used in pursuit of the rights and wishes of the individual. Not everybody gets everything they want, but advocacy can have a major impact by shifting the balance of power away from professionals and towards service users. For these reasons it is essential that awareness-raising tools and training in advocacy skills are made available to the widest possible range of people, not least to older people themselves.

FURTHER READING

Atkinson, D. (1999) *Advocacy: A Review*. Brighton: Pavilion Publishing and Joseph Rowntree Foundation
This is a highly accessible analysis of the strengths and weaknesses of the advocacy sector in the UK, with some useful recommendations about the possible future direction for advocacy.

Dunning, A. (2005) *Information, Advice and Advocacy for Older People: Defining and Developing Services*. York: Joseph Rowntree Foundation
This report was the result of a major consultation exercise looking at the powerful role that information, advice and advocacy services can play in the lives of older people.

Henderson, R. and Pochin, M. (2001) *A Right Result? Advocacy, justice and empowerment*. Bristol: Policy Press
A core text on independent advocacy that explores definitions and models of advocacy as well as setting out a framework for the delivery of high quality advocacy services to vulnerable groups.

Wells, S. (2007) *Developments in Dementia Advocacy*. London: WASSR
This book offers the reader a practical guide to the development and delivery of effective advocacy support to people with dementia and contains a useful guide to non-instructed advocacy.

Useful websites

www.actionforadvocacy.org.uk
Action for Advocacy

www.wassr.org/dementia
Dementia Advocacy Network

www.opaal.org.uk
Older People's Advocacy Alliance

www.elderabuse.org.uk
Action on Elder Abuse

www.counselandcare.org.uk
Counsel and Care

www.helptheaged.org.uk
Help the Aged

www.ageconcern.org.uk
Age Concern England

REFERENCES

Action for Advocacy (2002) *The Advocacy Charter*. London: A4A
Action for Advocacy (2006) *A Code of Practice for Advocates*. London: A4A
Action on Elder Abuse and Action for Advocacy (2005) *Elder Abuse Advocacy Toolkit*. London: Action on Elder Abuse
Age Concern Cymru (2007) *Advocacy Counts: A report on advocacy provision in Wales*. Cardiff: Age Concern Cymru
Asist (2007) *The Watching Brief*. Staffordshire: Advocacy Services in Staffordshire (ASSIST)
Atkinson, D (1999) *Advocacy: A Review*. Brighton: Pavilion Publishing and Joseph Rowntree Foundation
Department of Health (2005) The Mental Capacity Act. London: HMSO

Department of Health (2006) *Our Health, Our Care, Our Say*. London: HMSO

Dunning, A (2005) *Information, Advice and Advocacy for Older People: Defining and Developing Services*. York: Joseph Rowntree Foundation

Get Heard Consultancy (2007) *Commissioning Advocacy for Older People*. Southport: Get Heard Consultancy

Harding, T. (1997) *A Life Worth Living: The Independence and Inclusion of Older People*. London: Help the Aged

Henderson, R. and Pochin, M. (2001) *A Right Result? Advocacy, Justice and Empowerment*. Bristol: Policy Press

Henderson, R. (2006) 'Defining Non-instructed Advocacy'. *Planet Advocacy*, 18. London: A4A

Jones, J. (2004) *Adding Value Through Advocacy*. London: Westminster Advocacy Service for Senior Residents (WASSR)

Kapasi, R. and Silvera, M. (2002) *A Standards Framework for Delivering Effective Health and Social Care Advocacy for Black and Minority Ethnic Londoners*. London: King's Fund

Kileen, J. (1996) *Advocacy and Dementia*. Edinburgh: Alzheimer Scotland – Action on Dementia

Kitchen, G. (2006) *Mapping Older People's Advocacy in the English Regions*. Southport: Get Heard Consultancy and OPAAL

OPAAL UK (2006) *Making a Difference*. Stoke on Trent: Older People's Advocacy Alliance and Beth Johnson Foundation

Scottish Executive (2000) *Adults with Incapacity (Scotland) Act*. Edinburgh: TSO

Solle, D. (2006) *With Us in Mind: Service User Recommendations for Advocacy Standards in England*. London: Mind Publications

The Social Exclusion Unit (Cabinet Office Task Force) (2006) *A Sure Start to Later Life: Ending Inequalities for Older People*. London: Office of the Deputy Prime Minister

Wells, S. (2006) *Developments in Dementia Advocacy*. London: WASSR

Chapter 10

Victims or Survivors?
The Protection of Older
Vulnerable Adults

Joy Gauci

Learning outcomes

Reading this chapter will enable you:

- to form an evidence-based approach to the theme of old age oppression founded on research evidence, practice knowledge and media awareness;

- to develop a critical awareness of legal and policy guidelines for intervention and safeguarding, recognising the ethical complexity of responses to legal definitions of vulnerability;

- to create a framework for therapeutic work with older survivors of oppression and abuse.

INTRODUCTION

In the last 15 years, there has been a growing awareness of the protective rights of older people, and their particular vulnerability to harm, exploitation and abuse. Recognising the research indications that older people who have dependency needs are particularly exposed to oppression, this chapter invites an exploration of the status of victimhood for vulnerable older people who access welfare support services both in their own homes and in a range of social and living contexts. Legal definitions of need and vulnerability are explored with their formal emphasis on the call for responsive, accountable welfare practice. A range of anti-oppressive, rights-based and protective legislation is considered, with a central focus on *No Secrets* (Department of Health, 2000) as a valuable guide for inter-agency protective practice.

This chapter challenges the concept of victimhood, and the images we have of older people who are dependent on welfare. The article, *Granny Battering* (Baker, 1975) presented the first significant image of old age victimisation in the UK, designed to raise media awareness and springboard legal and policy reform. The focus on the experience of a frail, older woman exposed to physical hardship deeply challenges our conception of social justice, and calls for raised societal recognition of, and sensitivity to, the rights of older people.

Is this the image we hold of older people from our experience of welfare practice? Baker's article is now frequently challenged as a narrow, stereotypical and gendered image of old age victimhood. Accountable welfare practice has a responsibility to challenge entrenched social constructions of older people as frail and dependent, as research suggests that negative associations of dependency can also result in victimhood. In reality, in our welfare practice we are often faced with as many images of old age dignity and resourceful resilience as images of frail dependency. It is this sense of shared connectedness, empathy and value that sustains our motivation in a sensitive and challenging context of practice.

This chapter recognises the ethical dilemmas for welfare practitioners who have to make accountable protective responses while also responding to the diversity of experience of older people and their individual levels of resourcefulness and independent capacity. A focus on active citizenship rights and empowerment theory is presented as a fundamental challenge to societal oppression and a valuable guide for welfare practice.

The importance, yet complexity, of the welfare practitioner's role in responding appropriately to such a challenging issue is considerable. It raises various questions which the chapter seeks to address. Why are vulnerable older people exposed to particular harms? How do we interpret a harm or violation and who decides on appropriate thresholds and responses? The chapter addresses these issues and proposes a framework for practice that can be both technically accountable and therapeutically responsive to the individual.

THE ACCOUNT OF OLD AGE VICTIMHOOD – A SOCIO-CULTURAL PERSPECTIVE

The particular hardships experienced by older people exposed to abuse or direct exploitation have been emphasised in 'vulnerable adult' research from the late 80s in particular, with early writers coining the term 'elder abuse' to suggest specific old age associations with vulnerability to oppression and exploitation.

An early study highlighted the high risk of older people to physical and financial abuse (Lau and Kosberg, 1979). Brown and Stein's (1997) study identified the disproportionate vulnerability of older people among the vulnerable adult care sector. Specific themes have been the prevalence of elder abuse in the community, with an estimate of one in 20 subjected to some form of abuse by informal carers (Ogg and Bennett, 1992); the association of 'elder abuse' and domestic violence/spouse abuse (Pillemer and Finkelhor, 1989); the focus on old age and financial/sexual exploitation (Ramsey-Klawsnik, 1991) and the prevalence of sexual assault for people using mental health services (Schoener, 1989).

The dominant research focus in the 1980s and 1990s on the high risk of abuse in institutional and group living contexts has been increasingly challenged by an emphasis on particular risks in community contexts. *No Secrets* responds to abuse and neglect as the specific core of old age oppression in care, pinpointing the dominant themes of physical, sexual, emotional and financial abuse. These types of abuse are also highlighted for other vulnerable adult groups, including adults with learning disabilities and adults with mental health needs. However, the age factor suggests a high risk of multiple abuses and oppressions.

Research identifies the significance of old age abuse as a contemporary social problem and one which UK welfare services have a responsibility to recognise and to challenge. Clearly it is not a UK-specific issue and a sample of the significant studies includes those from Canada (Pillemer and Finkelhor, 1989), Holland (Comijs, 1999) and Israel (Siegel-Itzkovich, 2005). Acknowledging the limitations of current knowledge and research, the Department of Health has commissioned a prevalence study of the mistreatment and abuse of older people in the UK (Department of Health, 2007). Its initial findings will be drawn on in this chapter.

Research of old age abuse has three dominant themes:

A. Exploitation in informal care relationships.
B. Hardship and oppression in formal welfare care.
C. General old age oppression in a socio-cultural context.

A. Victimhood in the context of informal care relationships

Since 1990, there has been a legislative focus on informal care as part of the state promotion of community care for older people (NHS and Community Care Act 1990). While it is important to acknowledge and value informal carers, this direct policy emphasis creates additional risk factors as the informal carer role is often involuntary and can result in long-term care scenarios with complex emotional dynamics (Ungerson, 1987). Particular risks include over-protection, the 'overwhelmed carer' syndrome, and the complications of financial dependency (Bonnie and Wallace, 2002).

Initial images of old age victimhood suggested isolated cases where an informal carer was reacting to the burden of their care responsibility (Eastman, 1984; Hugman, 1994). Hugman (p. 493) presented abuse resulting from the 'stresses of poorly supported long term caring'. These early images of inadequate care by an informal carer suggested the risk of unintentional harm or neglect and this is still a relevant message for practice. A failure to fully recognise the importance of an older person's recreational needs or independent dignity can clearly result in a significant harm. However, it is highly sensitive to charge an informal carer, who may have involuntarily adopted their carer role, with caring inadequately or failing to meet the 'textbook' view of appropriate care. Early research also focussed on carer associations with mental health issues and alcohol dependency. It is appropriate to acknowledge, but to make a cautious response to, these early informal carer images because of the risk of stereotyping and inappropriately judging.

Equally relevant identity factors of informal carers include gender, ethnicity and migrant status. Evidence suggests a high proportion of carers are female – and although there have been recent government campaigns to support female carers in juggling family and work commitments, little attention is given to the demands of caring for an older family dependant where the predominantly female care force may have their own age and health-related needs (Hirst, 2004).

Cultural migration and resettlement is also a significant theme in the context of informal care (Cook *et al.*, 2004). There is a need for recognition of the complexity of a reliance on adult sons and daughters to act as interpreters, and the tensions in families where the children have 'anglicised', creating a gulf between them and older parents. One Chinese woman observed:

> I have children who speak English, but they are not able to explain to me in Chinese in a way that I can understand.
>
> (Cook *et al.*, 2004: 89)

Many of the informal care scenarios explored in this section feature unintentional harm, but it is important to distinguish motive and to acknowledge the increasing research focus on intentional exploitation and abuse. Similar outcomes may result from intentional or unintentional harm; for example, to deny an older relative adequate social engagement might be intended or unintentionally result from lack of awareness. However, the emotional vulnerability of the informal care relationship must be acknowledged. Action on Elder Abuse defined abuse as a violation of a relationship of trust:

> . . . a single or repeated act or lack of an appropriate action occurring within any relationship where there is an expectation of trust which causes harm or distress to an older person.
>
> (*Action on Elder Abuse*, 2000: 2)

This definition raises the severe emotional damage resulting from the direct abuse and exploitation of a relationship of trust. This is an important recognition – yet welfare practice must be cautious of a judgement which could be based on just one lack of an appropriate action by an informal carer.

The reality is that the dominance of care is provided informally in a community context and this does expose older people to particular risks of harm and exploitation. In the UK National Prevalence Study (2006–2008) the older people consulted identified frustration of the caregiver as a frequent motive for abuse. However, it is important to recognise the support needs and vulnerability of informal carers rather than to scapegoat and to judge. Bennett and Kingston (1993: 18) found 79 per cent of carers to have associated mental health and emotional needs, and 45.2 per cent to be alcohol dependent. Studies of sexual abuse perpetrated by men with learning disabilities emphasise the vulnerability of perpetrators also (Churchill *et al.*, 1997). The Carers National Strategy

(Department of Health, 1999) identifies the need for support to enable informal carers to sustain consistent care relationships, with a focus on their right to a say in formal support services and recognition of their claim for quality of life.

Summary

There are evident concerns about particular risks in community contexts because of a reliance on informal care. To focus on old age exploitation and harm at the hands of an informal carer, however, risks scapegoating the carer and detracting from a sense of societal responsibility.

Messages for practice

- Awareness of stress scenarios for informal care relationships and the complexity of having to respond to both parties where there are competing needs.
- Recognition of the practice complexity of having to avoid judgemental reactions to informal carers. Risk of partiality can be prevented by two workers having involvement in the scenario of conflict. This allows one worker to specifically promote the needs of the carer.

B. Oppression in formal welfare

Oppression in formal welfare contexts can be recognised both within personal helping relationships and on a structural level.

Welfare and the helping relationship

The connection between institutional care and oppression, and the risk of hardship resulting from power imbalances between the care recipient and formal care giver was highlighted as early as the 1960s (Goffman,1968) and is now universally acknowledged. There has been significant press coverage of institutional scandals in the last few years, for example, the newspaper and television coverage of the ill-treatment and neglect of 6 patients including the attempted poisoning of 2 older people in an English care home (Gregory, 2004) and reports regarding institutional abuse of older people in an NHS ward in Manchester (CHI, 2003). Goffman's reference to 'spoiled identities' highlights the threat of institutional care to a person's sense of individual identity and self-esteem. The concept of 'whole person' care is a challenge to promote in any large group care context where there is a complex relationship between vulnerability, care processes and outcomes. Even where, as with informal care scenarios, the harm is unintended, there is still a high risk of oppression in formal care contexts. In such contexts of formal care with emphasis on health and safety accountability, it is difficult to avoid a risk-dominated focus and risk factors such as cognitive impairment and high risk of falls may result in physical restraints or use of psychotropic medicines (Arling *et al.*, 2005).

Risk of exploitation and harm must be balanced, however, with a recognition of positive examples of formal and even 'institution' type care. Yahnke (2005) provides a glimpse of the quality of dignified care in a palliative care unit in Toronto, conveying a strong sense of individualised and compassionate care.

Increasingly the service-user movement has challenged state control in welfare and individual professional power (Beresford, 2003; Cree and Davis, 2007). A wealth of authors focus on the abuses of professional power: indirect power as abuse of authority or failure to respond in an anti-oppressive manner and direct power such as exploitation, abuse and coercion (Dominelli, 2002; Banks, 2004; Thompson, 2002).

There is increased legal protection of standards of care in the formal welfare sector. Currently, the Nursing and Midwifery Council (NMC) and the General Social Care Council (GSCC) provide legally accountable standards of care for nurses and social workers. All organisations that are regulated by the Commission for Social Care Inspection (Care Standards Act 2000) have a responsibility both to protect care standards and to acknowledge or 'whistle-blow' where neglect, harm and abuse occur. The Care Standards Act also established the POVA (Protection of Vulnerable Adults) Register (implemented in 2004), which enforces the disclosure of criminal records held by potential care workers. Multi-agency public protection duties are established in the Domestic Violence, Crime and Victims Act 2004, the Mental Capacity Act 2005 and the Safeguarding Vulnerable Groups Act 2006.

Welfare and structural oppression

Formal welfare provision at a structural level risks further creating deprivation and inequalities due to political tensions in boundaries and priorities between the individual, family and the state. Despite a vision of integrated service approaches and responsive, individual care initiatives to allow older people to remain living at home (NHS and Community Care Act, Department of Health, 1990), there is still a risk that older adults are 'victimised' by separate and competitive services.

The competitive dimension can create rivalry between agencies supplying care (Wistow and Hardy, 1996). The complexity of market principles are evidenced and challenged in the recent modernisation agenda for older people – emphasized in 1997 and 2001 (Department of Health, 1997; Department of Health, 2001). Initiatives in intermediate care services and a variety of integrated care projects generated through Primary Care Trusts do allow for greater innovation.

Challenge of indiscriminate health and welfare services

It is important to advocate for individuality of response to older people as service users, promoting an understanding of their cultural identities and beliefs, social circumstances, and health needs and concerns. It is crucial to place a recognition of need in a holistic framework. It is important, for example, to recognise the importance of culture and religion when working with older people in rehabilitation or hospice care (Coxon, Billings and Alaszewski, 2005) and to acknowledge the different gendered expectations and experiences of care and dependency (Gilligan, 1982).

Kayser-Jones (1981) provided an important challenge of uniform and basic services for older people, viewing assembly line services as a form of 'abuse'. This was, arguably, in 1981 a radical line, but still provides a necessary challenge to services that fail to provide choices and individuality of response for older people. Another term derived from this definition of abuse is 'dehumanisation' – 'attacking the older person's privacy and capacity to assume responsibility for their own lives' (Kayser-Jones, 1981: 51). The recent focus on quality of life and active ageing has allowed for a radical challenge of standardised or 'dehumanised' service responses to older people. However, there is a delicate line to be drawn in welfare practice with older people – radical enough to challenge the oppressive forces identified, but not extreme enough to destabilise welfare and disrupt the security often required in older age.

C. Old age victimhood in a socio-cultural context

Section A above explored the early research focus on stress factors for informal carers. While it is important to recognise particular risk scenarios in welfare for older people, this needs to be placed in a broader socio-cultural context that moves away from blaming the informal carer to a broader acknowledgement of ageist forces in society (Tinker, 1996). Kingston and Penhale (1995) and Leroux and Petrunik (1990) raised caution about the early research perspectives of old age abuse and harm, suggesting isolated cases of pathological injustice. Biggs and Phillipson

(1992) suggested the traditional image of the 'abused elder' fits an existing stereotype emphasising the marginalisation of older people. A recent Quality of Life study (Biggs *et al.*, 1995) highlighted inequalities of quality of life for older people – identifying the impact of deficits of income, health and social participation. Older people are potentially casualties of wider social structures that operate in systematically unjust ways, and we have a responsibility to recognise the political, social and personal barriers that inhibit older people from becoming more active citizens.

There is also a risk of too strong an association of old age with a biological process that causes societal devaluing and also allows the older person to consider themselves unworthy of respect. Some writers identify cultural interpretations of identity and value in older age, challenging the dominance of the Western model of the nuclear family opposed to the Eastern model of extended family systems, where the elderly person has a respected authoritative voice (Qureshi, 1991). In ethnicity-based studies of ageing, ethnic minorities are disadvantaged in income and health, but can have stronger levels of social support (Nazroo *et al.*, 2003) and a meaningful role (Tsang *et al.*, 2004).

Reflection

Although there is a lack of definitive studies, it is important to recognise that images of race, gender and disability will add to the level of old age oppression. Social participation in old age has been found to be linked to gender, ethnicity, class and regional variation (Davidson *et al.*, 2005).

Summary

Research indicates the clear links between old age vulnerability and exploitation, and suggests older people who receive welfare services are particularly 'at risk'. However, while striving to identify high risk patterns and causes of abuse, *No Secrets* (Department of Health, 2000) has recognised the complexity of the picture and the need to avoid neat patterns that risk further stereotyping in welfare responses.

Different views of victimhood will determine different practice responses. The difference between a 'scientific' (Gelles and Loseke, cited in Biggs *et al.*, 1995) and a 'social activist' approach is that the latter perspective places the concept of old age oppression at our feet – as carers of older people, as relatives or neighbours, as welfare practitioners, and as members of a society that is intrinsically ageist.

Messages for practice

- The professional welfare relationship has a particular tension as having a protective duty but also seeking to promote the independent rights and dignity of older people.
- Practitioner responsibility to recognise the risks of harmful interactions, acknowledging not only risk of intentional exploitation (in formal and informal welfare) but the unintentional harms of an over-protective stance and uniform responses.
- There is a high risk of a conspiracy of silence in informal care relationships where the abused person can be reluctant to acknowledge abuse and risk destabilising their potential to remain living independently in the community.
- People from minority ethnic groups are generally less likely to either be aware of, or to be offered, health and social care services than white British people (Ahmad, 2000; Butt and Mirza, 1996). It is important for us not to assume their own informal welfare networks will protect them from oppression and exploitation.

Case study 1

Steve Johns and Claire Wainwright have lived together for five years in a flat attached to a supported living group home for adults with learning difficulties. Steve (74) has epilepsy and a mild learning impairment but has a high level of independent skills and has lived alone previously. Claire (69) lived in institutions in early adulthood but was part of a resettlement project that supported her to develop independence skills and move into a supported flat in the community eight years ago. She has managed to sustain community living with a level of support and monitoring, but tends to lack confidence and underestimate her independent capability. Claire has a moderate learning difficulty although she is more physically robust than Steve, who relies on her when his epilepsy causes health issues.

The warden has expressed a concern about Steve's heavy handed nature when interacting with Claire. She has often heard him shouting at Claire and feels the relationship is too intense. The warden has tried talking about her concerns with Claire, but has found Claire to be defensive of Steve and the warden feels unsure how to protect her.

- What concerns you in this scenario and who is exposed to oppression?
- What is the nature and what are the causes of oppression?
- What factors make the individual(s) vulnerable to harm or hardship?
- Do you think it is appropriate to intervene to support Claire?
- What intervention would you propose?
- What messages from research and knowledge of the stresses in informal care relationships are relevant, and how do these guide you in your response to Steve?
- What are the socio-cultural factors you would take into account?

Case study 2

Kazia Staciwa makes an appointment to see her GP to discuss her level of anxiety and need for help. She and her mother, Henia, cared for Kazia's father who had been disabled with MS. Sadly, since his death 10 months ago, her mother, Henia, has gone into physical and emotional decline and Kazia has needed to give her mother increasing support. Henia has been socially withdrawn, neglectful of self-care and quite disorientated, relying heavily on Kazia for prompts and general monitoring.

Kazia is a single mother of two young boys, and indicates that working part-time, caring for her sons and trying to meet her mother's increasing support needs is a greater responsibility than she can manage. She is sleeping and eating poorly and getting increasingly tense and frustrated when interacting with her mother.

The social worker at the GP surgery contacts Kazia at her GP's request, to propose a home visit to talk with her and her mother and see what support might be available for them. Kazia indicates that the social worker is welcome to do a home visit but it would be best if she did not spend significant time with her mother as this could agitate her. Kazia suggests there is a language barrier. Her mother is Polish and lacks confidence speaking in English. In the last few months, Henia has withdrawn socially and is refusing to communicate in English unless essential. Kazia feels the social worker's visit could distress her mother and there would be little opportunity for dialogue anyway because of the increased language barrier between Henia and her outside world.

- Do you think there are potentially any protective issues in this scenario and what are the factors of vulnerability?
- What socio-cultural factors do you consider to be relevant?
- Do you feel there might be competing needs and, if so, how do you propose intervening with recognition of a responsibility to respond to both Kazia and Henia?
- What factors would you focus on to provide a safeguard against oppression or harm?

Activity 1

In each of the case studies:

- Do you feel it is essential to take the individual's gender, ethnicity and class into account?
- What particular aspects of identity are relevant in the circumstances presented?
- Would it add to the experience of oppression if a practitioner took a uniform approach, not taking into account aspects of class, gender and race?

Reflection on Case Study 2

The 'stressed carer' syndrome of early research has validity in this scenario, and it is important for the welfare practitioner to focus on this in their plan of intervention. However, it is crucial to hold a broader socio-cultural framework of analysis. This will prevent a judgemental response to Kazia as perpetrator of the abuse, and allow for a more objective recognition of her emotional needs and claim for support, both in her carer role, and in her identity as a wife and active citizen.

LEGAL DEFINITIONS OF VULNERABILITY, HARM AND ABUSE TO GUIDE PATERNALISTIC ACTION

Legislation has acknowledged the particular vulnerability of older people who use welfare services. There is, however, a tension in legislative guidance between a) a traditional paternalistic duty to protect, emphasising vulnerability, dependency and welfare responsibility and b) an increasing recognition of the duty to promote empowerment rights of individual participation, choice and control. The legal definition highlights the vulnerability associated with traditional groups of service users:

> Community Care means providing services and support which people who are affected by the problems of ageing, mental illness, mental handicap or physical or sensory disability need to be able to live as independently as possible in their own homes, or in 'homely' settings in the community.
> (White Paper, *Caring for People*, Department of Health, 1989: 3)

Currently UK Legislation clearly links those who use community services with vulnerability to abuse. However it is important to recognise that a much wider range of people are vulnerable to abuse or oppression for a wide variety of reasons, including alcohol and drug addiction, homelessness, immigration status and sexual identity. As this is the case it has been suggested by the Joint Committee on Human Rights (2007) that the government and other public bodies should champion understanding of human rights principles in an effort to transform health and social care services. They also suggest that the Department of Health make the Human Rights act integral to policy making and to all the care they provide (Joint Committee on Human Rights, 2007).

Duty to respond to need and material hardship

Traditionally, the legal system connects old age and vulnerability in its broadest sense as an indication of its duty to provide services to respond to need and hardship:

- National Assistance Act 1948 (s.29 – promotion of welfare, s.21 – provision of residential care).
- Health Services and Public Health Act 1968 (s.47 – arrangements for the welfare of older people).
- Chronically Sick and Disabled Persons Act 1970 (s.2 – assessment to provide services).

- National Health Service and Community Care Act 1990 (this Act continues the legal tradition of responding to vulnerability with service provision but does have a stronger value base promoting choice and control for the service user).

An increasing focus on the promotion of rights

The rights of the individual are promoted in the Anti-Discriminatory Laws (Race Relations Act 1976; Sex Discrimination Act 1975 and 1986; Disability Discrimination Act 1995) and in the Human Rights Act 1998. These are general rights-based laws that do not identify traditional vulnerable groups of welfare recipients but have a general application to promote freedom from harassment and discrimination in societal contexts. The increasing legal focus on citizenship rights and empowerment suggests a challenge to traditional paternalistic responses, emphasising welfare duty on the basis of vulnerability and dependency.

Protective safeguards – a stand against the harm of neglect and abuse

The third legal perspective acknowledges the specific responsibility of welfare services to protect older people against harm, neglect and abuse (Department of Health, 2000). This is a particular interpretation of vulnerability as exposure to neglect and abuse, promoting a clear paternalistic stance against abuse and neglect:

> There can be *No Secrets* and no hiding place when it comes to exposing the abuse of vulnerable adults.
>
> (Department of Health, 2000)

A White Paper offering guidance rather than a legally binding duty to act, *No Secrets* (Department of Health, 2000) requires local authorities to have policies in place to protect vulnerable adults from abuse. It advocates interprofessional working but emphasises the key role of social services in co-ordinating protective responses.

NO SECRETS AS A TEMPLATE FOR PROTECTIVE ACTION

No secrets is the most significant legal guide for practice to date in the UK Law, recommending responses to vulnerable adults at risk of neglect and abuse in particular.

Characteristics of *No Secrets*:

A. Identification of a vulnerable adult:

> Anyone of 18 years and over who is or may be in need of community care services by reason of mental or other disability, age or illness and who is or may be unable to take care of himself or herself, or unable to protect himself or herself against significant harm or serious exploitation.
>
> (Department of Constitutional Affairs, 1997)

Note that vulnerability in this context is interpreted as vulnerability to harm and the phrase 'significant harm' is a deliberate echo of the Children Act 1989, suggesting a strong protective baseline for interventions.

B. Principles of approach *(No Secrets*, 4.3):

> Practice will actively promote the 'empowerment and wellbeing' of the vulnerable adult, supporting the 'rights of the individual to lead an independent life based on self determination and personal choice'.

C. A working definition of abuse (*No Secrets*, 2.5):

> Abuse is the violation of an individual's human and civil rights by any other person or persons.

D. Different categories of harm as abuse and neglect (*No Secrets*, 2.7):

- physical abuse;
- sexual abuse;
- psychological abuse;
- financial or material abuse;
- neglect and acts of omission;
- discriminatory abuse.

E. Process for interventions (*No Secrets*, Section 3):

- identification of need/harm/abuse;
- interpretation and recognition of a duty to protect/intervene;
- intervention/identification adult protection plan;
- relevance of a formal hearing;
- interprofessional working;
- decision about criminal proceedings;
- safeguarding/monitoring and review process.

A summary of *No Secrets*

- *No Secrets* would appear to be a just and appropriate legal response to the increasing recognition of the extent of old age oppression. It echoes the Children's Act 1989 with its categorisation of types of abuse and baseline for intervention on the basis of 'significant harm'. Categories and scales of harm are important in allowing practitioners to make precise, informed responses to potential victims. The clear protective stance and acknowledgement of vulnerability is balanced with a recognition of the need to respond to vulnerable adults with respect for their individual dignity and right to autonomy. The definition of abuse in *No Secrets* is based on a rights-based focus: the human and civil rights of vulnerable people.
- *No Secrets* works in conjunction with existing legislation. It promotes an integrated approach to anti-abuse welfare work by placing it within the broader framework of protective welfare work – specifically in the context of the 'needs-led assessment' identified in the National Health Service and Community Care Act (1990). This is vitally important to prevent isolated reactive interventions where possible. The value of the monitoring and review system is that where abuse is identified but a vulnerable adult chooses to continue in the 'at-risk' situation, the risk can be monitored in a non-directive style of intervention over a period of time.
- It promotes an inter-agency framework (*No Secrets*, 3.1) and provides a framework for agencies to recognise how to deal with disclosure and the handling of sensitive and confidential information (*No Secrets*, 5.5–5.10).

Case study 3

Adam and Elisabeth Davies
Adam (aged 78) and Elisabeth (aged 64) have been married for 39 years and have two adult children, both married and living away. Adam retired from the army in his late 40s and worked as a postman until he was 60. Elisabeth undertook secretarial training and worked as an administrator after their children finished their primary school years. Elisabeth has had intermittent clinical depression over the last five years. Adam's health remained robust until a year ago when he suffered a stroke, which has resulted in left-side weakness, particularly in his lower body, so that he needs help with transfers. He moves about indoors with a wheeled trolley. The stroke also caused a level of memory impairment. Elisabeth

provides all Adam's care except on Tuesdays when Adam attends a local day centre to release Elisabeth from her carer responsibility so that she can participate in an art class.

Adam has been attending the day centre for three months when he asks to speak with a care worker and asks if respite care can be arranged for him that day, as he is tired of his wife's rough handling and shouting, and he wants to go somewhere where he can feel safe. The care worker talks with Adam's key worker, who confirms that Adam has indicated before that his wife resents having to care for him and can show her resentment in her handling of him.

Intervention using guidance from *No Secrets*

The definitions in *No Secrets* would suggest that Adam Davies is potentially a victim of abuse; he appears to be exposed to physical abuse (rough handling) and psychological abuse (the exposure to anger and seeming resentment of his wife to provide for his physical care needs). The cause can be interpreted on different levels: on a micro level, the cause appears to be the stresses in the informal care relationship where Adam is physically demanding to be cared for and Elisabeth resents her carer role, finding it emotionally exhausting as well as physically exacting. In a socio-cultural framework, there are pressures created by an assumption that Elisabeth will care as her duty as a wife. As an older woman there has been little focus on her active citizenship rights to social participation and fulfilment: her carer role has been the dominant focus in her recent life. Similarly, Adam has lost his identity as a physically strong, independent man and is struggling to keep his self-esteem in a role where he is physically dependent and where he feels a burden because of his wife's resentment. Both partners have a sense of guilt and sadness at the radical changes in the quality of their lives. Both feel their rights have been diminished, but are uncertain how far this is just the circumstances of ageing, and how far they have a right to take a stand against it.

Legislation indicates that Adam's vulnerability promotes protective intervention and staff have a responsibility to respond to his request. However, the Carers (Recognition and Services) Act 1995 would emphasise Elisabeth's right also to an assessment for her support needs. There could be a conflict of competing needs and rights.

No Secrets promotes interprofessional working practice. This would allow for a social worker to take the lead role with Adam to undertake an assessment (National Health Service and Community Care Act, 1990) provide support and monitor his level of vulnerability. A member of the nursing staff at the day centre could work with Elisabeth to ensure her support needs are also met.

ACCOUNTABLE PRACTICE: RIGHTS-BASED INTERVENTIONS

Traditionally, vulnerability has been seen to be associated with old age hardship and need and, with the advent of *No Secrets*, specifically associated with harm, abuse and neglect. An earlier definition of abuse provides more specific guidance:

> Ill-treatment (including sexual abuse and forms of ill-treatment that are not physical); the impairment of, or an avoidable deterioration in, physical or mental health, and the impairment of physical, emotional, social or behavioural development.
> (Department of Constitutional Affairs, 1997)

Although the *No Secrets* framework has a clear perspective on service user rights, its dominant pitch is paternalistic with a focus on accountable processes and outcomes that alleviate risk. There is an undeniable welfare duty both to be aware of the prevalence of old age oppression and to take a proactive stand. This is appropriate, as there is an on-going risk that experiences of oppression in older age remain unrecognised by the individual, the worker, or the community in which the older person lives and functions (Rose, Peabody and Stratigeas, 1991). In the UK National Prevalence Survey (2006–2008) older people identified a common risk of fear, denial and shame preventing older people from acknowledging the abuse.

As practitioners, we hold clear images of responsible action based on case law and cultures of welfare practice. For example, inappropriate invasion of physical body space, overdosing or failure to give prescribed medication, deprivation of food, warmth, continence needs. However, many of the practice judgements about risk and harm have a complexity of interpretation relating to our individual views of what constitutes quality of life for older people.

Practice dilemmas:

- In a group living context, when does restraining one resident to protect another become abusive?
- Could a daughter or son caring for their older relative with dementia at home be charged with 'serious neglect' if they are not providing adequate social stimulation?
- Is it neglect if a worker fails to provide a Bengali interpreter at a community art club for older people in a multi-ethnic urban community?
- Is dressing an older resident or patient in borrowed clothes as theirs are lost in the laundry system, a form of abuse?

The challenge of a harm focus

No Secrets (Department of Health, 2000) defines abuse as the 'violation of an individual's human and civil rights' – a valuable definition in highlighting aspects of social stigma and discrimination as potential causes of the abuse of an individual's dignity, status and function in a societal context. It is an equalising definition, presenting a victim as any person whose citizenship rights are transgressed. It potentially draws on a range of legal rights:

- Right to respect for human dignity, choice and freedom of expression (Human Rights Act 1998).
- Right to a needs-led assessment to identify need and monitor risk (NHS and Community Care Act 1990).
- Respect for the individual's right to choose whether there is a welfare intervention, and to control what type of intervention is chosen unless the adult has a level of incapacity that would prevent them making autonomous decisions (Mental Capacity Act, 2005).
- Right to privacy in family and private life (Human Rights Act 1998).
- Right to appropriate exchange and disclosure of personal information (Data Protection Act 1998).
- Right to quality of care provision, accountability and monitoring (Care Standards Act 2000).

Examining the range of rights covered, how do we recognize injustice? We need to avoid having a narrow frame of reference for our judgements by focussing on empowerment and citizen's rights for older people; how would we feel if we were expected to dress in the clothes of another person without our permission being sought? Would we not view this as a breach of our rights to dignity and identity? Does this then constitute harm?

An awareness of the causes and definitions of oppression and abuse will determine the type of intervention required. Bennett and Kingston (1993) identify a range of interventions on a spectrum from 'passive' to 'aggressive' with aggressive intervention including the formal legal system, police and court of protection and passive intervention including advocacy, empowerment, carer support and education. The promotion of education is significant – as older people, practitioners and members of the public, we need to understand an individual's experience of oppression in a framework of active citizenship rights. Note the difference this perspective makes in responding to Steve Johns, Claire Wainwright (Case Study 1) and Kazia and Henia Staciwa (Case Study 2).

The only legal justification of particular protection is where the older person has a level of mental incapacity that would affect their ability to make rational choices about level of risk and quality of life. Even then, the Mental Capacity Act 2005 clearly emphasises that an adult with mental incapacity should be protected to make decisions as fully as possible and that welfare practitioners should adopt a 'presumption for capacity' unless otherwise proven. Where intervention is proposed, it should involve the 'least restrictive' action. I would argue that an active citizenship perspective is particularly important in practice with older people with mental incapacity, to promote their participation and control as far as is possible.

Messages for practice

- It is important to recognise that each vulnerable adult will hold different views of the extent of risk they wish to live with.
- The practitioner needs to judge what level of intervention is appropriate, recognising the individual's level of mental capacity and respecting their right to make individual choices based on their view of quality of life.
- A narrow harm focus limits the response to an older person and potentially diminishes an interpretation of their citizenship rights.

VICTIMS OR SURVIVORS: THE CHALLENGE OF IMAGES OF DEPENDENCY

On one level, it would seem appropriate to recognise, and even emphasise, difference and the particular vulnerability of older adults who are dependent on welfare to claim protective responses (Department of Health, 2000: 2.3). However, an active citizenship claim promotes not only rights but responsibility; a challenge to the images of passive victimhood suggested above.

It is clear that older people are very wary of being considered dependent and reliant on services. In fact they don't want to be considered as service users at all but would rather be viewed as individuals with lives that do not revolve around ill-health and the input of services. The UK National Prevalence Study (Mowlam *et al.*, 2007) made clear that those subjected to abuse and maltreatment should be interviewed in a manner that allows them to relate their experiences in the wider context of their life experience. For example, an older man who was victimised and disempowered because his formal carer had subjected him to financial abuse, wants the social worker and the police officer to recognise that his need for a formal care service was only one piece of his identity. He was also chairman of the local choral society and needed this part of his identity and the skills it involved to be valued and acknowledged in the protective welfare response that followed.

The value of an active citizenship claim is that it equalises. It challenges traditional categories of service users and reminds us that we are all potentially victims of oppression in a societal context. Any one of us could be financially exploited by a formal carer or employee.

Penhale and Parker (2008: 156) portray oppression as a 'continuum running from oppression and exploitation through to empowerment and emancipation'. The image of a spectrum is helpful; I would view experiences of abuse and neglect as one part, the extreme end of the spectrum, within the larger picture of old age oppression. The concept of victimhood has particular connections with concepts of abuse and neglect, but has negative associations suggesting passivity and vulnerability.

Survivors, by contrast, are people who have moved through their experience of trauma to an 'emancipated' or liberated state. This is, potentially, an empowering experience that allows people to regain a sense of control and sense of their own autonomy in life. It could potentially mean not only the restoration of former strength of personhood but an enhanced resourcefulness, that could be channelled to help other older people by providing peer counselling and support.

Within this spectrum, however, it is important to recognise that there will be those who need support to regain this emancipated state, and this is the potential role of the skilled welfare practitioner.

Active citizenship and the empowerment model

If oppression, of any type, is created in a socio-cultural context, part of the journey to recovery will be through understanding the person's experience and renewing their sense of social identity. Banks (2004) identifies three levels of empowerment as a force for promoting the rights of service users. They range from a conservative interpretation of a service user's right to involvement and participation, to a radical approach that promotes the service user's right to active involvement and control. Active citizenship emphasises the right to human value and connectedness, the right to an identity rooted in its socio-cultural context. This is the value of a 'nurturing system' (Chestang, 1972) where the family and community provide space for the individual to develop or regain a sense of self, develop coping strategies and being provided with the resources to counteract 'negative valuations' placed on him or her by the dominant culture (Hopps, Pinderhughes and Shanker, 1995; Ahmad, 1993). This holistic perspective of healing has spiritual dimensions – giving an older person who might be frail, institutionalised or oppressed a sense of wholeness and worth (MacKinlay, 2001), and placing their experience in a context which has meaning and value. McKevitt, Redfern, Mold and Wolfe (2005) considered the change in self-esteem of older people experiencing disability and their experience of continuities and discontinuities. Where self-esteem remained high, people connected this with 'inner resources' such as 'religious faith, a sense of humour or long-established ability to cope'.

To view older people as victims is to emphasise their protective rights. To view older people as survivors is to acknowledge their resourcefulness and right to participation. This is not to deny or diminish the experience of trauma, but to find different ways of viewing loss and change. This perspective challenges a societal view of difference and dependency. Walmsley (1993) promotes the idea that we are all dependent and that this should be viewed as a common and equalising bond of humanity rather than the promotion of a community separation between independent and dependent people. This concept introduces the value of reciprocity; an important challenge to the image of passive victimhood.

Messages for practice

- Older people may, within reason, choose to continue living with risk.
- Pain and hardship is part of the life experience and that through surviving trauma individuals will experience growth and will have gained insight.
- Response to victims should recognise their capacity and resourcefulness.

THERAPEUTIC MODELS IN WORK WITH SURVIVORS

A therapeutic framework allows us a) to recognise the individual's psychological experience and b) to draw on their insight and resourcefulness to balance distortion and find meaning through trauma and loss. Again, this is arguably a radical approach – the therapist as a 'quiet revolutionary' (Rogers, 1979). The role of the therapist has a basis in humanistic principles that convey both empathic understanding and respect for the individual's capacity to use their resourceful energy for development and growth. In welfare terms, this promotes the principle of self ownership or 'self-actualisation' (Rogers) for people who might have been previously viewed as 'vulnerable'.

A project providing support for abused and neglected older people in Washington DC (Cabness, 1989) identified as its primary aim the facilitation of 'the recovery of the residents' self-esteem and optimum levels of psychosocial functioning'. The project provides an example of this model of therapeutic interaction. It includes supportive counselling, health promotion, peer interaction and transgenerational activities as a combat to the dislocation caused by trauma.

This balance of power is provided in therapeutic helping relationships like counselling, which respect the individual's personal experience and 'life story'. However, such techniques are also valid and valuable in mainstream welfare helping relationships as a person-centred or strengths-focussed approach. A 'strengths' perspective focusses on people's own ability to define their interaction with their environment (Salesby, 1992 cited in Payne: 273). In this context, I would emphasise its value in allowing older people to recognise their ability to draw on their own strength and to redefine the experience of victimhood.

CONCLUSION: PRACTICE GUIDE TO THERAPEUTIC INTERVENTIONS WITH OLDER SURVIVORS

- Respect the individual identity of the person and the individuality of their experience.
- Listen to the individual's story in their own words, valuing their insight and recognising the uniqueness of their experience.
- Respond with empathy, demonstrating respect for and belief in their resourcefulness and skills of survival.
- Understand both their level of capacity and their level of independent resourcefulness and provide support as appropriate.

- Minimise the intrusiveness of interventions and recognise the potential stigma of welfare dependency.
- Respond to the person holistically, recognising the impact of their socio-cultural context and working within their context of support.
- Develop a therapeutic helping relationship that acknowledges the impact of their experience of victimhood.
- Recognise the needs and vulnerabilities of perpetrators and respond accordingly.
- Acknowledge responsibility to challenge ways in which individuals and organisations create disempowerment and oppression towards older people.
- Develop heightened skills of reflective practice, recognising the sensitive and complex nature of work with survivors and consistently appraising own practice.

REFERENCES

Action on Elder Abuse (2000) *Listening is Not Enough*. London: Action on Elder Abuse

ADSS (2005) Safeguarding Adults: A National Framework of Standards for Good Practice and Outcomes in Adult Protection Work. London: ADSS

Ahmad, W.I.U. (1993) Race and Health in Contemporary Britain. Basingstoke: Open University Press

Ahmad, W.I.U. (ed) (2000) *Ethnicity, Disability and Chronic Illness*. Buckingham: Open University Press

Arling, G., Kane, R., Lewis, T. and Mueller, C. (2005) 'Future development of NH Quality Indicators'. *The Gerontologist*, 45 (2): 147–56

Baker, A. (1975) 'Granny Battering'. *Modern Geriatrics*, 5 (8): 20–4

Banks, S. (2004) *Ethics, Accountability and the Social Professions*. Basingstoke: Palgrave Macmillan

Bennett, G. and Kingston, P. (1993) *Elder Abuse: Concepts, Theories and Interventions*. Harlow: Longman

Beresford, P. (2003) *Citizen Involvement: A Practical Guide for Change*. Basingstoke: Macmillan

Biggs, S., Phillipson, C. and Kingston, P. (1995) *Elder Abuse in Perspective*. Buckingham: Open University Press.

Biggs, S. and Philipson, C. (1992) *Understanding Elder Abuse: A Training Manual for Helping Professions (Social Science Training Manual)*. London: Longman

Bonnie, R. and Wallace, R. (2002) *Elder Abuse, Neglect and Exploitation in Aging America*. Washington, DC: National Academy Press

Brown, H. and Turk, V. (1992) 'Defining sexual abuse as it affects adults with learning disabilities'. *Mental Handicap*, 20: 44–55

Brown, H. and Stein, J. (1997) 'Sexual abuse perpetrated by men with intellectual disabilities: a comparative study'. *Journal of Intellectual Disability Research*, 41 (3): 215–24

Butt, J. and Mirza, K. (1996) *Social Care and Black Communities: A Review of Recent Research Studies*. London: Her Majesty's Stationery Office

Cabness, J. (1989) 'The emergence shelter: a model for building self esteem of abused elders'. *Journal of Elder Abuse and Neglect*, 1 (2): 71–82

Carers National Strategy (1999) *Caring for Carers*. London: Department of Health

Chestang, L.W. (1972) *Character Development in a Hostile Environment (Occassional Paper 3)*. Chicago: University of Chicago Press

Churchill, H., Brown, A., Craft, A. and Horrocks, C. (1997) *There are no Easy Answers: Service Needs of People with Learning Disabilities Who Sexually Abuse Others*. Chesterfield/Nottingham: ARC/NAPSAC

Comijs, H.C. (1999) *Elder Mistreatment: Prevalence, Risk Indicators and Consequences*. Amsterdam: Vrije Universiteit

Commission for Health Improvement (CHI) (2003) *Investigation Into Matters Arising From Care on Rowan Ward, Manchester Mental Health and Social Care Trust*. Norwich: The Stationery Office

Cook, J., Maltby, T. and Warren, L. (2004) 'A participatory approach to older women's quality of life' in Walker A. and Hagan Hennessey, C. (eds) *Growing Older: Quality of Life in Old Age*. Maidenhead: Open University Press/McGraw-Hill

Coulthard, M., Walker, A. and Morgan, A. (2002) *People's Perceptions of their Neighbourhood and Community Involvement: Results from the Social Capital Module of the General Household Survey 2000*. London: The Stationery Office

Coxon, K., Billings, J. and Alaszewski, A. (2005) 'Providing integrated health and social care for older persons in the UK' in Leichsenring, K. and Alaszewski, A. (eds) *Providing Integrated Health and Social Care for Older Persons: A European Overview of Issues at Stake*. Aldershot: Ashgate

Cree, V. and Davis, A. (2007) *Social Work: Voices from the Inside*. Abingdon: Routledge

Davidson, K., Warren, L. and Maynard, M. (2005) *Social Involvement: Aspects of gender and ethnicity* in Walker, A. and Hennessey, C. (eds) *Understanding Quality of Life in Old Age*. Maidenhead, Open University Press/McGraw-Hill

Department of Constitutional Affairs (1997) *Who Decides: Making Decisions on Behalf of Mentally Incapacitated Adults*. A consultation paper issued by the Lord Chancellor's Department. London: HMSO

Department of Health (1989) *Caring for People*. London: Department of Health

Department of Health (1990) *NHS and Community Care Act*. London: Department of Health

Department of Health (1997) *The New NHS: Modern, Dependable*. London: Department of Health

Department of Health (1999) *The Carers National Strategy*. London: Department of Health

Department of Health (2000) *No Secrets: Guidance on Developing and Implementing Multi-agency Policies to Protect Vulnerable Adults from Abuse*. London: Department of Health

Department of Health (2001) *National Service Framework for Older People*. London: Department of Health

Department of Health (2007) *Modernising Adult Social Care*. London: Department of Health

Dominelli, L. (2002) *Feminist Social Work: Theory and Practice*. Basingstoke: Palgrave Macmillan

Eastman, M. (1984) *Old Age Abuse*. Mitcham: Age Concern

Gilligan, C. (1982) *In a Different Voice: Psychological Theory and Women's Development*. London: Harvard University Press

Goffman, E. (1968) *Asylums: Essays on the Social Situations of Mental Patients and Other Inmates*. London: Penguin

Gregory, J. (2004) *Taywood Review Closing Report*. Norfolk: Norfolk Constabulary and Norfolk County Council

Hirst, M. (2004) *Hearts and Minds: The Health Effects of Caring, Research Summary*. Glasgow: Carers Scotland

Hudson, B. (2002) 'Interprofessionality in health and social care: The achilles' heel of partnership?' *Journal of Interprofessional Care*, 16 (1): 8-17

Hopps, J.G., Pinderhughes, E. and Shankar, R. (1995) The Power to Care. Clinical Practice Effectiveness with Overwhelmed Clients. New York: Free Press

Hugman, R. (1994) *Ageing and the Care of Older People in Europe*. Basingstoke: Macmillan

Joint Committee on Human Rights (2007) *The Human Rights of Older People in Healthcare. Eighteenth Report of Session 2006–2007. Volume 1 – Report and Formal Minutes*. London: The Stationery Office

Kayser-Jones, J. (1981) *Old, Alone and Neglected: Care of the Aged in the United States and Scotland*. London: University of California Press

Kingston, P. and Penhale, B. (1995) *Family Violence and the Caring Professions.* Basingstoke: Macmillan

Lau, E. and Kosberg, J. (1979) 'Abuse of the elderly by informal care providers'. *Ageing*, September/October: 11–15

Leroux, T. and Petrunik, M. (1990) 'The construction of Elder Abuse as a social problem: A Canadian perspective'. *International Journal of Heath Service*, 20 (4): 651–63

MacKinlay, E. (2001) *The Spiritual Dimension of Ageing*. London: Jessica Kingsley

McKevitt, C., Refern, J., Mold, F. and Wolfe, C. (2004) Qualitative Studies of Stroke: a Systematic Review. *Stroke*, 35, 1499–1505

Mowlam, A., Tennant, R., Dixon, J. and McCreadie, C. (2007) *UK Study of Abuse and Neglect of Older People: Qualitative Findings*. London: National Centre for Social Research, Kings College London

National Health Service and Community Care Act (1990) Office of Public Sector Information, Available at: **http://www.opsi.gov.uk/ACTS/acts/1990/ukpga_19900019_en_1** (Accessed 23/12/2008)

Nazroo, J.Y., Bajekal, M., Blane, D., Grewal, I. and Lewis, J. (2003) *Ethnic Inequalities in Quality of Life at Older Ages: Subjective and Objective Components.* GO Findings 11, Sheffield: Growing Older Programme, University of Sheffield

Ogg, J. and Bennett, G. (1992) Elder Abuse in Britain. *British Medical Journal* 305 (October), 998–9

Penhale, B. and Parker, J. (2008) *Working With Vulnerable Adults*. Abingdon: Routledge

Pillemer, K.A. and Finkelhor, D (1989) 'Causes of Elder Abuse: Caregiver Stress Versus Problem Relatives'. *American Journal of Orthopsychiatry* 59 (2): 179–87

Protection of Vulnerable Adults (POVA) index – Care Standards Act 2000, s.81

Qureshi, B. (1991) 'Traditions of ethnic minority groups' in Squires, A. (ed.) *Multicultural Health Care and Rehabilitation of Older People* London: Age Concern

Ramsey-Klawsnik (1991), 'Interviewing elders for suspected sexual abuse: guidelines and techniques'. *The Journal of Elder Abuse and Neglect*, 5 (1): 5–19

Rogers, C.R. (1979) The Foundations of the Person-Centred Approach. *Education*, 100, (2) 98–107

Rose, S., Peabody, C. and Stratigeas, B. (1991) 'Undetected abuse among intensive case management clients'. *Hospital and Community Psychiatry*, 42: 499–503

Schindler, R. (1999) 'Empowering the aged – a post-modern approach'. *International Journal of Aging and Human Development*, 49 (3): 165–77

Schoener, G.R. (1989) *Psychotherapist's Sexual Involvement with Clients: Interviews and Prevention*. Minneapolis, MN: Walk in Counseling Center

Salesby, J. (1992) Cited in Payne, M. (1992) *Modern Social Work Theory: A Critical Introduction*. Basingstoke: Macmillan

Siegel-Itzkovich, J. (2005) 'A fifth of elderly people in Israel are abused'. *British Medical Journal*, 330: 498

Thompson, N. (2002) *Loss and Grief: A Guide for Human Services Practitioners*. Basingstoke: Palgrave Macmillan

Tinker, A. (1996) *Older People in Modern Society* (4th edn). Harlow: Addison Wesley Longman

Tsang, E., Liamputtong, P. and Piersonn, J. (2004) 'The views of older Chinese people in Melbourne about their quality of life'. *Ageing and Society*, 24 (1): 51–74

Ungerson, C. (1987) *Policy is Personal: Sex, Gender and Informal Care*. New York: Tavistock

Walker, A. and Hennessey, C. (eds) (2004) *Growing Older: Quality of Life in Old Age*. Maidenhead: Open University Press/McGraw-Hill

Walmsley, J. (1993) *Contradictions in Caring: Reciprocity and Interdependence*. Disability and Society, 8 (2), 129–41

Warr, P., Butcher, V. and Robertson, I. (2004) 'Activity and psychological well-being in older people'. *Aging and Mental Health*, 8: 172–83

Whittaker, T. (1995) 'Violence, gender and elder abuse: towards a feminist analysis and practice'. *Journal of Gender Studies*, 4 (1): 35–45

Wistow, G. and Hardy, B. (1996) 'Competition, collaboration and markets'. *Journal of Interprofessional Care* 10 (1): 5–10

Yahnke, R. (2005) 'Dying at grace'. *The Gerontologist*, 45 (12)

Chapter 11

Interprofessional Working

Michelle Cornes

Learning outcomes

Reading this chapter will enable you:

- to understand the policy background underpinning interprofessional working;

- to understand the different co-ordinating mechanisms which underpin interprofessional practice;

- to be aware of some of the challenges of achieving interprofessional working in practice.

INTRODUCTION

This chapter explores interprofessional working in the context of delivering integrated health and social care services for older people. The first section introduces the policy background to interprofessional working in the UK and considers the evidence base for integrated care. The second section considers the co-ordinating and integrating mechanisms that underpin interprofessional practice. The third section addresses the barriers to achieving good practice and the issues these raise for older people and their carers. As there is no agreed definition of what constitutes 'interprofessional working' this chapter approaches the topic in the broadest sense recognising (not unproblematically) that a wide range of terms are often used interchangeably (for example, multiprofessional working, multi-disciplinary working, interdisciplinary working, joint working, partnership working, integrated working, collaborative working).

Helpfully, Finch (2000) suggests that the Department of Health's vision of interprofessional collaboration requires practitioners:

- to 'know about' the roles of other professional groups;
- to be able to 'work with' other professionals, in the context of a team where each member has a clearly defined role;
- to be able to 'substitute for' roles traditionally played by other professionals, when circumstances suggest that this would be more effective;
- to seek flexibility in career routes: 'moving across'.

THE POLICY BACKGROUND

Integrated working between health and social care has risen up the political agenda of European governments and represents one response to the demographic challenge of population ageing and long-term care (Coxon *et al.*, 2005). As Dowling *et al.* (2004) point out, it is difficult to find a contemporary policy document or set of good practice guidelines that does not have collaboration as a central strategy for the delivery of welfare. There are, however, significant differences in policy developments across the UK. In Northern Ireland, health and personal social services have been delivered within an integrated structure of Health and Social Services Trusts since 1973 (Challis *et al.*, 2006). Joint health and social services trusts provide community services and the full range of social care services including the purchase of residential and nursing home beds. However, studies suggest that although integration is in place, services 'separate out' beneath the top levels (Petch, 2008).

In England and Wales, care is provided through NHS Trusts, which are responsible for providing hospital and community-based health services in conjunction with general practitioners. Social care services such as home support and the purchase of residential care are provided or commissioned mainly by local government.

In England, the 'flexibilities' contained in Section 31 of the Health Act 1999 have put in place the legal frameworks for 'pooled budgets' and 'care trusts'. Care trusts are a new level of primary care organisation that can commission both health and social care services, while the rationale for pooled budgets is that resources contributed to the pool by partner organisations will lose their distinctive health and social care identity (Glasby and Peck, 2004). These are optional structures that local health and social care economies can choose to put in place locally. The recent White Paper, *Your Health, Your Care, Your Say* (Department of

Health, 2006), sets out a vision for services that will support people to take greater control over their own lives, allowing everyone to enjoy a good quality of life, so that they are able to contribute fully to their communities. Services should be seamless, proactive and tailored to individual needs. It is acknowledged that there needs to be a greater focus on prevention and the early use of low level support services. In unlocking this vision, interprofessional working and integration is recognised as key. This is especially the case when it comes to meeting the needs of older people with long-term conditions and complex needs. The government is encouraging the development of multi-disciplinary networks and teams at Primary Care Trust and local authority level. They will be expected to use a Common Assessment Framework, with prompt and ongoing access to an appropriate level of specialist expertise for diagnosis, treatment and follow-up. The networks will need to operate on a sufficiently large geographic scale to ensure the involvement of all the key players, including social services, housing, and NHS primary, voluntary and secondary care services. The implication is that services for older people should not stand alone.

In Scotland, care is provided by 14 health boards. Here, a key feature has been the development and implementation of the Joint Future Agenda (Hubbard and Themessl-Huber, 2005; Petch, 2008). In terms of 'rebalancing care of older people' (Scottish Executive, 2001) this stipulated that every local authority area should have in place a comprehensive joint hospital discharge/rapid response team and a comprehensive, joint intensive home support team by mid-2002. Improving joint working is to be facilitated by five key elements: single assessment; intensive care management; information sharing; equipment and adaptations; and occupational therapy services.

Effective liaison between agencies and professionals across the UK is assumed to be vital for several reasons but, particularly, to ensure that scarce resources are used economically to meet genuine need (Swift, 2002). The Audit Commission (1998) sees partnership working as having a particular role to play in tackling so called 'wicked issues' such as avoidable admission to hospital for older people. Huxham (1996) talks of 'collaborative advantage' and the possibility of better outcomes for service users and carers. However, others have pointed to the lack of robust empirical evidence about the cost, efficiency or the effectiveness of integrated care (Coxon *et al.*, 2005). According to Petch (2008), while the process of partnership working allows enhanced understanding of the roles and rationale of other professionals and working cultures, the evidence base in support of partnership working delivering more effective outcomes is flimsy. Brown *et al.* (2003) compared two integrated health and social care teams for older people in Wiltshire with a traditional non-integrated team and concluded that the research did not produce any findings that suggested that the former is more clinically effective than the latter. Kharicha *et al.* (2004) make the point that while collaborative (or joint) working between social services and primary health care continues to rise up the policy agenda, current policy is not based on sound evidence of benefit to either patients or the wider community. They conclude that the underlying assumption that a greater degree of integration provides benefits to users and carers is a perspective that at times obscures the issue of resource availability, especially in the form of practical community services such as district nursing and home help. Greig and Poxton (2001) pose the question of integrating care, 'Nice process, but did it change anyone's life?'

CO-ORDINATING AND INTEGRATING MECHANISMS IN INTERPROFESSIONAL CARE

According to Swift (2002), the activities of any one discipline, whether it be medicine, nursing, allied health professions, social work, voluntary agencies, may at best be wasted or at worst harmful if they are not related to an assessment and planned programme of care. Across Europe and North America, interprofessional working is nearly always underpinned by care or case management (Leichsenring, 2004). In England, for example, the National Service Framework for Older People (Department of Health, 2001a) introduced the 'Single Assessment Process' (SAP). This built on the earlier guidance for Community Care Assessment (Department of Health, 1990) that proposes a 'single door' approach to community care service delivery. In this model, social services are identified as 'lead agents' responsible for assessing all care needs and, where appropriate, inviting other agencies to assist by commissioning from them specialist assessments of one form or another (for example, the specialist assessments of the consultant physician, nurse, physiotherapist, occupational therapist, speech and language therapist, podiatrist, nutritionist, dentist, pharmacist, optometrist, audiologist, etc.). The potential contributions of those working in housing (Foord and Simic, 2005) and in the voluntary and community sector (Cornes and Manthorpe, 2005) should also be included where appropriate. Finally, it is expected that the 'care manager' will co-ordinate the information that has been generated through the various specialist assessments in to an 'integrated care plan' (Department of Health, 2006). With the full involvement of older people and their families, this should set overarching goals (rooted in rehabilitation and the promotion of independence and wellbeing) that all the different agencies and professionals can work toward achieving together. It is recognised that interprofessional team working is most valuable when members work together with a common purpose to achieve a consistent quality of service within resources available (Hastings, 2002). Summing up the Single Assessment Process, Ormiston (2002: 39) notes:

> It may be helpful to think of 'unified' rather than 'single assessment' . . . It is intended that staff make sure that relevant information about a person is brought together whenever treatment or care decisions are made, streamlining practices and reducing duplication for service users.

Discussing developments across nine European Countries, Billings *et al.* (2005) observe that the efforts made in the selected countries to tackle evident problems at the interfaces between health and social care systems are usually in the form of 'model projects'. Because such model projects are dependent on the existing cultural, professional and social policy traditions, they conclude that there cannot be a 'ranking' of the different models and neither can a general 'recipe' be provided for integrating services. In Scotland and England, model projects launched under the banners of 'rapid response' and 'intermediate care', are at the forefront of attempts to redraw the boundaries between health and social care. Intermediate care often brings different professionals together in multi-disciplinary teams and aims to promote faster recovery from illness, prevent unnecessary acute hospital admissions, support timely hospital discharge and maximise independent living (Department of Health, 2001b). Although intermediate care is not specifically targeted on older people, this group forms the great majority of its users. In describing the proliferation of intermediate care teams across the UK an early progress report by the Department of Health (2002) referred to the 'blooming of a thousand flowers'.

> Intermediate care, by its very nature, cannot be the sole preserve of any single profession, organisation or sector. It is not just about health care, nor social care, nor housing – it is about all of these things and more and how professions and organisations can work together to make the core principle of delivering person centred care a reality . . . It is, quintessentially, about partnerships between organisations and professions and this is another key area where development is needed, so that services become fully integrated.
> (Department of Health, 2002: 3)

Case study

This case study shows how interprofessional care might be provided to an older person following surgery for a hip fracture and subsequent referral to an intermediate care team.

You are 86 years old. You live in the UK alone in a large semi-detached house. Your daughter lives in Australia. You have had a stroke and have been in hospital for ten days. You can walk a few metres with the help of one person. Your speech has been affected. You feel low and depressed and you wonder how you will cope when you return home. The social worker is coming to see you.

Activity 1

- What do you expect from this person?
- What are your goals and objectives?
- How will these be achieved?
- Which professionals will be involved?

Incorporate your ideas on the care plan below.

Goals and expected outcomes	Planned action to achieve goals	Roles and responsibilities

BARRIERS TO ACHIEVING INTERPROFESSIONAL WORKING

While the benefits of enhanced interprofessional working have long been obvious, widespread implementation and maintenance have remained elusive (Pullon, 2008). Based on their evidence from nine European countries, Coxon *et al.* (2005) argue that while there is often a concerted effort to achieve integration between health and social care agencies, the reality is that, in most countries, these agencies are structurally divided and struggle to work together in an integrated manner. The most recent review of the National Service Framework for Older People (Healthcare Commission, Commission for Social Care Inspection and the Audit Commission, 2006) suggests that there are still too many mismatches between needs and provision of services and that care for older people is still not sufficiently integrated.

Most discussions of the barriers to interprofessional working begin by acknowledging the historical divide between different occupational groups. Glasby (2003) describes how in England there are separate agencies responsible for meeting the health and social care needs of the population and how the underlying assumption is that it is possible to distinguish between people who are ill/injured (health needs) and people who need lower-level support due to frailty or disability (social needs). The difficulties associated with this are reported by Cornes and Clough (2000) when they describe the distinction that is to be made as to whether someone needs a bath for medical or social reasons. If the reason for the bath is the relief of a medical problem, then the bath is to be undertaken by nursing staff, paid for from health budgets and provided free for the individual user. On the other hand, if the bath is necessary because people want to be clean and cannot bathe themselves, then the bath is provided through social care staff, and paid for by the individual or the social services department dependent on levels of financial resources of different people. It needs little imagination to realise that there are boundary areas where a bath could be defined as either medical or social, nor to understand that staff may complete an assessment to achieve a desired end result. The language of official documents is full of terms like 'integrated commissioning' and 'seamless services'. The expectation is that agencies will work together in the interests of service users. Yet there are questions as to how organisations, which have separate structures and separate (and limited) funding, can co-operate effectively. Ware *et al.* (2003) found that separate budgets for health and social care undermined joint working. Indeed, it might be suggested that additional funding outside normal finance arrangements, such as funding provided for intermediate care teams, in part succeed because they avoid the problems of how rationing within and between organisations is to take place (Cornes and Clough, 2001)

Based on practice observations, Cornes and Clough (2004) demonstrate that social workers, district nurses and most other professionals in community care maintain their own separate arrangements for assessment and care management in order to 'gate keep' access to resources and services:

> **Researcher:** [Discussing implementation of 1990 Community Care Act] So in the beginning there was a 'joint assessment' for everyone?
>
> **Social Worker:** Yes, but it wasn't joint – the district nurses would do their assessment and we would do ours. Although we sort of approached it in a holistic way, it didn't really work like that.
>
> **Researcher:** So, in the beginning you made visits together, but when you were there you did your own thing?
>
> **Social Worker:** Yes, well that's how I view it. What is a 'joint assessment'? I don't think anybody's sussed that one out yet . . .
> (Quoted in Cornes and Clough, 2004: 7)

The study also suggests that social work practitioners do not have time to act as care managers in the way that was originally intended by the 1990 NHS and Community Care Act. Because they were so busy with the bureaucracy of social care there was little time left to orchestrate the in-puts of other professionals and agencies. Where needs were identified that were perceived to fall outside the specific professional domain then the process was one of 'passing the baton' and 'referring on' for further assessment by another agency:

> Seen from the perspective of older people and their families, accessing all or part of the total care system depends on service users and their families negotiating a maze of multiple assessment and a labyrinth of bureaucracy. The maze is dynamic and, depending upon the nature of the 'presenting problem' or 'episode', can configure in different ways; opening some pathways, shutting off others. The engine which drives the maze is the relationships between different professionals and organisations as expressed in the process and practice of 'referring on'.
> (Cornes and Clough, 2004: 9)

Multiple assessment and the involvement of lots of different agencies and professionals in the care of the older person should not, however, be mistaken as being part of the problem. As Manthorpe *et al.* (1996: 153) point out, different perspectives, generated by different professional groups in the process of assessment, need not sit contra to the spirit of joint working given that it can be beneficial to have a fuller picture of the uncertainties rather than being led by any one apparent consensus. Rather it is the unco-ordinated and fragmented nature of this input that causes distress for users and professionals alike.

Nazorko (1996) makes the point that interprofessional working is a time-consuming exercise. But the number of nurses, doctors and other professionals has not been increased to take account of the rising numbers of people over the age of 85 who require comprehensive assessment. The priority is seen as freeing beds to enable others to be treated. Busy clinicians often hand matters over to a care manager and do not become involved in the care management process. As a result, in most parts of the UK, multi-disciplinary assessment and case conferences are rare.

Interprofessional relationships

Hudson (2002: 7) suggests that, while much attention has been focussed on inter-organisational working, much less attention has been paid to interprofessional relationships:

> To some extent the assumption seems to be that if inter-agency partnership policies, processes and structures are established, then front line partnerships between a range of traditionally separate professionals will fall into place. Such belief is contrary to the received sociological wisdom that professions are essentially self-interested groupings.

Nolan and Caldock (1996) argue that 'professional protectionism' – the tendency to defend that area of practice to which a discipline lays claim – and 'professional reductionism' – the tendency to reduce the focus of assessment or activity to a set of problems consistent with a particular professional paradigm – are two major factors that are 'alive and well'. Professional reductionism was first identified in a famous study by Runciman (1989) that asked different professional groups to watch the same video footage of an older person chatting to an assessor. The person in question was described variously as being cheerful to depressed, apathetic to dogmatic, proud to lonely, neat to unkempt; a multitude of needs were identified; and the solutions offered varied significantly according to the professional group. Dalley (1989) understands 'professional identity' in terms of distinct behaviours and attitudes that can sometimes lead to defensive tribalism and promotion of tribal ties at the expense of looking outwards. In a study of assessment practices, Wirth (1998) highlights the considerable mutual suspicion that can exist between social workers and district nurses about the adequacy of each other's work. Each viewed their own profession more positively than the other's and as being the key figure in assessment of need and co-ordination of services. Indeed, a key debate to emerge in the interprofessional literature has been around who should act as the 'care' or 'case' manager. More recent policy guidance has tended to shift responsibility away from social services to health personnel with the introduction of 'case management' for the management of long-term conditions (Cochrane and Fitzpatrick, 2005). Pollard (2008) reports findings from a qualitative study exploring pre-qualifying health and social care students' experiences of interprofessional learning and working in practice placement settings. The findings show that some staff in placement settings experienced problems when working with colleagues from other disciplines and that, consequently, through processes of non-formal learning and unconscious role modelling, some students learned inappropriate behaviours with regard to interprofessional working.

NEW APPROACHES TO INTERPROFESSIONAL WORKING

Focussing on one locality in England, Doyle and Cornes (2006) describe how a wide range of 'model projects' have evolved to facilitate partnership working around the needs of older people and how these have recently been brought together under the umbrella of the 'Community Older Persons Team' (COPT). The COPT comprises 53 professionals working in seven distinct services across three broad areas: intermediate care; prevention and wellbeing; and hospital discharge. Members of the COPT currently include: social workers, therapists, a pharmacist, health visitor, podiatrists, district nurses, health and social care support workers, accident prevention staff and a GP with 'special interests'. Staff working under the COPT umbrella are line managed by a single manager. To facilitate professional development and prevent isolation from peers all staff have access to a manager from their own discipline. On a less positive note, despite the integrated management structure, the wider organisation still functions as two separate employers when it comes to systems for IT, finance and human resource support.

The King's Fund suggest that while partnership working may be more easily facilitated in the context of intermediate care and other model projects such as the COPT, encapsulating small subsets of the system in isolated and protected enclaves will not address the intractable problems in the wider health and social care system (Harries *et al.*, 1998). According to Stevenson (2005), the challenge is how to mainstream interprofessional working. It is suggested that this might be achieved through the creation of 'locality teams' that would eventually eradicate the need for project-style services, such as the thousand flowers that have bloomed around intermediate care. The argument is that mainstream care managers should have sufficient skills and resources at their disposal to be able to 'step-up' and 'step-down' a person's care package without having to hand them over to an interim care manager:

> The pattern of future care, especially for older people, will be one in which joint commissioning arrangements (and greater partnership working) commission well-resourced health & social care locality teams. Such teams could bring together a full range of professions and skills, generalists and specialists, underpinned by a large number of trained rehabilitative support workers, able to respond flexibly and quickly to people's changing needs, and offer continuity of care. With a single point of contact, an open door approach, pro-active and shared assessment and reassessment, access to rapid diagnostics, assistive technology, and good care planning and care management we may see a revolution in care for older individuals.
>
> (Stevenson, 2005: 4)

For Petch (2008: 83), the more pressing concern is the extent to which partnership working will remain key to the policy agenda:

> There is a new focus on personalisation, on the individual service users becoming the key driver in determining the network of support they access. The logic of such an approach would suggest that the agencies that will thrive are those that are favoured by service users and their support brokers . . . Perhaps the destiny of partnership working, the waxing and waning of different models is destined to provide a constant organisational backcloth while front stage more immediate initiatives are brought to the fore.

THE VIEWS OF OLDER PEOPLE AND THEIR FAMILIES

Blickem and Priyadharshini (2007) describe how older people on a stroke rehabilitation ward experienced interprofessional practice delivered through a multi-professional team comprising doctors, nurses, physiotherapists, occupational therapists, speech and language therapists and senior house officers. They report that older people often experienced a sense of bewilderment as a result of the complex range (and sometimes conflicting) professional priorities that needed to be negotiated and satisfied. Older people and their families reported that they were often expected to relay messages on behalf of professionals and that miscommunication was commonplace. They describe how a stroke can have a devastating effect on an individual's sense of self and how most illness that incapacitates or necessitates change in everyday routine requires emotional rehabilitation, that involves some kind of identity reconstruction and restoration of self. However, many older people on the ward felt that being subject to a range of professional perspectives was akin to dissection of self and that this could ultimately lengthen the process of reconstructing and asserting a coherent new identity.

Based on interviews with 230 service users (including older people) who had direct experience of receiving care through one of 15 health and social care partnerships, Cook *et al.* (2007: 4) make the following practice recommendations:

- In the planning and commissioning of services, agencies should ensure that they are responding to the outcomes defined by service users. Asking about outcomes can help partnerships come up with more creative solutions to supporting service users.
- Partnerships should be delivering on all the outcomes identified. Standard assessment and review processes may not pick up on the extent to which these outcomes are being delivered and they need to be reviewed to ensure that they focus on outcomes.
- Links with other statutory sectors and with the voluntary and social enterprise sectors (outside of the immediate partnership) can help partnerships work creatively to deliver on the desired outcomes.
- Outcome focussed monitoring should be the key component of quality assurance in partnership development.

CONCLUSION

This chapter has explored interprofessional working in the context of delivering integrated health and social care services to older people. Integrated working has risen on the political agenda and represents one response to the focus on population ageing and long term care. Despite commitment to interprofessional working across the UK, the evidence base for its effectiveness is weak especially as regards outcomes for older people and their carers. Interprofessional working is often underpinned by assessment and care management but there are many barriers that prohibit good practice. For the most part, interprofessional working is often confined to intermediate care or other 'model projects' rather than mainstream services. The reality is that, in most countries, agencies are structurally divided and struggle to work together in an integrated manner. The consequence for service users and carers is often fragmented and uncoordinated care which does not always meet all their needs.

More recently, there has been a renewed focus on interprofessional working in the context of health promotion, illness prevention and the management of chronic disease. Most challenging perhaps will be the implementation of the personalisation agenda. Currently, it is unclear as to the role that service users and their carers will be expected to play in co-ordinating and managing their own 'multi-disciplinary' care. While health services are increasingly promoting the potential of 'case management' in the management of long term conditions, social care is moving away from such models in favour of advocacy and brokerage. Only time will tell if this emerges as a new conceptual 'Berlin Wall'.

> Many of those receiving a personal budget for social care also have a long-term health condition, yet the NHS only rarely allocates services though a personal budget.
>
> (Leadbetter *et al.*, 2008: 72)

FURTHER READING

Glasby, J. (2007) *Understanding Health and Social Care*. Bristol: The Policy Press
Provides a good introduction to the wider context of interprofessional working.

Squire, A. and Hastings, M. (eds) (2002) *Rehabilitation of the Older Person: A Handbook for the Interdisciplinary Team*. Cheltenham: Stanley Thornes
This book provides a practical insight to the contributions of the different professionals working in the interdisciplinary team.

Lank, E. (2006) *The Collaborative Advantage: How Organisations win by Working Together*. Basingstoke and New York: Palgrave Macmillan
Presents ideas on how collaboration might be managed for the benefit of separate teams or units within an organisation.

Billings, J. and Leichsenring, K. (eds) (2005) *Integrating Health and Social Care Services for Older Persons*. Aldershot: Ashgate
This book introduces a wide range of different approaches to interprofessional working and highlights the diversity in practice across Europe.

Useful websites

www.integratedcarenetwork.gov.uk
Integrated Care Network

www.csip.org.uk
Care Services Improvement Partnership

www.caipe.org.uk
Centre for Advancement of Interprofessional Education

www.scie.org.uk
Social Care Institute of Excellence

www.kcl.ac.uk/schools/sspp/interdisciplinary/scwru/index.html
Social Care Workforce Research Unit

REFERENCES

Audit Commission (1998) A *Fruitful Partnership: Effective Partnership Working*. London: Audit Commission

Blickem, C. and Priyadharshini, E. (2007) 'Patient narratives in interprofessional learning'. *Journal of Interprofessional Care*, 21 (6): 633–44

Billings, J., Leichsenring, K. and Tabibian, N. (2005) 'Elements for successful integration process in long-term care services. Some concluding remarks' in Billings, J. and Leichsenring, K. (eds) *Integrating Health and Social Care Services for Older Persons: Evidence from Nine European Countries*. Aldershot: Ashgate

Brown, L., Tucker, C. and Domokos, T. (2003) 'Evaluating the impact of health and social care teams on older people living in the community'. *Health and Social Care in the Community*, 11 (2): 85–95

Challis, D., Stewart, K., Donnelly, M., Weiner, K. and Hughes, J. (2006) 'Care management for older people: does integration make a difference?' *Journal of Interprofessional Care*, 20 (4): 335–48

Cochrane, D. and Fitzpatrick, S. (2005) 'What works in case management of high risk populations: identification of key components to improve effectiveness'. **http://www.goodmanagement-hsj.co.uk/pdf/Casemanagement_081205. pdf** (Accessed 23 September 2008)

Cook, A., Petch, A., Glendenning, C. and Glasby, J. (2007) 'Building Capacity in Health and Social Care Partnerships: Key Messages from a Multi-Stakeholder Network'. *Journal of Integrated Care*, 15 (4): 3–10

Cornes, M. and Clough, R. (2000) *Assessment in Community Care: Disputed Territory*. Lancaster: Lancaster University

Cornes, M. and Clough, R. (2001) 'The continuum of care: older people's experiences of intermediate care'. *Education and Ageing*, 16 (2): 179–202

Cornes, M. and Clough, R. (2004) 'Inside multi-disciplinary practice: challenges for single assessment'. *Journal of Integrated Care*, 12 (2): 3–13

Cornes, M. and Manthorpe, J. (2005) 'Someone to Expect Each Day'. *Community Care*, 8–14 December, 36–7

Coxon, K., Clausen, T. and Argoud, D. (2005) 'Inter-professional working and integrated care organisations' in Billings, J. and Leichsenring, K. (eds) *Integrating Health and Social Care Services for Older Persons*, Aldershot: Ashgate

Dalley, G. (1989) 'Professional ideology or organisational tribalism? The health service-social work divide' in Taylor, R. and Ford, J. (eds) *Social Work and Health Care*. London: Jessica Kingsley

Department of Health (1990) *The NHS and Community Care Act*. London: HMSO

Department of Health (2001a) *National Service Framework for Older People*. London: Department of Health

Department of Health (2001b) HSC 2001/1:LAC *Intermediate Care*. London: HMSO

Department of Health (2002) *Intermediate Care: Moving Forward*. London: Department of Health

Department of Health (2006) *Our Health, Our Care, Our Say: A New Direction from Community Services*. London: Department of Health

Dowling, B., Powell, M. and Glendinning, C. (2004) 'Conceptualising successful partnerships'. *Health and Social Care in the Community*, 12 (4): 309–17

Doyle, D. and Cornes, M. (2006) 'Mainstreaming Interprofessional Partnerships in a Metropolitan Borough'. *Journal of Integrated Care*, 14 (5): 27–37

Finch, J. (2000) 'Interprofessional education and teamworking: a view from education providers'. *British Medical Journal*, 321: 1138–40

Foord, M. and Simic, P. (eds) (2005) *Housing, Community Care and Supported Housing – Resolving Contradictions*. Totton: Chartered Institute of Housing

Glasby, J. (2003) *Hospital Discharge: Integrating Health and Social Care*. Abingdon: Radcliffe Medical Press

Glasby, J. and Peck, E. (eds) (2004) *Care Trusts: Partnership Working in Action*. Abingdon: Radcliffe Medical Press

Greig, R. and Poxton, R. (2001) 'Nice process – but did joint commissioning change anyone's life?' *Managing Community Care*, 9, 16–21

Hastings, M. (2002) 'Team working in rehabilitation' in Squire, A. and Hastings, M. (Eds) *Rehabilitation of the Older Person: A Handbook for the Interdisciplinary Team*. Cheltenham: Stanley Thornes

Harries, J., Fischer, M. Gordon, P. and Pamphling, D. (1998) *Projectitis*. London: King's Fund

Hubbard, G. and Themessl-Huber, M. (2005) 'Professional perceptions of joint working in primary care and social care services for older people in Scotland'. *Journal of Interprofessional Care*, 19 (4): 371–85

Hudson, B. (2002) 'Interprofessionality in health and social care: the Achilles' heel of partnership?' *Journal of Interprofessional Care*, 16 (1): 7–17

Healthcare Commission, Commission for Social Care Inspection and the Audit Commission (2006) *Living Well in Later Life: A Review of Progress Against the National Service Framework for Older People*. London: Healthcare Commission

Huxham, C. (ed) (1996) *Creating Collaborative Advantage*. London: Sage

Kharicha, K., Levin, E., Illiffe, S. and Davey, B. (2004) 'Social work, general practice and evidenced-base policy in the collaborative care of older people: current problems and future possibilities.' *Health and Social Care in the Community*, 12 (2): 134–41

Leadbeater, C., Bartlett, J. and Gallagher, N. (2008) *Making it Personal*. London: Demos

Leichsenring, K. (2004) 'Providing integrated health and social care for older persons – A European overview' in Leichsenring, K. and Alaszewski, A. (eds) *Providing Integrated Health and Social Care for Older Persons – A European Overview*. Aldershot: Ashgate

Manthorpe, J., Stanley, N., Bradley, G. and Alaszewski, A. (1997) 'Working together effectively? Assessing older people for community care services'. *Health Care in Later Life*, 1 (3): 143–55

Nazorko, L. (1996) 'The right staff to fit the bill'. *Nursing Times*, 31.7.96, 44–5

Nolan, M. and Caldock, K. (1996) 'Assessment: identifying the barriers to good practice'. *Health and Social Care in the Community*, 4 (2): 77–85

Ormiston, H. (2002) 'The single assessment process'. *Managing Community Care*, 10 (2): 38–43

Petch, A. (2008) *Health and Social Care: Establishing a Joint Future?* Edinburgh: Dunedin Academic Press

Pollard, K. (2008) 'Non-formal learning and interprofessional collaboration in health and social care: the influence of the quality of staff interaction on student learning about collaborative behaviour in practice placements'. *Learning in Health and Social Care*, 7 (1): 12–26

Pullon, S. (2008) 'Competence, respect and trust: key features of successful interprofessional nurse–doctor relationships'. *Journal of Interprofessional Care*, 22 (2): 133–48

Runciman, P. (1989) 'Health assessment of the elderly at home; the case for shared learning'. *Journal of Advanced Nursing*, 14 (2): 111–19

Scottish Executive (2001) *Better Care for All Our Futures*. Edinburgh: Scottish Executive

Stevenson, J. (2005) 'Intermediate care – how will it contribute to meeting current national priorities and supporting local service redesign?' **www.changeagentteam.org.uk/_library/Intermediatecaretheway forwardfinal0505.doc** (Accessed 5 May 2008)

Swift, C. (2002) 'Disease and disability in older people – the effectiveness of specialist interdisciplinary health-care services' in Squire, A. and Hastings, M. (eds) *Rehabilitation of the Older Person: A Handbook for the Interdisciplinary Team*. Cheltenham: Nelson Thornes

Ware, T., Matosevic, T., Hardy, B., Knapp, M., Kendall, J. and Forder, J. (2003) 'Commissioning care services for older people in England: the view from care managers, users and carers'. *Ageing and Society*, 23: 411–28

Wirth, A. (1998) 'Community care assessment of older people: identifying the contribution of community nurses and social workers'. *Health and Social Care in the Community*, 6 (5): 382–6

Part Three

Chapter 12

Healthy Lifestyles: Influencing Patterns of Premature Mortality and the Causes of Morbidity

F. J. Raymond Duffy

Learning outcomes

Reading this chapter will enable you to:

- understand the important role played by social determinants of health on the lifestyles adopted by older people;

- be aware of the principle causes of mortality and morbidity in older people in the UK;

- appreciate the difference between modifiable lifestyle factors (those that you can exercise some control over) and those that you have little control over;

- outline a number of interventions that may be used to improve what older people eat; increase their activity levels; help them to consider the impact of the substances they consume (particularly alcohol and tobacco); reduce the risks taken with eyesight and hearing; may help them to avoid dementia-causing illness and depression;

- examine the role of government and health care professionals in promoting preventative care and making healthy choice easier.

INTRODUCTION

Meeting the needs of an ageing society is one of the main challenges that we face this century. One of the most important of these needs is maintaining the health and wellbeing of older people. However, it is very difficult to determine what we mean by having good health and wellbeing because, although good health is something that everyone desires, health does not have a universal meaning. Health on an individual level is a concept that is not defined medically, but one that is affected by a wide range of factors such as personal experiences, attitudes, perceptions about health, the degree of autonomy and the availability and robustness of your social support network (Cowley, 2006). Significantly though, there is little doubt that our situations in later life depend a great deal on what has occurred earlier in life, and not all the determinants of our health in old age can be attributed to any of the life choices that we have made. When examining the evidence around the factors that determine health in old age there are many factors that the individual has little control over. These factors include:

- genetic and biological factors;
- age;
- gender;
- socioeconomic status;
- poverty;
- access to education and educational attainment;
- inadequate housing;
- living in a socially deprived community;
- religion, cultural patterns and beliefs;
- exposure to environmental pollution;
- availability of, and access to, transport;
- discrimination on the grounds of age.
        (Naidoo and Wills, 2000; Squire, 2002; Ewles and Simnett, 2003)

All the factors mentioned above affect the lives of older people. However, these factors alone, although they are contributing significantly to mortality and morbidity, do not directly cause them. There is also no doubt that the socioeconomic determinants listed above lead to inequalities in health throughout life that continue in old age (Grundy and Sloggett, 2003). Disadvantage can give rise to, or exacerbate, health-damaging behaviours such as smoking and poor nutrition and so health behaviours (lifestyle determinants) are difficult to separate from their social context (Naidoo and Wills, 2000). Improving people's health means addressing the social, environmental and economic factors that affect their health, as well as their individual behaviours and lifestyle. The route to improving the health of the population overall is probably through tackling the socioeconomic and environmental determinants of health, which will reduce health inequalities (Ewles and Simnett, 2003).

However, tackling these determinants is a societal and governmental task. What we can all do is try to attempt to live as healthy a life as possible by making healthy lifestyle choices when we can. In order to get an idea of the contribution that lifestyle choices may make to health and wellbeing it is worth considering the major causes of mortality and morbidity in older people.

MORTALITY (WHAT KILLS OLDER PEOPLE PREMATURELY?)

In terms of mortality, the three major causes of death in the UK in rank order, (highest to lowest), in those aged over 65, are:

- circulatory diseases (heart disease and stroke);
- cancer (particularly lung, prostate, breast and colorectal cancer);
- respiratory diseases (particularly pneumonia and COPD).

(House of Lords Science and Technology Committee 2005, Office of National Statistics, 2006)

Deaths from circulatory disease and respiratory illness all increase significantly with age. Cancer is less age dependent but, according to Cancer Research UK (2006a), over 170 000 people over 65 are diagnosed with cancer every year, amounting to 64 per cent of all cancers diagnosed in the UK, and over 107 000 people over 65 die of cancer every year. In the over 65s age group the most common are lung, prostate, breast and colorectal cancers. Survival rates from lung and breast cancer are particularly strongly age-related, diminishing greatly in the over 70 age group. Survival rates for prostate and colorectal cancers begin to diminish markedly only past the age of 80 (Cancer Research UK, 2006b).

MORBIDITY (WHICH ILLNESSES AFFECT THE HEALTH OF OLDER PEOPLE?)

Looking at morbidity, a third of adults in the UK (around four million people) aged 65–74, and almost half of adults aged 75 and over (about two million people), report having a limiting long-standing sickness or disability. The proportion of people reporting a limiting long-standing illness or disability has remained broadly stable over the last decade

(Office of National Statistics, 2004). The impact of socioeconomic health determinants, particularly poverty, is worth noting. Adults aged 65–74 on below-average incomes are more likely to have a limiting long-standing illness or disability than those on above-average incomes. Those aged 65 and over who had routine or manual jobs are also more likely to suffer a long-standing illness or disability than those with non-manual work histories (Palmer, MacInnes and Kenway, 2007). So what causes all this long-standing illness and disability? The four most prevalent causes of morbidity involve:

- the heart and circulatory system (particularly CHD and stroke);
- the musculoskeletal system (particularly osteoarthritis, rheumatoid arthritis and ankylosing spondylitis);
- endocrine and metabolic functions (particularly diabetes and thyroid disorders);
- the respiratory system (principally COPD and Chronic Asthma).
      (House of Lords Science and Technology Committee, 2005)

Other illnesses affecting predominantly older people include opthalmic complaints. In the UK there are close to two million people aged over 65 who have a sight loss that significantly affects their daily life. This equates to one in five of the over-65 age group. Many have either glaucoma, which may affect about 2 per cent of the population over 40, or macular degeneration associated with ageing, which may affect up to 8 per cent of those over 65; a further 50 per cent may have an untreated refractive error and cataracts. All of these conditions may respond to current treatments (Tate *et al.*, 2005). The prevalence of sight loss increases with age and there is growing concern that the numbers of older people with sight problems will increase dramatically, not just because we have an ageing population but because the incidence of some key underlying causes of sight loss such as obesity and diabetes are also increasing (Royal National Institute for the Blind (RNIB), 2008). Sight loss not only impacts significantly on an older person's quality of life. There are also significant adverse health impacts associated with sight loss, such as an increased risk of depression and falls. Older people with sight problems are 1.7 times more likely to have a fall and at 90 per cent higher odds of multiple falls than a person with no visual impairment. People with sight problems are also likely to have additional disabilities and are likely to live alone (Bosanquet and Mehta, 2008).

Another significant cause of morbidity is hearing loss. In the UK there are approximately nine million people who have a significant hearing impairment, 6.5 million of who are over 60 (Royal National Institute for the Deaf (RNID), 2006). Hearing loss is the commonest of the sensory impairments suffered in old age and is experienced by half of people over 60. Even more so than sight loss, it has long been regarded as an inevitable consequence of growing old, not only by health care professionals but also by the general public, so very often people do not complain about it as much as they should. Social withdrawal is, for many people, the main consequence of hearing loss, particularly as there is a stigma attached to hearing impairment. Glasses can be regarded as fashion accessories, but the same is not true of hearing aids (House of Lords Science and Technology Committee, 2005).

Other significant causes of morbidity are the dementia-causing illnesses. Dementia-causing illnesses affect over 21 per cent of everyone in the UK who is over 85 (Alzheimer's Society, 2007).

Finally, another illness that merits mention is depression. This is the most common mental health problem in later life with up to 2.4 million older people in the UK having depression severe enough to impair their quality of life (Lee, 2006). This number is expected to increase in future years, with the World Health Organisation (WHO) predicting that by 2020 depressive disorders will become the second most frequent cause of ill-health worldwide (WHO, 2004a). In terms of premature mortality depression is strongly linked to suicide, but it has also consistently been linked to mortality following a myocardial infarction; it significantly increases the risk of heart disease, even when other risk factors like smoking are controlled (Van der Kooy *et al.*, 2007). Although it is suspected that around 50 per cent of all people with depression in the community do not present to their GP (National Institute for Clinical Excellence (NICE), 2004), it is still the third most common reason for consultation in GP practice (NHS Centre for Reviews and Dissemination, 2002).

THE EFFECT OF LIFESTYLE: CAN PATTERNS OF MORTALITY AND MORBIDITY BE ALTERED?

Looking at the previous sections of this chapter, the major causes of morbidity and mortality are well known. Two significant risk factors for many of them that cannot be modified are your age and your genetics (WHO, 2005). The impact of the social determinants of health such as poverty and poor housing, poor access to transport, etc., are also well recognised, but require a concerted effort by both government and society to tackle them (Scharf *et al.*, 2002; Palmer, MacInnes and Kenway, 2007). Therefore, the most important modifiable risks (those we may have some personal control over) relate to:

- what we eat;
- how active we are;
- what substances we take (particularly alcohol and tobacco);
- the risks we take with our eyesight and hearing;
- what we do to try to avoid dementia-causing illnesses;
- what we do to avoid depression.

What we eat: nutrition and diet

Tackling obesity

The focus of government and health care efforts in this area has been on tackling the growing problem of obesity in UK adults and children. There has never been more than general advice given on what a healthy diet for older people is (Food Standards Agency, 2008). However, the advice given to adults is considered to be appropriate in most cases. This is particularly true when considering the need to discourage an unhealthy diet with low fruit and vegetable consumption and excessive energy intake. The National Institute for Health and Clinical Excellence (2006) states that every adult should aim to maintain or achieve a healthy weight, to improve their health and reduce the risk of diseases associated with obesity. Assessment of the health risks associated with being overweight and obesity in adults should be based on a body mass index (BMI) and waist circumference as follows (see Figure 1):

Classification	BMI (kg/m²)
Healthy weight	18.5–24.9
Overweight	25–29.9
Obesity I	30–34.9
Obesity II	35–39.9
Obesity III	40 or more

Figure 1 NICE: CG43: Obesity: Classification system for determining overweight or obese category

BMI and waist circumference

- For men, waist circumference of less than 94 cm is low, 94–102 cm is high and more than 102 cm is very high.
- For women, waist circumference of less than 80 cm is low, 80–88 cm is high and more than 88 cm is very high.

Note that BMI may be a less accurate measure of adiposity in adults who are highly muscular, adults from Asia who have smaller skeletal frames and therefore would have higher body fat percentage than Caucasian adults of same height. As a result Asians with a BMI above 23 should be considered overweight (WHO Expert Consultation, 2004) and older people where the presence of a number of factors, like loss of height, reduction in lean body mass with age and the presence of chronic disease can lead to problems with both with measurement and interpretation. Health care professionals should exercise clinical judgement when considering risk factors in these groups. (Adapted from NICE, 2006.)

NICE (2006) also suggests that adults should follow these strategies, which may make it easier to maintain a healthy weight:

- base meals on starchy foods such as potatoes, bread, rice and pasta, choosing wholegrain where possible;
- eat plenty of fibre-rich foods – such as oats, beans, peas, lentils, grains, seeds, fruit and vegetables, as well as wholegrain bread and brown rice and pasta;
- eat at least five portions of a variety of fruit and vegetables each day, in place of foods higher in fat and calories;
- eat a low-fat diet and avoid increasing your fat and/or calorie intake;
- eat as little as possible of: fried foods; drinks and confectionery high in added sugars; other food and drinks high in fat and sugar, such as some take-away and fast foods;
- eat breakfast;
- watch the portion size of meals and snacks, and how often you are eating;
- minimise the calories you take in from alcohol.

Additionally, you should aim to be active by:

- making activities – such as walking, cycling, swimming, aerobics and gardening – part of everyday life;
- minimise sedentary activities, such as sitting for long periods watching television, at a computer or playing video games;
- build activity into your day – for example, by taking the stairs instead of the lift, taking a walk at lunchtime.

This simplistic advice though fails to acknowledge that tackling obesity involves a variety of difficult behavioural changes, which include what may be challenging alterations to diet, changes in shopping behaviour, increases in exercise, different transport choices, reductions in alcohol consumption and other life-altering measures (Government Office for Science, 2007).

A more helpful view may be to make the first objective the prevention of further weight gain. Once weight is stabilised, the second objective is to achieve some level of weight loss. Weight loss goals should be realistic and achievable. For many older obese people achieving a body mass index in the ideal range and within a reasonable time is hard. However, a weight loss of 5 kg (11 lbs) is equivalent to a loss of some 6 per cent in body weight for a man or woman of average height with a BMI of 30, the boundary between the overweight and obese categories. This degree of weight loss can reduce back and joint pain, breathlessness, the frequency of sleep apnoea and improve lung function. It may also result in psychological benefits, such as the alleviation of depression and anxiety (Royal College of Physicians, 1998). It is also worth noting that, in older adults, effective interventions associated with even modest weight loss have been shown to reduce the health care costs arising from associated chronic diseases such as diabetes (Knowler et al., 2002; Lindstrom et al., 2006).

There is a great need to tackle poor diet and obesity in older people with some urgency, but more research into successful methods for bringing about dietary behavioural change is required (Government Office for Science, 2007). Tackling the root causes of poor diet and obesity are even more complex than trying to alter the behaviour of the individual. Obesity can be linked to broad social developments and shifts in values, such as changes in food production, use of motorised transport and alterations in our work/home lifestyle patterns. An understanding of the contribution of these causes of obesity is critical to any plan to improve the national diet (Government Office for Science, 2007). The Government Office for Science (2007) goes on to caution that the priority is not to be over-reliant on any single approach. No 'magic pill' or technological fix for obesity that is sustainable and cost effective is likely to be found.

Malnutrition

Although obesity may be the dominant public health issue, for a minority of older people malnutrition is a significant issue. Finch *et al.* (1998) indicated that even among less frail community-dwelling older people, 3 per cent of men and 6 per cent of women are underweight. Those on a low income, the very old, many people with chronic conditions like heart failure and COPD and those living in care homes and hospitals are specifically at risk from nutritional inadequacy (Finch *et al.*, 1998). Indeed, if those who are undernourished eat what is considered a healthy diet by the majority of people, they may experience further weight loss as they may not consume enough calories and may suffer deficiency of other nutrients. Those who are underweight need to consume sufficient energy and protein to maintain or improve their body weight. An indication of the amount of calories and protein they require to avoid protein energy malnutrition can be gauged from the information in Figure 2.

Estimated Average Requirements (EAR) for Energy (kcal/day)

	Males	Females
60–64 years	2380	1900
65–74 years	2330	1900
75+ years	2110	1810

Reference Nutrient Intakes (RNI) for Protein (g/day)

	Males	Females
60–64 years	~53.3	46.5
65–74 years	~53.3	46.5
75+ years	~53.3	46.5

Figure 2 Estimated average energy and protein requirements of older people (adapted from the MedicDirect: Fitness and Wellbeing Elderly Diet page. Available at: **www.medicdirect.co.uk/lifestyle/default.ihtml?pid=864&step=4**)

Older people suffering from malnutrition need to consume at least these amounts to prevent further deterioration and may need to exceed them to recover.

How active we are: physical activity and exercise

In the UK, lack of physical activity is a growing problem for the whole population and one that even affects people of normal weight. Among adults, 41 per cent of women and 35 per cent of men put their health at risk by being inactive. By age 75, this has risen to 70 per cent of men and 80 per cent of women (Department of Health Physical Activity, Health Improvement and Prevention, 2004; Bromley, Sproston and Shelton, 2005).

WHO (2002) suggested that countries should develop culturally appropriate guidelines for physical activity for older men and women and promote regular moderate physical activity for people as they age. To this end, for Europe and other Westernised countries, they produced the *Heidelberg Guidelines for Promoting Physical Activity Among Older Persons* in 1996. These suggested the types of activity that would be appropriate for older people. The current advice given in the UK is that adults:

- Should achieve a total of at least 30 minutes a day of at least moderate intensity physical activity on five or more days of the week. The recommended levels of activity can be achieved either by doing all the daily activity in one session, or through several shorter bouts of activity of 10 minutes or more. The activity can be any exercise that is performed as part of everyday life such as climbing stairs or brisk walking; or structured exercise or sport; or a combination of these.
- More specific activity recommendations for adults are made for beneficial effects for individual diseases and conditions. All movement contributes to energy expenditure and is important for weight management. It is likely that for many people, 45–60 minutes of moderate intensity physical activity a day is necessary to prevent obesity. For bone health, activities that produce high physical stresses on the bones are necessary.
- The recommendations for adults are also appropriate for older adults. Older people should take particular care to keep moving and retain their mobility through daily activity. Additionally, specific activities that promote improved strength, co-ordination and balance are particularly beneficial for older people.

(Department of Health Physical Activity, Health Improvement and Prevention, 2004)

Bromley, Sproston and Shelton (2005) showed that only 21 per cent of men and 15 per cent of women aged 65–74 years undertook this minimum recommended level. If older people can be encouraged to be moderately active the benefits include reduced risk of premature death, reduced risk of developing the major chronic diseases such as coronary heart disease, stroke, diabetes and cancers, delayed functional decline, better mobility, reduced risk and incidence of falls, increased bone health and lower blood pressure (WHO, 2002; Department of Health Physical Activity, Health Improvement and Prevention, 2004).

Exercise also has benefits for older people's mental health because active living improves mental health and often promotes social contacts (WHO, 2002). Being active can help older people remain as independent as possible for the longest period of time. It can also reduce the onset of chronic diseases in both healthy and chronically ill older people. For example, regular moderate physical activity reduces the risk of cardiac death by 20 to 25 per cent among people with established heart disease (Merz and Forrester, 1997). It can also substantially reduce the severity of disabilities associated with heart disease and other chronic illnesses (Department of Health Physical Activity, Health Improvement and Prevention, 2004). Exercise in later life can be both enjoyable and beneficial. Even in extreme old age, exercise can restore function in ways that make the difference between being safely independent at home and losing that independence (Expert Group on the Health of Older People, 2002).

What substances we take: smoking and alcohol

Smoking

WHO (2002) argue that smoking is the most important modifiable risk factor of all and state that action needs to be taken to encourage older people not to smoke and to provide older people with help to quit smoking. In the UK substantial effort has been made in the last 30 years to reduce smoking prevalence with some success. One effect of this is that the over 60s are more likely than younger people to have smoked at some time in their lives. However, they are also more likely than younger people to have given up. Only 12 per cent of over-65s smoked in 2006, the smallest proportion for any age group (Office of National Statistics, 2008). The Expert Group on the Health of Older People (2002) states that older smokers should be encouraged to try to stop and high-risk groups such as those with heart disease should be targeted for extra help in giving up smoking. Giving up, even in old age, still improves respiratory function and reduces the risk of stroke, heart disease and lung cancer. It seems that it is never too late to give up (Expert Group on the Health of Older People, 2002).

Alcohol

The relationship between alcohol intake and health outcomes is complex. It is clear though that the problems associated with hazardous or harmful alcohol consumption are numerous. Prolonged excessive alcohol intake contributes to liver disease, high blood pressure and some specific cancers (Wood and Bain, 2002). In addition, an increased risk of developing breast cancer, problems with sexual activity, an increased risk of contracting sexually transmitted disease, and being involved in an accident, are all forms of physical harm associated with lesser levels of consumption (WHO, 2004b). Insomnia, depression, anxiety, suicide, amnesia and dementia are all psychological forms of harm that can be caused by alcohol (Wood and Bain, 2002).

By contrast, there is some evidence that moderate, regular drinking can have some health benefits for men over the age of 40 and post-menopausal women (Wood and Bain, 2002). For example, Mukamal *et al.* (2003) reported that men who consumed alcohol on three or four days of the week had approximately one third the risk of a heart attack compared with those who drank alcohol less than one day per week. Alcohol use and abuse is clearly a health concern, but is it of relevance to older people? A number of related factors have combined to make this subject increasingly a matter of clinical and health research interest. The factors involved are:

- the increasing numbers of older people within the population (this alone will mean that there will be an apparent increase in older people involved in hazardous or harmful alcohol use);
- the fact that those who are involved in alcohol misuse are likely to survive beyond age 65 because of better treatment;
- the increasing amount of alcohol and substance abuse in those who are not yet over 65.

As a result it is expected that in future generations there will be increasing numbers of older people suffering the effects of hazardous or harmful alcohol use (Derry, 2000).

For several years now, reported statistics on harmful and hazardous drinking have been based on the recommended safe limit for alcohol consumption being 21 units of alcohol per week for men and 14 units of alcohol for women (Department of Health, 1995). It has been estimated that 17 per cent of men over 65 and 7 per cent of women over 65 exceed this amount (Alcohol Concern, 2007). Current recommendations, however, recommend consuming less than this, suggesting that men should not consistently drink more than three to four units of alcohol per day and women should drink no more than two to three units of alcohol per day. Most health agencies also recommend two or three alcohol-free days every week (NHS Quality Improvement Scotland, 2008). In the UK a unit of alcohol contains 8 g (10 ml) of ethanol. This is approximately the amount of alcohol contained in half a pint of 3.5 per cent beer or lager, or one 25 ml pub measure of spirits. A small (125 ml) glass of average strength (12 per cent) wine contains 1.5 units (SIGN, 2003).

WHO (2002) has also stated that efforts should be made to attempt to prevent and reduce alcohol and drug misuse in older people. This requires that health professionals should be able to identify and be aware of the possibility of problem drinking and substance misuse in older people and be ready to help. As the abuse of alcohol is a national concern, all four countries of the United Kingdom have policies aimed at reducing alcohol problems across society that health care professionals should be aware of. The current policies are listed in the recommended reading.

The risks we take with our eyesight and hearing

Avoiding sight loss

Sight loss is now a major health issue, affecting about two million people in the UK. Significant numbers of people also live with irremediable or certifiable sight loss estimates suggest that there could be around 980 000 (RNIB, 2008). Evidence suggests that over 50 per cent of sight loss is due to preventable or treatable causes; in the older population this figure may be as high as 70 per cent (Tate et al., 2005). The leading causes are age-related macular degeneration (AMD), glaucoma and diabetic retinopathy. The incidence of all three is increasing but the most marked increase is in diabetic retinopathy, where numbers have almost doubled since 1990 (Bunce and Wormold, 2006).

Clearly, priority needs to be given to reducing preventable vision loss and treating eye disease. The key to doing this is to improve diagnosis and early intervention because, detection of disease at an earlier stage, it enables more to be done to delay progression of disease. Early referral to an ophthalmologist, for example, is particularly important for patients with type 2 diabetes and those at risk of retinopathy, because laser treatment is associated with a 50 per cent reduction in the risk of severe visual loss

(Bosanquet and Mehta, 2008). The most effective thing that older adults can do to increase the likelihood of the early detection of eye problems is to have an eye test annually. An eye test can identify conditions such as glaucoma and AMD at an asymptomatic stage, allowing for early treatment and the avoidance of significant sight loss. However, only two-thirds of the adult population in the UK are having a regular eye test. Of particular concern is that, among those at increased risk of eye disease (those aged over 60), one in five has not had an eye test within the past two years (RNIB, 2006).

Also of concern is the low level of understanding of eye health issues and the purpose of an eye test. Of those people who have not had a test in the past two years, 64 per cent stated that this was because 'they did not have a problem with their eyes'. Failure to recognise the importance of regular eye testing is a symptom of a larger problem. Most people are unaware that there are risk factors that contribute to their chances of developing eye disease and that some of these risks can be reduced. The most obvious of these risk factors are smoking and obesity (RNIB, 2006).

Avoiding hearing loss

One in seven people in the UK is deaf or hard of hearing and most are older people who are gradually losing their hearing as part of the ageing process. More than 50 per cent of people over the age of 60 have some degree of hearing loss. A few have conductive hearing impairment (impairment related to abnormality in the external or middle ear), which can be caused by obstruction of the auditory canal by wax, which is easily treatable. For many though, it is permanent damage caused by infection, as occurs in Chronic Otitis Media (Tolson and Swan, 2006). Most age-related hearing impairments though are sensorineural losses (Tolson and Swan, 2006). Sensorineural hearing loss is related to damage to the inner ear, auditory nerves and particularly damage to the hair cells in the cochlea. Age-related hearing loss, also called Presbycusis, has a genetic component. Therefore, for some at risk of hearing loss as they age, there may be little that can be done at present. However, for many, their hearing loss is probably due to environmental factors (House of Lords Science and Technology Committee, 2005). The most significant factor is noise exposure. Most commonly in older people this has been noise pollution at work. However, growing numbers of people, including older people, have subjected their ears to potentially damaging noise by listening to music via personal headphones or from loud noise at concerts, noisy bars, clubs or discos. This damage builds up gradually and the effects may not be noticed until years later. The likelihood is that the number of older people affected by recreational noise will increase in future. You can prevent deafness due to noise by taking sensible, practical steps like using noise limiters or noise filters in audio devices to protect your hearing, and by reducing the length of time you listen to very loud sounds (RNID, 2008a).

Other factors that we are aware of that increase the risk of age-related hearing loss are drugs, infection and osteoporosis. A significant number of drugs are ototoxic and may cause damage to the inner ear, resulting in hearing loss, balance problems and tinnitus. Some antibiotics, aspirin and loop diuretics, for example furosemide and bumetanide, can cause deafness and tinnitus. Reducing drug use and avoiding the use of ototoxic drugs outside life-threatening situations may help some people avoid hearing loss. Bacterial and viral infectious diseases such as measles, cytomegaloviral disease, whooping cough, meningitis and acute otitis media (severe middle ear infection) can also cause mild to severe hearing loss. These may not be avoidable in old age but encouraging vaccination could have an impact on future numbers (Macnair and Hicks, 2008).

Age related hearing impairment develops slowly and people may be unaware that it is occurring until it begins to affect their daily lives. Therefore, it is important for all older people to be aware that if they think they have a hearing loss, the first thing they need to do is go to the GP. The hearing impairment they have may be easily treatable. If it is not, the GP will probably arrange an appointment at an audiology clinic (RNID, 2008b).

Nothing can be done at present to 'cure' deafness or hearing loss caused by ageing, but modern hearing aids can make a huge difference, making it possible to communicate with less stress and take a full part in everyday life. A hearing aid cannot give you perfect hearing, but wearing a hearing aid will make a real difference to an older person's quality of life. It should help them hear everyday sounds like the telephone and make it much easier for them to follow conversations. As a result, their confidence in talking to people should improve. However, only one in three people who could benefit from a hearing aid actually has one (House of Lords Science and Technology Committee, 2005).

What we do to try to avoid dementia-causing illnesses

The most significant risk factor for dementia is age and that, unfortunately, is unavoidable. There are, however, some things that can be done to reduce the risk of dementia-causing illnesses. Indications are that people who are obese are considerably more likely to develop dementia in later life. Therefore, if you adopt a healthy lifestyle and diet, one which reduces the risk of heart disease, hypertension and diabetes, you reduce the risk of developing a dementia (Gow and Gilhooly, 2003).

Staying mentally active and stimulated also appears to help. Activities that exercise and challenge, such as puzzles, playing games, learning new skills and even social activities that provide stimulation, may help stave off Alzheimer's disease, although the mechanism for this is unclear (Scarmeas et al., 2001). Activities that combine mental, physical and social stimulation may be even better, particularly since the maintenance of social networks and having an extensive social network seem to protect against dementia (Berkman, 2000).

Stopping smoking and participating in regular physical activity also appears to have an impact. This probably relates to reducing the risk of hypertension, heart attack, stroke and diabetes, which are all known risk factors for dementia (Gow and Gilhooly, 2003; Alzheimer's Scotland, 2006). Finally, avoid drinking excessive amounts of alcohol, as alcohol use is a known cause of some dementia illnesses and is also associated with vascular disease that can lead to vascular dementia (Ruitenberg et al., 2002). It is worth noting that these suggestions only reduce the risk of developing dementia; they will not mean that the person will definitely avoid it, particularly since two of the most significant risk factors are age and genetics. Furthermore, in order to have a significant impact on reducing overall risk, people are likely to have to make these changes from middle age (Gow and Gilhooly, 2003).

What we do to avoid depression

Older people live through lots of losses that can be contributory factors to depression. They may lose skills such as being able to drive and have physical illnesses, hearing or sight problems that prevent them from playing an active role in the community. They may also have lost loved ones, which can lead to their social network breaking down and lead them to becoming socially isolated (Department of Health, 2005). Depression can also occur because of sudden bereavement, retirement and separation factors such as loss of family contact or family disputes, a reduction in day-to-day callers, loss of functioning and mobility, fear due to increase in crime, and as a consequence of negative attitudes towards older people all of which reduce their levels of esteem (National Council on Ageing and Older People, 2005). Because of all these contributing factors, many older people accept depression as an inevitable part of ageing and, as a result, are less likely to seek help. They also have a poor perception of the help they are likely to receive (Department of Health, 2005). This is despite the fact that most depression responds well to current treatments (NICE, 2004).

Depression is a female-dominated illness but this is likely to be exaggerated because women are more likely to report depression than men, even though depression is undoubtedly the most common functional disorder affecting ageing males. Despite the slight predominance of women in terms of those affected by depression, it is men who are most successful at committing suicide. Indeed, suicide rates tend to rise with age so that, worldwide, the highest rates are seen in males over the age of 75 (WHO, 2001). Depression is often under-diagnosed and under-treated, particularly in older men who are less likely to seek professional help because of psychological problems (Baldwin *et al.*, 2002).

Perhaps the first action that needs to be taken then, with regard to the prevention of depression is more awareness of the nature of depression's signs, symptoms and management in older people, within the general population and throughout health professionals. Older people and health care professionals need to be aware that depression is not a normal part of ageing, should not be stigmatised and that it is very treatable (Hughes, 2006).

The second action to prevent depression is participation by the sufferer in regular physical exercise. A higher prevalence of depression is significantly associated with no regular physical exercise. Involvement in physical exercise is effective in the treatment of clinical depression and can be as successful as psychotherapy or medication, particularly in the longer term (Department of Health Physical Activity, Health Improvement and Prevention, 2004). It may also help people with generalised anxiety disorder, phobias, panic attacks and stress disorders, which may all feature in depressive illness. It can also help people feel better about themselves through improved physical self-perceptions and can improve self-esteem, particularly in those with initial low self-esteem. Physical activity also helps reduce physiological reactions to stress, particularly loss of sleep (Department of Health Physical Activity, Health Improvement and Prevention, 2004). Andrews (2001) points out that the social benefits of group exercise activities in later life should not be underestimated in a population where social isolation and loneliness may be common.

A third action for an older person to consider is to examine the level of social support that is available to them. Depression is less common in older people who have higher levels of social support. Having family and friends available for support and assistance can enhance coping and offer a buffer against stress and subsequent depression. This is probably because older people who have supportive friends or family have opportunities to discuss their difficulties and feelings with others (Vanderhorst and McLaren, 2005).

A fourth action for an older person to consider is the significance of their alcohol intake. Alcohol is a known depressant drug and can be another factor that predisposes people to depression. To avoid depression it would appear wise for the older person to restrict alcohol intake to the recommended limits (Bird and Parslow, 2002).

HEALTH AND WELLBEING IS NOT JUST ABOUT HEALTHY LIFESTYLE CHOICES

Health and wellbeing, however, is not just a question of making efforts to avoid the major causes of ill-health. In order to feel that you have good health and wellbeing you need to have autonomy, the will to live, have a meaning and purpose in life, be able to express your self creatively, feel a part of a greater whole, be aware of your own individuality and have vitality and energy (Rijke, 1993).

In recent years there has been great interest in what older people feel contributes positively to their health and wellbeing and quality of life (Audit Commission and Better Government for Older People, 2004; Gabriel and Bowling, 2004; Bowers et al., 2005; Age Concern and the Mental Health Foundation 2006). The findings of such reports have been very similar in that older people highlight the need to:

- maintain good health and physical functioning;
- maintain self-efficacy and have a sense of control over one's life;
- engage in a range of social activities and feel supported;
- have an adequate income;
- live in an area with good community facilities and services including transport;
- feel safe in one's neighbourhood.

It is clear from these findings that although looking after our health is important, what we do to stay active within our community in old age also has an impact on our health. Avoiding exclusion from social relations, civic activities and neighbourhood inclusion are all associated with good mental health and wellbeing (Scharf, Philipson and Smith, 2005). Participation in society can reduce older people's isolation, make them feel secure and increase their self esteem. Older people need to have a meaningful role in life that can provide a sense of purpose and identity, a reason to get out of the bed in the morning and something to care about (Age Concern and the Mental Health Foundation, 2006). Often older people want to make contributions to society but face barriers to participation in many areas of public and private life. For example, compulsory retirement results in a loss of role and a reduction in their social networks (Age Concern and the Mental Health Foundation, 2006). Fear of crime can also restrict activities and encourages social isolation, compromising mental health as a result (Stafford, Chandola and Marmot, 2007).

Older people want to maintain good health; they see this as fundamental to ensuring their quality of life (Gabriel and Bowling, 2004). Failing health may be an inevitable consequence of growing older, but many of the determinants of poor health can be avoided and preventative health care as a result has a huge role to play in reducing the burden of ill-health in older people (WHO, 2002).

PREVENTATIVE CARE

In order to have an impact on the chief health determinants that affect older people there has to be effective partnership working at all levels. This begins at government level. They have a particularly important role to play in adopting policies that reduce poverty, improve transport, tackle poor housing and prevent socially isolating poorer communities in particular (Department of Social Security for the Inter-Ministerial Group for Older People, 2001). Their policies have to make choosing healthy choices throughout life easier. That also requires the co-operation of food producers and the retail sector, transport and trade and therefore legislation and regulation is also required (WHO, 2005). There also has to be effective working between public health, health and social services, education, the voluntary sector and the general public in order to create partnerships and alliances that tackle social health determinants, not just for our older people but for us all (Age Concern and the Mental Health Foundation, 2006). WHO (2002) in their 'Healthy Ageing' policy document suggests a route to achieving this that involves wholesale changes in the way that we all consider old age at a personal, societal and governmental level, to which the EU and the UK Government need to remain committed. Health and social care professionals also need to work at a local level, consult with older people and allow older people to be involved at all levels of this process. Professionals need to understand older people's needs, their priorities and address their concerns. It is only by valuing their knowledge and skills and engaging with them, that we can hope to invest in improving their health and, consequently, our future health (Better Government for Older People, 2000). To alter older people's lifestyles significantly for the good, they have to be involved.

CONCLUSION

Health and wellbeing depends on your age, your genetics and a range of socioeconomic health determinants. These are factors that older people may have little control over, but are factors that society should address on their behalf. Health and wellbeing also depends on avoiding social exclusion (including ageism), maintaining control of decision making, having a role in society and adopting a healthy lifestyle (early enough to maintain your health in later years). This chapter has explored some of the major causes of morbidity and mortality and suggests some actions that individuals can take to maintain their health in later years. However, although adopting a healthy lifestyle can help, WHO (2002) have suggested that we need to go further and governments and health care professionals ought to pursue an agenda that promotes the idea of 'active ageing'. This involves wholesale changes in the way that we all consider old age at a personal, societal and governmental level. Health and social care professionals play an important role in this process. The WHO charges them with the task of providing appropriate health promotion to the over-50s and to champion the plight and the rights of older people worldwide. Health and social care professionals should view improving the health and wellbeing of older people as a noble purpose of benefit to us all. The lessons learned now will not only benefit the current generation, but have the potential to vastly improve the lives of future generations as they follow on the same journey.

FURTHER READING

Department of Health (2004) *Making Healthy Choices Easier*. London: The Stationery Office
This UK Government White Paper sets out the key principles for supporting the public in England to make healthier and more informed choices in regards to their health. It also details the NHS's role in this.

HM Government (2005) *Opportunity Age: Volume 2 A Social Portrait of Ageing in the UK*. London: HMSO
What is it like to grow old in the UK and what might be the experiences of the generation to follow? Drawing on a variety of research and statistics, this volume provides a snapshot of some of the key evidence on ageing

today in the UK and – where information is available – explores future trends.

World Health Organisation (2002) *Active Ageing; A Policy Framework*. Geneva: World Health Organisation Noncommunicable Disease Prevention and Health Promotion Ageing and Life Course. Downloadable from: **www.who. int/ageing/publications/active/en/index.html**

World Health Organisation (2005) *Preventing Chronic Diseases: A Vital Investment: WHO Global Report*. Geneva: WHO.
Downloadable from: **www.who.int/topics/chronic_disease/en**

The UK Alcohol Harm Reduction Strategies. In England, the national alcohol harm reduction strategy was first published in 2004. Currently, the Department of Health policy published in 2007 is called *Safe, Sensible, Social: The Next Steps in the National Alcohol Strategy*. The Scottish Government policy is the Scottish Executive (2007) *Plan for Action on Alcohol Problems (Update)*. *The Plan for Action on Alcohol Problems* (in Scotland) was originally published in 2002. Northern Ireland's policy is called the *New Strategic Direction (NSD) for Alcohol and Drugs 2006–2011*. The Welsh alcohol harm reduction policy is called *Working Together to Reduce Harm: The Substance Misuse Strategy for Wales 2008–2018*.

Useful websites

www.bgop.org.uk/home.aspx
Better Government for Older People: began in 1998 and aims to aid in the development of new approaches to enable public services in the UK to meet the needs of an ageing population.

www.poverty.org.uk
The Poverty Site: this is a UK site that holds UK statistics on poverty and social exclusion. This site is particularly relevant if you wish to explore issues surrounding the socioeconomic determinants of health.

www.mhilli.org
The UK Inquiry into Mental Health and Wellbeing in Later Life.

www.euro.who.int/ageing
The World Health Organisation Regional Office for Europe: Healthy Ageing Site.

www.healthyaging.net
The Healthy Aging Website: the site of a US-based campaign to provide an opportunity for organisations and individuals to help spread the word about successful ageing. The site provides a regular update of new tips and techniques for positive ageing.

REFERENCES

Age Concern and the Mental Health Foundation (2006) *Promoting Mental Health and Well-being in Later Life: A First Report from the UK Inquiry into Mental Health and Well-Being in Later Life.* London: Age Concern

Alcohol Concern (2007) *Factsheet: Alcohol Misuse Among Older People.* London: Alcohol Concern

Alzheimer's Scotland (2006) *Dementia – How to Reduce your Risk.* Edinburgh: Alzheimer's Scotland

Alzheimer's Society (2007) *Dementia UK: A Report into the Prevalence and Cost of Dementia Prepared by the Personal Social Services Research Unit (PSSRU) at the London School of Economics and the Institute of Psychiatry at King's College London, for the Alzheimer's Society.* London: Alzheimer's Society

Andrews, G.R. (2001) Promoting Health and Function in an Ageing Population. *British Medical Journal,* 322: 728–9

Audit Commission and Better Government for Older People (2004) *Older People – Independence and Well-being: The Challenge for Public Services.* London: Audit Commission

Baldwin, R.C., Chiu, E., Katona, C. and Graham, N. (2002) *Guidelines on Depression in Older People: Practising the Evidence.* London: Martin Dunitz

Berkman, L. (2000) 'Which influences cognitive function: Living alone or being alone?' *The Lancet,* 355: 1291–2

Better Government for Older People (2000) *All Our Futures: The Report of the BGOP Steering Committee.* Wolverhampton: Better Government for Older People Programme

Bird, M.J. and Parslow, R.A. (2002) 'Potential for community programmes to prevent depression in older adults'. *Medical Journal of Australia,* 177 (7 Supplement): S107–S110

Bosanquet, N. and Mehta, P. (2008) *Evidence Base to Support the UK Vision Strategy.* Essex: Vision 2020 UK **www.vision2020uk.org.uk/news.asp?new sID=1140&section=000100050006** (Accessed 21 May 2008)

Bowers, H., Eastman, M., Harris, J. and Macadam, A. (2005) *Moving Out of the Shadows: A Report on Mental Health and Well-being in Later Life.* London: Help and Care Development Ltd

Bromley, C., Sproston, K. and Shelton, N. (2005) *The Scottish Health Survey 2003: Volume 2: Adults.* Edinburgh: Scottish Executive Health Department

Bunce, C. and Wormold, R. (2006) 'Leading causes for certification of blindness and partial sight in England and Wales'. *BMC Public Health,* 6: 58.

Cancer Research UK (2006a) *Cancer Stats – Incidence – UK.* London: Cancer Research UK. **http://publications.cancerresearchuk.org/epages/crukstore. sf/en_GB/?ObjectPath=/Shops/crukstore/Categories/BrowseByType/ CancerStatsReport** (Accessed 26 March 2008)

Cancer Research UK (2006b) *Cancer Stats – Mortality – UK.* London: Cancer Research UK **http://publications.cancerresearchuk.org/epages/crukstore. sf/en_GB/?ObjectPath=/Shops/crukstore/Categories/BrowseByType/ CancerStatsReport** (Accessed 26 March 2008)

Cowley, S. (2006) 'Health promotion for older people' in Redfern, S.J. and Ross,

F.M. (eds) *Nursing Older People* (4th edn). Edinburgh: Elsevier/Churchill Livingstone

Department of Health (1995) *Sensible Drinking. The Report of an Inter-Departmental Working Group.* London: Department of Health

Department of Health (2005) *Better Health in Old Age.* London: Department of Health

Department of Health Physical Activity, Health Improvement and Prevention (2004) *At Least Five a Week: Evidence on the Impact of Physical Activity and Its Relationship to Health: A Report from the Chief Medical Officer.* London: The Stationery Office

Department of Social Security for the Inter-Ministerial Group for Older People (2001) *Building on Partnership: The Government Response to the Recommendations of the Better Government for Older People Programme.* Hayes: Welfare Reform

Derry, A.D. (2000) 'Substance use in older adults: A review of current assessment, treatment and service provision'. *Journal of Substance Use*, 5: 252–62

Expert Group on the Health of Older People (2002) *Adding Life to Years: Report of the Expert Group on the Healthcare of Older People.* Edinburgh: Scottish Executive

Ewles, L. and Simnett, I. (2003) *Promoting Health: a Practical Guide* (5th edn). Edinburgh: Bailliere Tindall

Finch, S., Doyle, W., Lowe, C., Bates, C.J., Prentice, A., Smithers, G. *et al.* (1998) *National Diet and Nutrition Survey: People Aged 65 years and Over.* London: The Stationery Office

Food Standards Agency (2008) E*at Well, Be Well: Ages and Stages: Older People.* **www.eatwell.gov.uk/agesandstages/olderpeople** (Accessed 27 November 2008)

Gabriel, Z. and Bowling, A. (2004) 'Quality of life from the perspectives of older people'. *Ageing and Society*, 24: 675–91

Grundy, E. and Sloggett, A. (2003) 'Health inequalities in the older population: the role of personal capital, social resources and socioeconomic circumstances'. *Social Science and Medicine*, 56: 935–47

Government Office for Science (2007) *Foresight: Tackling Obesities – Future Choices: Project Report (Second Edition).* London: Department of Innovation, Universities and Skills

Gow, J. and Gilhooly, M. (2003) *Risk Factors for Dementia and Cognitive Decline.* Edinburgh: NHS Health Scotland

HM Government (2005) *Opportunity Age: Volume 2 – A Social Portrait of Ageing in the UK.* London: HMSO

House of Lords Science and Technology Committee (2005) *Ageing: Scientific Aspects: Volume I, Report.* London: The Stationery Office

Hughes, C. (2006) 'Chapter 25: Depression in older people' in Redfern, S.J. and Ross, F.M. (eds) *Nursing Older People* (4th edn). Edinburgh: Elsevier/ Churchill Livingstone

Knowler, W.C., Barret-Connor, E., Fowler, S.E., *et al.* (2002) 'Reduction in the incidence of Type 2 Diabetes with lifestyle intervention or metformin'. *New England Journal of Medicine*, 346 (6): 393–403

Lee, M. (2006) *Promoting Mental Health and Well-Being in Later Life: A First Report from the UK Inquiry into Mental Health and Well-Being in Later Life.* London: Age Concern and the Mental Health Foundation

Lindstrom, J., Ilanne-Parikka, P., Peltonen, M., *et al.* (2006) 'Sustained reduction in the incidence of Type 2 Diabetes by lifestyle intervention: Follow-up of the Finnish Diabetes Prevention Study'. *Lancet,* 368 (9548): 1637–39

Macnair, T. and Hicks, R (2008) Health Conditions: Deafness and Hearing Problems. **www.bbc.co.uk/health/conditions/deafness1.shtml** (Accessed 21 May 2008)

Merz, C.N. and Forrester, J.S. (1997) 'The secondary prevention of coronary heart disease'. *American Journal of Medicine,* 102: 573–80

Mukamal, K.J. Conigrave, K.M. Mittleman, M.A. Camargo, C.A. Stampfer, M.J. Willet W.C. and Rimm E.B.(2003) 'Roles of drinking pattern and type of alcohol consumed in coronary heart disease in men'. *New England Journal of Medicine,* 348 (2): 109–18

Naidoo, J. and Wills, J. (2000) *Health Promotion: Foundations for Practice* (2nd edn). Edinburgh: Bailliere Tindall

National Council on Ageing and Older People (2005) *Loneliness and Social Isolation Among Older Irish People.* Report no. 84. Dublin: NCAOP

National Institute for Clinical Excellence (2004) *Clinical Guideline 23: Depression: Management of Depression in Primary and Secondary Care.* London: NICE

National Institute for Health and Clinical Excellence (2006) *Clinical Guideline 43: Obesity: Guidance on the Prevention, Identification, Assessment and Management of Overwieght and Obesity in Adults and Children.* London: NICE

NHS Centre For Reviews and Dissemination (2002) 'Improving the recognition and management of depression in primary care'. *Effective Health Care,* 7 (5): 1–12

NHS Quality Improvement Scotland (2008) *Understanding Alcohol Misuse in Scotland: Harmful Drinking: Final Report.* Edinburgh: NHS QIS

Office of National Statistics (2008) *Society: Smoking Habits in Great Britain.* **www.statistics.gov.uk/cci/nugget.asp?id=313** (Accessed 20 March 2008)

Office of National Statistics (2004) *Living in Britain 2002.* London: Office of National Statistics

Office of National Statistics (2006) *Focus on Health: Mortality: Circulatory Diseases – Leading Cause Group.* **ww.statistics.org.uk/CCI/nugget.asp?ID=1337&Pos=24&ColRank=1000** (Accessed 27 November 2008)

Palmer, G., MacInnes, T. and Kenway, P. (2007) *Monitoring Poverty and Social Exclusion 2007.* York: Joseph Rowntree Foundation

Rijke, R. (1993) 'Health in medical science, from determinism towards autonomy' in Lafalle, R. and Fulder, S. (eds) *Towards a New Science of Health.* Abingdon: Routledge

Royal College of Physicians (1998) *Clinical Management of Overweight and Obese Patients with Particular Reference to the Use of Drugs.* London: RCP

Royal National Institute for the Blind (2006) *Campaign Report 25: Open Your Eyes: A Call for Action to Address the UK's Eye Health Crisis.* London: RNIB

Royal National Institute for the Blind (2008) *Research: Statistics: Numbers of People With Sight Problems by Age Group in the UK.* **www.rnib.org.uk/ xpedio/groups/public/documents/PublicWebsite/public_researchstats. hcsp#P216_14802** (Accessed 21 May 2008)

Royal National Institute for the Deaf (2006) *Information and Resources: Statistics.* **www.rnid.org.uk/information_resources/aboutdeafness/ statistics/statistics.htm#age** (Accessed 21 May 2008)

Royal National Institute for the Deaf (2008a) *Information and Resources: Noise.* **www.rnid.org.uk/information_resources/aboutdeafness/causes/noise** (Accessed 21 May 2008)

Royal National Institute for the Deaf (2008b) *Information and Resources: Hearing Tests.* **www.rnid.org.uk/information_resources/hearing_aids/ hearing_tests** (Accessed 21 May 2008)

Ruitenberg, A., van Swieten, J.C., Witteman, J.C., Mehta, K.M., van Duijn, C.M., Hofman, A. and Breteler, M.M.B. (2002) 'Alcohol consumption and risk of dementia: the Rotterdam study'. *The Lancet*, 359: 281–6

Scarmeas, N., Levy, G., Tang, M.X., Manly, J. and Stern, Y. (2001) 'Influence of leisure activity on the incidence of Alzheimer's Disease'. *Neurology*, 57: 2236–42

Scharf, T., Philipson, C., Smith, A.E. and Kingston, P. (2002) *Growing Older in Socially Deprived Areas: Social Exclusion in Later Life.* London: Help the Aged

Scharf, T., Philipson, C. and Smith, A.E. (2005) 'Social exclusion of older people in deprived urban communities in England'. *European Journal of Ageing.* 2 (2): 765–87

Squire, A. (2002) *Health and Wellbeing for Older People: Foundations for Practice.* Edinburgh: Bailliere Tindall

Stafford, M., Chandola, T. and Marmot, M. (2007) 'Association between fear of crime, and mental health and physical functioning'. *American Journal of Public Health*, 97 (11): 2076–81

Tate, R., Smeeth, L., Evans, J., Fletcher, A., Owen, C. and Rudnicka, A. (2005) *The Prevalence of Visual Impairment in the UK: A Literature Review.* London: Royal National Institute for the Blind

Tolson, D. and Swan, I.R.C. (2006) 'Hearing' in Redfern, S.J. and Ross, F.M. (eds) *Nursing Older People* (4th edn). Edinburgh: Elsevier/Churchill Livingstone

Vanderhorst, R.K. and Mc.Laren, S. (2005) 'Social relationships as predictors of depression and suicidal ideation in older adults'. *Aging and Mental Health*, 9 (6): 517–25

Van der Kooy, K., van Hout, H., Marwijk, H., Marten, H., Stehouwer C. and Beekman, A. (2007) 'Depression and the risk for cardiovascular diseases: systematic review and meta-analysis'. *International Journal of Geriatric Psychiatry*, 22: 613–26

Wood, R. and Bain, M.R.S. (2002) *The Health and Well-being of Older People in Scotland: Insights from the National Data.* Edinburgh: Information and Statistics Division, Common Services Agency for NHS Scotland

World Health Organisation (1996) *The Heidelberg Guidelines for Promoting*

Physical Activity Among Older Persons. Geneva: WHO Ageing and Health Programme

World Health Organisation (2001) *Men, Ageing and Health. Achieving Health Across the Lifespan*. Geneva: World Health Organisation Noncommunicable Disease and Mental Health Cluster, Non-communicable Disease and Health Promotion Department and the Ageing and Life Course Unit

World Health Organisation (2002) *Active Ageing: A Policy Framework*. Geneva: World Health Organisation Noncommunicable Disease Prevention and Health Promotion Ageing and Life Course Unit

World Health Organisation (2004a) *The World Health Report*. Geneva: WHO

World Health Organisation (2004b) *Global Status Report on Alcohol 2004*. Geneva: World Health Organisation, Department of Mental Health and Substance Abuse.

World Health Organisation (2005) *Preventing Chronic Diseases: A Vital Investment: WHO Global Report*. Geneva: WHO

WHO Expert Consultation (2004) Appropriate Body-mass Index for Asian Populations and its Implications for Policy and Intervention Strategies. *The Lancet*, 363 (10): 157–63.

Chapter 13

Promoting Mental Health and Wellbeing

Billy Mathers

Learning outcomes

Reading this chapter will enable you to:

- have an understanding of what mental health and wellbeing is and why it is necessary in everyday practice;

- have an understanding of how to apply strategies for mental health promotion in practice;

- have a better understanding of possible triggers of mental health problems in the older adult.

INTRODUCTION

The issues discussed in this chapter are important not least because of the changing demographics of the UK. As described in Chapter 2, according to the UK Government's standard documents the population is expected to live longer.

One of these documents also indicates that people over 50 begin to experience circumstances that may adversely affect their mental health. For example, many people start to change their working patterns and some cease employment completely. This can have the effect of lowering their self-esteem and sense of achievement as well as reducing their financial independence. Children may leave home, which reduces the older adult's influence within the family, another possible trigger of reduced self-esteem. They may also be required to assume caring responsibilities for their older relatives, perhaps for the first time. In addition they may become more likely to develop long-term or even terminal health conditions. As people age, the chances of losing a spouse or partner also increase, which may add the possibility of loneliness and social isolation. All these factors combine to increase the older adult's possibility of suffering from depression or suicidal ideation. It has been suggested that around 10–15 per cent of the population aged 65 and over will have depression at any given time (Department of Health, 2001a).

Thus, although mental illnesses such as the dementias are most commonly found in the older adult, it does not mean that older adults' mental health problems are restricted only to the dementias. This chapter will focus upon depression and its age-specific issues. Given the high incidence of mental health problems in old age and the growing older adult population, it is clear that mental health promotion strategies in everyday practice are of growing importance. In a recent report, the National Institute for Mental Health in England (2005) has stated that there is wide acknowledgement that the mental health and wellbeing of older people has been neglected across the spectrum of promotion, prevention and treatment services, which further underlines the need for strategies for health promotion in this age group.

REVIEW OF CURRENT LITERATURE

This literature review will briefly examine studies undertaken in the area of health promotion in mental health in the general population and will then proceed to focus more specifically on mental health promotion for the older adult. Key reports relating to mental health and wellbeing for the older adult and the conclusions drawn from these reports will be examined.

Mental health promotion in the general population

The terms mental health and mental illness are often used interchangeably but they are not the same. In this chapter the words mental health and wellbeing are used to emphasise the positive aspects of mental health. Recent UK legislation emphasises the priority that is being given to health promotion in the area of mental health and wellbeing. Standard One of The National Service Framework for Mental Health (Department of Health, 1999) included a clear remit to health and social services to promote mental health for all by working with individuals and communities. The Standard also states that these services should seek to combat discrimination against individuals and groups with mental health problems and to promote their social inclusion.

According to the UK guidance document on mental health promotion *Making It Happen – A Guide to Delivering Mental Health Promotion* (Department of Health, 2001b) the inclusion of Standard One in the National Service Framework for Mental Health puts mental health promotion centre-stage. The guide seeks to define mental health and mental health promotion and makes the case for investing in mental health promotion while showing how mental health promotion fits in with other policy initiatives.

Some research has offered insights into the essential components of mental health promotion. Mann *et al.* (2004) present evidence that a high level of self-esteem results in better health and social interaction, and that low self-esteem can result in wide-ranging mental health problems like depression, suicidal tendencies, eating disorders and anxiety, among others. In their discussion of the dynamics of self-esteem in relationships, they argue that an understanding of the development of self-esteem, its outcomes and promotion are necessary for the improvement of mental health. They also suggest that focussing on self-esteem is a central component of mental health promotion.

McElroy (2004) continues this theme as he stresses the need for self-esteem as a tool for mental health promotion.

> A person will value his or her self as they perceive others value or demean them. The end result is that individuals will conceive of themselves as having the characteristics and values that others attribute to them. Relationships are therefore a particularly important factor in the care of patients with low self-esteem. The interactions patients have with staff are integral to the enhancement, or otherwise, of their self-esteem. (p. 477)

The importance of positive self-esteem for good mental health is underlined by another health promotion theorist. 'The most basic task for one's mental, emotional and social health, which begins in infancy and continues until one dies, is the construction of his/her positive self-esteem' (Macdonald, 1994: 19).

Mental health promotion for the older adult

This theme of self-esteem as a mental health promotion strategy is continued by theorists of the care of the older adult. A study by Edwards and Chapman (2004) suggests that most interactions tend to be used by staff as a means of control, which results in a lack of self-esteem. Thus, the older adult remains dependent upon staff and lacks autonomy.

The same authors continue to suggest that mental wellness through self-esteem for older adults can be promoted through good communication. They present a four-component model of contemplating, caring, coping and conversing. They stress the importance of interpersonal communication processes in the care of older adults and some barriers to communication and mental wellness are briefly reviewed. This model challenges health professionals to develop awareness of their own care-giving styles and communication processes, and to assist others to communicate more effectively to advance mental wellness for older adults.

Self-esteem as opposed to low self-worth is a key component in research into mental health promotion for the older adult described by Bernard (2000). An effective teaching course in 'Mental Fitness' for the older adult is then described. This emphasises good communication leading to increased self-esteem. Hummert and Nussbaum (2001) have posited that there is a strong relationship between interpersonal communication and the maintenance of health during ageing and the process of communication is key to the ageing process.

A major UK-wide inquiry into mental health and the older adult, *Promoting Mental Health and Well-Being in Later Life*, has recently been completed by Age Concern, a leading pressure group (Lee, 2006). This inquiry examined existing evidence and gathered new information from a range of sources, including older people and carers. Together with the views of nearly 150 organisations and professionals, the findings in this report draw on the views of nearly 900 older people and carers on what helps to promote good mental health and wellbeing in later life. In addition to this evidence, focus groups with older people from minority groups were conducted.

The conclusions drawn from the evidence gathered in this inquiry were that there are five main areas that influence mental health and wellbeing in later life. These areas are described as discrimination, participation in meaningful activity, relationships, physical health and poverty.

The report continues to outline good reasons why society in general can benefit from the good mental and physical health of the older adult population. The majority of older people in the UK are healthy and happy and make valuable contributions to society and to the economy. Working people aged 50 and over contribute around a quarter of the total

British economy and their unpaid contributions as volunteers and carers contribute around 2.9 per cent of the nation's economic output. As the UK population ages, older people's contributions to the economy will become even more important, as will their contributions to their families and communities. Promoting good mental health and wellbeing in later life is essential to ensure that these contributions are maximised.

In contrast, the report goes on to outline the cost to the nation of poor mental health for older adults. For example, 0.5 per cent of people over 65 have some form of psychosis, 5 per cent have dementia and 20–25 per cent have depression severe enough to warrant intervention. Mental health problems among older people increase to 50 per cent in hospitals and 60 per cent in care homes. Thus, the report demonstrates the cost to the nation and, quite apart from the humanitarian aspects, argues that it is in the nation's economic interest to promote good mental health to prevent older adults from becoming unwell.

Case study

Iain MacLeod is a 75-year-old widower who lives alone in a council flat. He retired from his job as a van driver ten years ago. After retirement, he enjoyed regular involvement with his local bowls club, but this involvement has been greatly reduced since the death of his wife six years ago. He was prescribed anti-depressants shortly after this but his GP thinks he did not adhere to these for long. His low mood and depression worsened when he was diagnosed with diabetes five years ago. He administers his oral diabetic medication himself and is visited once a week by his District Nurse, Fiona, who advises on diet, monitors the effects and side-effects of his medication as well as his mental state and his social functioning. She also dresses Iain's leg ulcer, a side effect of his diabetes.

Fiona reports that currently Iain copes well with his medication but his low mood means he neglects his diet and social functioning. Most recently, she has noticed an increase in the amount of dirty dishes in the sink and suspects that Iain is not changing his clothes as often as he used to. He eats mainly takeaway meals or canned food, which he heats up on his electric stove. She feels Iain is depressed and potentially suicidal, although he has always denied suicidal ideation. Fiona has offered to bring a psychiatrist with her to assess his psychological functioning, but Iain has refused, saying he feels 'fine'.

Archie, the secretary from the bowls club, visits occasionally to encourage him to attend the club, but at the moment Iain shows no inclination, saying the fees are too expensive, although he says he enjoys Archie's visits. He enjoys a good relationship with his daughter, Alison, but she is married and lives 30 miles away, which means she can only visit once a week. Alison feels her father has never really recovered from the death of her mother. She also worries about his financial situation as he is only in receipt of the state pension. She tries to help him keep up-to-date with his bills but is aware that some of his mail lies unopened for long periods and results in 'final demands' for utilities having to be hurriedly settled, often by Alison herself. He collects his pension from the local Post Office himself and, although he has a small savings account in the local bank, he has little deposited in this as he finds it difficult to save on his state pension.

Reflection

- Depression is common among older adults. Referring to the information about depression in the older adult in the introduction section of this chapter, consider some of the factors in Iain's circumstances in the case study above which may cause him to be depressed.
- What steps do you think Fiona, the District Nurse, might take to promote a sense of mental health and wellbeing in Iain? You should think about interventions which she might carry out herself as well as referrals to other agencies. You can check your answers with the suggestions in the 'conclusions' section at the end of the chapter.
- One of the conclusions drawn from the evidence gathered in the Help the Aged report (Lee, 2006) was that there are five main areas that influence mental health and wellbeing in later life. One of these areas is described as 'discrimination'. Although there is no evidence from the case study that Fiona is discriminatory in her attitude to Iain, what aspects of her interactions with Iain might she need to pay particular attention to in order to ensure she avoids discriminatory behaviour? Once again, you can check your answer with the suggestions in the 'conclusions' section at the end of the chapter.

THE SERVICE USER'S PERSPECTIVE

It has become increasingly clear in recent years in the field of mental health that the service user's perspective is of vital importance. There is a growing realisation that individuals who have encountered mental health problems have a unique story to tell and this story needs to be listened to if these problems are to be addressed. One mental health service user talks about the need for psychiatric services to move from 'containment' towards 'therapeutic experience'. She calls for all health care professionals to be less mechanical in their interactions with mentally ill patients (Whitehill, 2003).

The consultation with older adult service users referred to in Chapter 1 provides some insights into how health professionals may need to change their approach in their communications with older adults. 'A professional approach, e.g., don't use my Christian name without asking me.' 'Whilst caring, talk to me, even though I feel I may not be able to reply. It isn't always possible to know what people may still understand.' 'More time to listen to my expectations and requirements and explore what is possible.' 'Listening ability without preconceived anticipation on conclusions about individual clients.' 'I value their time to listen and explain.'

The above comments are chiefly concerned with the need for effective communication. They remind us that good communication is particularly important with the older adult who may have mental health problems. This is because both the ageing process and psychological problems often curtail the individual's ability to communicate effectively. It is thus incumbent upon the health professional to pay particular attention to this aspect of the service user's care.

IMPLICATIONS FOR JOINT WORKING

Government guidelines like the National Service Framework for Mental Health (NSF) Department of Health (1999), emphasise the need for interdisciplinary working in the health service in general, and this is especially true in the mental health arena since there are so many contributing factors to mental disorder. The input of social workers is important because of the possible contribution of poor social conditions to the mental disorder of many people. The NSF (Department of Health, 1999) also indicates that the need for good housing and adequate finances is crucial and this is a major concern for social workers.

Occupational therapists assess the daily living skills of mentally ill patients. This has become especially important in recent years due to the move from institutions into the community. The ability to cook and budget for shopping is essential for community-based patients like Iain above and this is a key role for occupational therapists. Medical staff have a key role in the diagnosis and prescribing of medication. Nursing staff will administer intramuscular medication and monitor its effects and side effects and also assess and monitor mental and social functioning.

It is imperative that all disciplines communicate fully so that information is passed freely and a high standard of service can be provided. Furthermore, this is important for the safety of the public as there have been a number of patients suffering from mental illness involved in incidents of both homicide and suicide (Onyett, 2002). One strategy to facilitate this communication has been to develop Community Mental Health Teams (CMHTs). These are interdisciplinary and inter-agency in nature and feature all disciplines working together under one roof, offering a one stop seamless service to the mentally ill in the community. An evaluation by Simmonds *et al.* (2001) found such teams to be delivering many of the results which were desired – reduced inpatient stays, better engagement with services and reduction in suicides. Partnership working in such

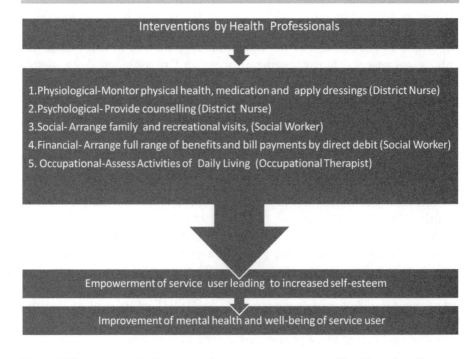

Interventions by Health Professionals

1. Physiological-Monitor physical health, medication and apply dressings (District Nurse)
2. Psychological-Provide counselling (District Nurse)
3. Social-Arrange family and recreational visits, (Social Worker)
4. Financial-Arrange full range of benefits and bill payments by direct debit (Social Worker)
5. Occupational-Assess Activities of Daily Living (Occupational Therapist)

Empowerment of service user leading to increased self-esteem

Improvement of mental health and well-being of service user

Figure 1 The ways in which joint working can promote mental health and wellbeing

teams requires flexibility and the willingness to share job descriptions to some extent for the team to work cohesively. Figure 1 illustrates the ways in which joint working could promote mental health and wellbeing in relation to Iain, the service user in the case study.

CONCLUSION

Older adults may have a wide range of mental health problems. These include:

- possible institutionalisation after a stay in a psychiatric hospital;
- negative symptoms of schizophrenia;
- dementia;
- depression which may be linked to suicidal ideation.

In this chapter we have focussed on depression in the older adult and have noted that health professionals have a key role in promoting mental health and wellbeing with such individuals. The case study demonstrates that the older adult is at high risk of depression due to a variety of demographic factors and health determinants.

There is a wide range of interventions that the health professional in the case study, Fiona, would have been able to carry out in her role as a district nurse to promote mental health and wellbeing. She would also have been able to make referrals to other agencies to achieve this.

Fiona's main role is in monitoring the effects of Iain's medication and diet in controlling his diabetes. Where this is done effectively, it will have the effect of improving his physical health, which, in turn can have a positive effect on self-esteem and promotion of mental wellbeing. During her visit, Fiona could also spend time talking to Iain about his problems and allow him to give vent to his feelings, which may lift his mood, knowing that someone is interested in his problems. The use of Rogerian counselling skills like open-ended questioning (Rogers, 2002) would help to facilitate this.

There are many other issues that Fiona could address indirectly by referral to other agencies. The lack of finance is often a challenge to an older adult's self-esteem and can greatly limit their social interaction due to inability to pay fees and cover travel and meal costs. Referring Iain to a social worker might result in him receiving further state benefits to which he is entitled but which at present he is not receiving like, for example, attendance allowance. This extra finance could allow Alison, his daughter, to visit more often and lengthen her visits, as it is possible for individuals to receive attendance allowance even when they live alone.

The social worker might also be able to arrange for Iain's bills to be paid by direct debit through his bank if a current account could be opened. This might result in greater peace of mind for Iain and raise his mood as result. The general improvement in his finances overall might also allow him to socialise more, for example, at the bowls club, which he has complained was too expensive for him in the past. Such social networks are extremely important in promoting mental wellbeing.

Fiona could also refer Iain to social services for home carer visits. The home carers would be able to provide help with general household chores such as washing dishes and laundry, promoting both Iain's physical and mental wellbeing as a result. Help with cooking and the choice of meals could also be offered, thus improving his diet, another key factor in mental health promotion.

Fiona could also safeguard herself against age discrimination in her interactions with Iain by some simple strategies, such as showing self-awareness. Self awareness is being able to view ourselves from another person's perspective and is a key component in interpersonal relationships (Donnelly and Neville, 2008). For example, she could think about her manner and tone of voice with Iain to guard against a patronising approach.

A humanistic approach, believing that the individual has the ability to solve their own problems within a supportive relationship, would also help (Rogers, 2002). Too often a paternalistic 'top down' approach has been adopted by health professionals and this is especially true when the individual is older. Fiona should remember that Iain still has the capacity to make many choices for himself and should encourage this whenever possible and appropriate.

This chapter outlines the unique challenges presented by the older adult with mental health problems. It acknowledges that the older adult may be at higher risk of depression than the general population. Such problems require specific and skilled interventions from mental health professionals including health promotion strategies such as those discussed.

FURTHER READING

Barker, P. (1997) *Assessment in Psychiatric and Mental Health Nursing – In Search of the Whole Person*. Cheltenham: Stanley Thornes
A standard text on assessment in mental health.

Barker, P. (2004) *Psychiatric and Mental Health Nursing: The Craft of Caring*. London: Hodder Arnold
This is a comprehensive mental health textbook and contains useful chapters from a mental health service user perspective.

Norman, I. and Ryrie, I. (2004) *The Art and Science of Mental Health Nursing*. Maidenhead: Open University Press/McGraw-Hill
This text contains chapters in key areas in mental health including a chapter on mental health promotion.

Stuart, G.W. and Laraia, M.T. (2005) *Principles and Practice of Psychiatric Nursing*. St. Louis, MI: Elsevier/Mosby
A well-respected mental health textbook containing a section on mental health promotion.

Useful websites

www.ageconcern.org.uk
A general website for the older adult, including mental health issues.

www.psychology.wichita.edu/surl/usabilitynews/61/older_adults.htm
A website focussing upon psychological issues in old age.

www.nihseniorhealth.gov
A more general older adult website but with information about mental health issues.

www.oasisnet.org
A website focussing upon psychological issues in old age.

www.aging.pitt.edu/seniors/resources/general.asp
A more general older adult website but with information about mental health issues.

REFERENCES

Bernard, M. (2000) *Promoting Health in Old Age*. Buckingham: Open University Press
Department of Health (1999) *National Service Framework for Mental Health*. London: Department of Health

Department of Health (2001a) *National Service Framework for Older People*. London: Department of Health

Department of Health (2001b) *Making It Happen: A Guide to Delivering Mental Health Promotion*. London: Department of Health

Donnelly, E. and Neville, L. (2008) *Communication and Interpersonal Skills*. Exeter: Reflect Press

Edwards, H. and Chapman, H. (2004) 'Contemplating, caring, coping, conversing: a model for promoting mental wellness in later life'. *Journal of Gerontological Nursing*, 30 (5): 16–21

Hummert, M.L. and Nussbaum, J. (2001) 'Introduction' in Hummert. M.L. and Nussbaum, J. (eds) *Successful Aging, Communication and Health*. Mahweh, NJ: Lawrence Erlbaum Associates

Lee, M. (2006) *Promoting Mental Health and Well-Being in Later Life: A First Report from the UK Inquiry into Mental Health and Well-Being in Later Life*. London: Help the Aged

Mann, M., Hosman, C., Schaalma, H.K. and de Vries, N. (2004) 'Self-esteem in a broad spectrum approach for mental health'. *Health Education Research*, 4 (10): 357–72

Macdonald, G. (1994) 'Self-esteem and the promotion of mental health' in Trent, D. and Reed, C. (eds), *Promotion of Mental Health*. Aldershot: Avebury

McElroy, A. (2004) 'Suicide prevention and the broad-spectrum approach to health promotion'. *Health Education Research*, 19, (4): 476–80

National Institute for Mental Health in England (2005) *Making it Possible: Improving Mental Health and Well-Being in England*. London: National Institute for Mental Health in England

Onyett, S. (2002) *Teamworking in Mental Health*. Basingstoke: Palgrave

Rogers, C.R. (2002) *Client-Centred Therapy*. London: Constable.

Scottish Executive (2007) *All Our Futures: Planning for a Scotland with an Ageing Population*. Edinburgh: Scottish Government

Simmonds, S., Coid, J., Joseph, P., Marriott, S. and Tyrer, P. (2001) 'Community mental health team management in severe mental illness: a systematic review'. *British Journal of Psychiatry*, 178: 497–502

Whitehill, I. (2003) 'The concept of recovery', in Barker, P. (ed.) *Psychiatric and Mental Health Nursing: The Craft of Caring*. London: Hodder Arnold

Chapter 14

Promoting Physical Health

Graham Harris

Learning outcomes

Reading this chapter will enable you to:

- explain the current emphasis on health promotion in later life and identify the opportunities that may exist to promote older people's physical health;

- discuss the knowledge, skills and qualities required to promote older people's health and how these may differ from those needed for other age groups;

- explain the kinds of health promoting interventions that are likely to be successful when working with older people;

- apply your knowledge and skills to a specific case study and highlight a range of measures to enhance older people's physical health and wellbeing.

INTRODUCTION

The promotion of health and active living has long been identified as a priority in the care of older people. Recent British health policy continues with this emphasis – indeed it is evident in publications such as the Scottish *Let's Make Scotland More Active* Strategy (The Stationery Office, 2003) and the Welsh and English National Service Frameworks (NSF) for Older People (Department of Health, 2001; Health Care Alliance, 2003). In fact, in the latter, promoting health and an active life is the ultimate standard to be achieved (Department of Health, 2001).

However, according to Squire (2002), in practice, health promotion is often neglected or dismissed as being of little value. Sometimes, it seems, there is an attitude of '*why bother?*' where older people are concerned and, despite considerable progress over the past decade, much remains to be done to get across the message that health promotion is as important in old age as at any other time within the life span.

Of course it must be acknowledged that later life may bring many challenges. For some, there are significant health issues. Long-term conditions are more common and health threats increase, sometimes arising from changes linked to the ageing process and sometimes from social factors such as financial difficulties following retirement (Nettleton, 1995; Woodrow, 2002; Siegrist *et al.*, 2004; Bowker *et al.*, 2006). Nevertheless, as many initiatives show, much can be done to preserve health and wellbeing and to maintain independence. There are, in fact, very few areas of later life that cannot be enhanced in some way by appropriate health-promoting activity.

With this in mind, this chapter discusses a number of key areas for promoting older people's physical health: considering where opportunities exist, the knowledge, skills and qualities required, and the kinds of interventions and actions likely to be successful. Detailing a range of recent projects, the concept of health promotion is briefly explored, and a case study examined, to demonstrate how, by often simple measures, later life can be enhanced and physical health improved.

REVIEW OF THE LITERATURE

Setting the scene

A literature search for the topic 'health promotion', even if narrowed to just British sources over the past ten years – results in an overwhelming list of references, from textbooks and journals, to media news items and internet sites. Add the words 'older people' to the search criteria and although the number of citations is vastly reduced, a huge amount remains. Much is, it seems, already being done to address older people's health promotion needs with topics like nutrition, exercise, the prevention of obesity, smoking cessation and the moderation of alcohol consumption already high on the agenda.

Clearly, these topics are relevant to all age groups. This raises a question then: should health promotion for older people be considered and even delivered separately to that provided for other adults? Put more simply, what makes health promotion for older people different?

Within the literature, answers to this question are generally vague. Evans (2000), for example, highlights a debate over integrating older people into mainstream health promotion, but never really clarifies his position. Andrews (2001) similarly argues that significant health gains can be achieved if older age groups are targeted but does not explain why all age groups cannot be targeted together. The question remains: what makes health promotion for older people different to that of other age groups?

The issue underlining the need for a different approach is essentially one of attitudes and beliefs – in particular the damaging effects of negative attitudes to ageing and indeed older people themselves. At the centre of such beliefs there is a popular stereotype portraying older people as frail, vulnerable and disabled individuals, shuffling their way through a muddled and lonely existence, from which health is little more than an illusive, rapidly fading memory and the spectre of death an almost eagerly awaited friend (Slater, 1995; Evans, 2000; Iliffe and Drennan, 2000).

Imagery like this is everywhere around us. Of course, it is not always so melodramatic. On the contrary, it is usually more restrained and commonplace. A road sign near an older people's residential home, for example, will display two hunched figures, one walking with a stick, the other holding on to their partner (see Figure 1) (TSO, 2007). While the caution is valid, it can lead to a false assumption that all older people are 'doddery' or disabled. Even birthday and retirement cards can be stigmatising, rarely depicting old age as more adventurous than sitting, feet up, taking a 'well-deserved' rest. While we may recognise these ideas

Figure 1 British Road Sign Warning of Likelihood of Older People Crossing (TSO, 2007).

are exaggerations and not generally representative, it is easy to see how the constant, often subtle cues lead to false assumptions that become common belief.

Within the literature, there is a huge body of evidence to challenge such beliefs. Indeed, numerous authors point out that the prevalence of both acute and chronic disease is far less than many people would anticipate (Illife and Drennan, 2000; Marmot, 2001; Bowker *et al.*, 2006). Further, as Evans (2000) states, the vast majority of older people report being in good health even though there is a difference between the 'young old' (those over retirement age but not yet 75 years old) and the 'older old' (those over 75 years).

So then, how does this relate to promoting health for older people? If they are healthier or less disabled than generally believed, what should be addressed? Logically, it would seem the principal goal would be to maintain or enhance the health picture; correcting public beliefs would not seem urgent. However, it is important not to underestimate the impact of negative attitudes; they must be tackled as a priority (Squire, 2002).

To strengthen this point and put it into context, it is predicted that by 2020 the world's population will include more than 1 000 million people aged 60 years and over (Sanders, 2006). For these people, the aim is not just to add years to life but to add life to years (Evans, 2000). To do so, the starting point is accepting that it is not only desirable but indeed entirely possible to maintain and enhance health in later life. With this belief in mind then, the next questions to ask are how does health promotion help and what is it about?

Activity 1

Think about the term 'health promotion'. What does it mean to you? Make a list of points that you would use to explain the term to a friend or colleague.

Promoting health: exploring the territory

Health promotion is a much debated concept so it is important to be clear what it actually means (Tannahill, 1985; Ewles and Simnett, 1999; Bernard, 2000; Naidoo and Wills, 2000). On the face of it, it is a perfectly straightforward term; simply a descriptor of any efforts to prevent illness and promote positive health; from education and advice giving to government policies and media campaigns (Brooker, 2003).

However, a whole 'professional' and 'academic' nomenclature surrounds the term, with associated concepts including health maintenance, health education, health gain, disease prevention, surveillance and screening. Underlying these concepts are various philosophical approaches and it is here the contention begins (Naidoo and Wills, 2000; Brooker, 2003; Laverack, 2007).

To illustrate, there is currently a debate about 'health gain', a concept that has appeared in the literature since the late 1990s. Specifically, the contention is that the concept is about 'curing disease and treating illness', traditionally the province of the medical profession (Nettleton, 1995; Haggart, 2000; Naidoo and Wills, 2000; Squire, 2002; Laverack, 2007). While this may seem quite reasonable, Squire (2002) is vehement that health promotion for older people should not be 'medically' focussed, suggesting that such an approach is about 'quick-fix' solutions that do not allow people to define health for themselves, imposing instead a disempowering professionally-set agenda that neglects the socio-cultural determinants of health such as social class or ethnic origin.

Interestingly, Uitenbroek (1996) argues in quite the opposite way. He asserts that a good medical knowledge is essential to develop effective health promoting interventions. Yet, Squire (2002) is adamant – older people explain health in their own terms and link it to their own life experience. Health for them, therefore, is not just about being free of a particular set of symptoms; it is about choice and control over as much of their lives as possible.

Sidell (2003) makes a similar argument for a 'positive health' model. She draws upon Antonovsky's (1996) 'salutogenic' approach, which focusses on the factors supporting human health. Using this approach, health promotion does not concentrate on problems like malnutrition, infections or falls. Quite the reverse; it is concerned with health and so, for instance, it is concerned with the ways in which exercise helps with safe mobility or how a balanced diet helps with physical activity.

Some authors are dismissive of these debates. Haughey (1995: 208) is particularly incisive, asserting 'all these extremely well meaning definitions of health and health education are remarkable if only for the fact that they are mainly held, or perhaps believed in, by health professionals. 'Experience', she continues, will make it clear that 'the ordinary man or woman in the street will report that being "healthy" to him or her means *not* being ill, or at least being able to carry on with normal everyday life for as long as possible'.

Type	Summary
Individual approaches	• often involve medical/nursing staff acting to ensure individuals are prevented from developing or protected against a disease-causing agent, e.g. immunisation or screening; • often involve educational input – giving information, helping a person to interpret evidence, etc. so they can make life choices; • can involve behavioural input – giving people information and support to help them cope, e.g. cigarette smoking cessation; • can be self-initiated, e.g. an individual's own choices.
Group approaches	• normally undertaken through a combination of educational and behavioural change approaches but can be community development focussed; • require a knowledge of group dynamics.
Community focussed approaches	Likely to involve one or a combination of the following: • **epidemiological focussed approach** – this is based on the prevalence/incidence of a condition within a geographical area (e.g. uses standardised statistical information to initiate initiatives such as TB prevention); • **social/societal change approach** – this includes initiating or lobbying for policy or legislation change, may be based on epidemiological evidence or expressed need within community (e.g. activity centre); • **community development** – this is where interventions are identified/carried out by the community. May involve health and other professionals empowering people to determine their own health promotion/ improvement needs, e.g. enabling people in a residential home to set up a residents' group.

Table 1 Types of health promotion (adapted from Drennan and Goodman, 2007)

Evidently, the arguments are complex but, then again, the territory is vast. Health promotion strategies range from individual and group projects – to community and even 'global community' initiatives (see Table 1) (Drennan and Goodman, 2007). The political, social, ecological and ethical implications are sometimes huge – even the smallest, most individual initiative may have consequences far wider than one person's behaviour. A discussion about healthy eating, for example, has implications for where and how foods are obtained, how they are transported, where and how they are grown or manufactured, how they are cooked, processed and so on.

Of course, the decision over which approach is adopted is not always an individual one and, in many cases, the principal concern is whatever will be effective. The fact is, regardless of approach, the charge to promote health is the same. This leads then to the next issues to be considered; opportunities to promote health and where future efforts might be meaningfully directed.

Activity 2

Review the contents of Table 1. For each approach identified, identify an example that relates to older people. If you are unable to think of a specific example for any of the approaches, ask yourself why this might be the case? Is any one approach used more widely than another? What are the implications of this for older people?

Opportunities for promoting health: possible future directions

Activity 3

Before reading the next section, make a list of the places where health promotion occurs and people you believe are actively involved in promoting older people's health.

Opportunities to promote health with older people exist wherever there are older people. This may seem a facile statement, but it is worth making since too often health promotion is thought of as something that occurs in hospitals or specialist centres. On the contrary, as the list provided by Ewles and Simnett (1999) shows (see Table 2), it is frequently unrelated to professional input. In fact, as Baltes and Baltes (1990) remind us, many everyday activities older people perform for themselves are health promoting; self help is undeniably one of the greatest health promoting influences of all.

In terms of getting information to large numbers of people, the mass media offers one of the best means. Indeed, it sometimes seems the media is bombarding us with health promoting messages – adverts and television (TV) programmes seem repeatedly focussed on 'self improvement' – from stopping smoking and eating the 'five-a-day' fruit and vegetables, to weight loss and exercise regimes.

Older people's health issues are, however, not always well represented by the media and, sadly, the wrong message is often given. An example of this relates to the issue of urinary continence. While it is excellent that this once 'hidden' topic is addressed on peak-time TV, it is disappointing that the adverts focus on incontinence pads when much more may be available with appropriate referral and advice (Heath and Watson, 2002; Bourne, 2003). In fact, there is a disproportionate amount of advertising given over to products for disabled older people, such as stairlifts or breaks in private respite facilities, perpetuating the negative stereotyping of later life.

• Mass media advertising campaigns.
• Campaigns on health issues.
• Educating people about health.
• Promoting self help.
• Measures to promote environmental safety.
• Development of public policy.
• Promoting physical health.
• Preventative and curative medical procedures.
• Codes of practice for health matters.
• Developing health-enhancing facilities for local communities.
• Designing and implementing workplace health policies.
• Providing social education.

Table 2 Health promoting activities (after Squire (2002) and Ewles and Simnett (1999))

Making more use of the media to show credible, healthy older people engaged in activities that maintain and enhance their health is critical for the future. To illustrate this using the previous example, advice about how oral fluids and pelvic floor exercises may contribute to treating continence needs could be publicised in ways other than leaflets in a doctor's waiting room or posters in an out-patients department.

Certainly, given current population and social trends, the health needs of all sections of the older population are becoming more diverse and complex (Hunt, 2005; Sanders, 2006). Hence, it is as important to consider the active older person who may be interested in different types of sports wear or skin care products, such as sun screens when going on holiday, as it is to consider a less active older person who may require advice and support with foot care and exercise maintenance (Penzer and Finch, 2001; Neno, 2007).

Indications for future health promoting activity are also found within a recent Department of Health publication that reviews progress in the development of older people's services (Department of Health, 2006). This stresses the importance of addressing the needs of 'excluded groups' such as the socially isolated, those living in poverty, those with mobility problems and those with sensory or cognitive impairments. Health and social care professionals may have opportunities within their daily practice to engage people from these groups. Indeed, as a major part of the role, resources should allow for such activity and there should be recognition for the work in terms of time allocation and education.

A recent research study undertaken by Runciman and her colleagues confirms the important work nurses undertake in this context. This study drew on the experience of over 370 NHS community nurses and clearly identified the wide scope of health-promoting activity, as well as the fact that much of it is embedded in daily practice and goes unrecognised (Runciman and Sander, 2006).

Of course, the vast majority of older people do not have or need regular contact with health professionals so other ways of providing support, advice and information must be considered. Government policy is critical here (for example, policy for cold weather payments) but so too are more localised efforts, such as information and activities provided by locality groups and informal carers.

As Tutton and Ager (2003) have highlighted, finding ways of promoting older people's participation is not always easy, but every encouragement should be given to those who wish to promote health for themselves and for others. More and more it is being recognised that it is better if professionals do not 'intervene' but 'facilitate' instead, in other words, when they enable others to take the lead for themselves (Toofany, 2007). This points then to the next section of this chapter: the qualities and skills needed to promote health.

Activity 4

Try to think of the last time you read a piece of health-promoting literature. What was it that you read? Were you already aware of the information or was it new to you? What did you learn? How was the information presented?

SKILLS AND QUALITIES FOR PROMOTING OLDER PEOPLE'S HEALTH

In all contexts, promoting health concerns relationships. Successful relationships require trust, respect and honesty (Hargie and Dickson, 2004). Older people are no different to any other group in terms of valuing respect, courtesy and genuine regard, nor are they unique in sometimes being subject to prejudice and discrimination. However, their experience of health and welfare services could so often be much improved just by the use of well-judged words and carefully thought out communications (McCabe and Timmins, 2006; O'Connell and Sutcliffe, 2007).

Communication to promote older people's health therefore needs to be sensitive, supportive and encouraging. Individually, the skills required include listening, self awareness and facilitation. Listening is key to understanding the nature of the situation, the person's beliefs and life experiences. Self-awareness is critical because it informs us of our own strengths and when we need to seek help. Facilitation skills are essential because, as already noted, the aim is to 'enable', not to impose or dictate what is right or wrong (see Table 3).

• Encourage autonomy by valuing the older person's knowledge and skills.
• Reduce dependency on professionals and enable self-determination.
• Build self-esteem and confidence by acknowledging choices.
• Encourage a partnership approach by listening and discussing information.
• Support independence by respecting informed decisions.
• Encourage older people to recognise their own coping strategies as expertise.

Table 3 Aims of facilitation in health promotion

The issue of not forcing our own beliefs on people needs some further discussion. It may seem obvious that the intention is neither to inflict opinions, nor to enforce particular behaviours. Nevertheless, some areas of health promotion policy do just that, the ban on smoking in public places being a good example. Trueland (2007) has highlighted the dilemmas care home staff face because of this. On one hand they try to get the message across that the care home is the resident's home but, on the other, they are telling residents that they cannot smoke there so an individual freedom is withdrawn.

Some argue the health effects of smoking warrant such an approach. Trueland (2007) cites a nurse who believes it is patronising to allow people 'little pleasures' just because they are old or near the end of life and firmly asserts that efforts should be made to tackle smoking habits. Here again, the issue of attitudes to later life rises to the fore but, in this case, the main issues seem to be ones of equity and, it could be asked, does the policy on smoking treat all individuals in a fair way?

Certainly, when undertaking health education activity, a more facilitative style is usually considered appropriate. As Drennan and Goodman (2007) point out, 'persuading' an unwilling person to make lifestyle changes will probably result in failure, leading to resistance to attempt the change at a later date. Similarly, it is recognised that 'lecturing' and multiple leaflets are likely to be ignored, even in situations where staff are well-intentioned, enthusiastic and well-informed. Enthusiasm may be contagious but an over-zealous approach can often inhibit and deter people.

The principles underpinning health education are generally the same in any situation: finding out what the person already knows, ensuring 'taught' content is up-to-date, accurate, relevant and logical, and regularly checking on understanding. This also applies to written materials like health education leaflets which should be jargon free, provide sufficient, current information and explain professional terms (Harris, 2005).

Finding user perspectives and evaluations of health promotion initiatives is difficult but increasingly it seems that, contrary to popular belief, health promotion services are popular among older people (Job, 2005; Department of Health, 2006). From the examples cited in the literature, it seems that those that involve a high level of activity and participation are especially effective.

However, for very frail older people living in isolation or poverty, much encouragement may first be needed to help them believe in themselves and their futures, and to help them see their own coping strategies as expertise (Cavanagh and McLafferty, 2007). As members of a society in which negative views of old age are common, it is unsurprising that many older people hold pessimistic beliefs about later life, seeing it as a time to expect and even accept deteriorating health, disability and loss of function (Hanlon, 1990; Slater 1995).

Great skill is needed to undo such thinking, especially when many health and social care professionals have been found to hold similar views (Phillipson, 1985; Chandler, 1986; Nettleton, 1995; Squire, 2002; Archibald, 2003). Nevertheless, continued efforts must be made to do so if health promotion is to address the needs of the broadest range of older people.

Activity 5

Reflect on your skills as a communicator. How would they help you to understand an older person's needs? How would you, or do you, convey respect when trying to give information or advice?

OLDER PEOPLE'S HEALTH: RECENT INITIATIVES AND ISSUES FOR DEVELOPMENT

As noted at the outset, a vast literature exists detailing various projects to promote older people's physical health and covering a wide range of topics. Sometimes, as with a project Squire (2002) describes, several issues are tackled at the same time. This project was called 'A Life in Retirement'. It was set up in 1993 and managed collaboratively by Age Concern and a local Community Health Trust. It addressed topics from healthy eating and oral health, sensible drinking and smoking cessation to increased mobility and exercise, and improved personal safety in and outside the home.

Falls and exercise

However, single focus projects are also common, with the literature providing countless examples, particularly in the area of falls prevention, an issue highlighted in the NSF (Department of Health, 2001). There are many reasons why falls appear to be one of the priorities here; among older people they are not just common, they are disabling and can be fatal.

Luxton and Riglin (2003) describe a project that uses professionals from health and social care agencies to help identify risk factors and prevent falls occurring. This includes a 'Walk Tall, Don't Fall' campaign targeting those in lunch clubs, church groups and sheltered housing. It also involves a one-off presentation on the causes of falls and an information pack developed locally so participants have details of resources nearby. One of the strengths of this project is that it also makes use of a community exercise group.

The exercise group is recommended as a very effective health promotion strategy for several reasons. There is considerable evidence to suggest that exercise for the majority of people is physically beneficial. Lane (1999) summarises this, stating that, for example, 30 minutes of exercise three or four times a week can prevent heart disease, help to avoid excess weight and put the necessary strain on the skeleton to induce bone formation. Furthermore, exercise increases muscle strength, flexibility, balance and posture, therefore reducing the risk of falls and fractures. It is not just the physical benefits that are important. Exercise is known to help people feel good emotionally and, when performed in groups, allows for peer support, interaction and companionship (Neno, 2007). In this respect, it is difficult to separate physical and mental health promotion; exercise serves both purposes.

Of course, setting up and sustaining enthusiasm for projects like these is not always easy. Uglow and Dewing (2004) describe how an exercise group for older people in a community hospital had to overcome numerous challenges to make the group successful. Staff shortages, holidays, commitment to the group, loss of volunteers and even, during the summer, excessive heat, all affected motivation. Further, some of the staff required time to build their confidence to lead sessions and it was concluded that they needed a real sense of ownership to maintain their enthusiasm.

The issue of feeling confident is significant. Health promoters must be certain that their work does no harm. Exercise tolerance, for example, will differ from person to person, so care is needed when identifying who may participate and the level of exercise to be promoted.

Mitchell (2006) has also discussed how a working group was set up to develop an education programme using local hospital and community services collaboratively. The group covered topics like eating and drinking for health, safety, mobility and walking aids, podiatry, tips on footwear and safety with medication, all delivered via a series of lectures and practical sessions. In this case the project was delivered by speakers very familiar with the information they were giving. Furthermore, they used clear evidence to support the project, including the NICE (2004) and RCN (2005) guidelines. Short (2006), in an article also discussing falls prevention, acknowledges the specialist nature of much health promotion and suggests that, before developing any initiatives, additional training may be needed.

The University of the Third Age

By contrast, there are many projects led by lay people and volunteers where less 'specialist' or professional knowledge is required. Midwinter (2004), for instance, reports on education programmes for older people involving the University of the Third Age, a self-help agency. This agency now has over 500 groups, all organised by the members themselves to provide education on subjects that members choose. There are no paid lecturers; the members work and learn together – learning is for the joy of learning itself! This may not seem an example of physical health promotion but, again, it involves activity that stimulates both physical and emotional wellbeing (Young, 2006).

Vigour

Another voluntary agency, this time a registered charity, is supporting a scheme helping to equip older people with skills needed to improve their employment prospects. The scheme, called 'Vigour', involves providing practical experience at work placements and training sessions (Suffolk Acre, undated). In effect it promotes the skills needed to undertake paid employment and there is substantial evidence that in so doing physical health and activity will be maintained (Siegrist *et al.*, 2004).

Sexual health

One area of health promotion with older people that has been neglected in the past is sexual health. Sadly, negative views of old age tend to impose a state of asexuality on anyone over retirement age, a myth which must be removed (Evans, 2000: 273). As Marshall (1997) states, an adult's sexual expression is not age dependent; all people, whatever their age, are sexual beings and will express their sexuality in whatever way they choose. In the past, it was suggested older people were generally reluctant to discuss sexual issues but this may be changing as the 'baby-boomer' generation is currently entering old age (Gott, 2006). Certainly, organisations like Age Concern are now offering advice about forming new intimate relations, an important development for several reasons (Sanders, 2006).

Grigg (2000) clearly identifies one of the reasons; the risks of sexually transmitted infections. Too often, it seems, these risks are dismissed as minimal when the reverse is actually true. Since the chances of pregnancy decline, older people tend not to use contraception including barrier methods when engaging in sexual activity. However, the immune system is often less robust so infection is easily transmitted. Furthermore, infections like HIV tend to be more aggressive in older people, and older women can contract the virus more easily because their vaginal walls are thinner.

Disease aside, a reason why a more permissive approach to older people's sexuality is to be welcomed is because of the taboos surrounding the topic. Intolerance and a misplaced sense of propriety have for too long produced guilt and shame about sexuality when, for many, it is an important source of pleasure and comfort, and can enhance physical wellbeing. Acknowledging that there may be some changes in libido and arousal times, there really is no reason why older people should not enjoy fulfilling sexual lives, nor should their concerns be dismissed if difficulties arise (Grigg, 2000; Harris, 2004).

Promoting learning

Other areas for life enhancement that have seen recent development include an initiative described by Sanders (2006) aimed at promoting learning for older people in an acute hospital. It was recognised that leisure activities are often neglected in hospitals and yet they are significant to recovery. Hence, a programme of learning and socialising was put in place either on a one-to-one basis or within a group. Supported by managers and nurses, the project includes mind-stimulating activities like participating in art classes and social interaction (Sanders, 2006).

It seems that the potential for the promotion of older people's physical health is almost boundless. Although resources and training costs are always significant, the greatest barriers to overcome are those of public attitudes. Changing attitudes is notoriously difficult and yet the beginnings of a shift in the culture may be appearing (Duffin, 2006). It is to be hoped that momentum will be gained and the benefits of healthy, active living will become more widespread in the older population.

HEALTH PROMOTION IN PRACTICE

Case study

Alice Thomas is a 78-year-old widow who lives alone in a bungalow in a small town. Although she has had osteoarthritis in her hips and hands since her late 50s, she believes her condition is well controlled by medication and describes her health as good. Gregarious and witty, she enjoys both reading and, until recently, an active social life – eating out, shopping and visiting her family who live nearby.

About five years ago, Alice fell while at home and broke her hip. She underwent surgery and made a good recovery. However, she now uses a stick when walking and has been left with a slight limp. Over the past year, she has had two further falls – one at home and one while out shopping with her daughter. Although she suffered no major injuries, the falls have affected her confidence and she has become more sedentary. She found the second fall particularly embarrassing because it was witnessed by strangers. In fact, when her daughter came to assist her, Alice was quite abrupt, resenting 'fuss and attention' and snapping that she wanted to be left alone. Alice's daughter is concerned her mother is becoming 'unsafe' to look after herself and Alice is dismissive of what she perceives as unnecessary interference.

More recently, Alice has noticed that she has 'put on weight' – she finds the effort of housework increasingly tiring, and her social life has reduced. Her daughter visits more frequently but Alice misses going into town and meeting friends.

Activity 6

Having read through the preceding case study, list the areas you feel raise issues for health promotion. What would you tackle as a priority and how do you think this could be managed? What type of help do you think Alice would accept? What health promoting actions might she undertake for herself?

Reflections on the case study

In Alice's case, a number of issues for health promotion are quickly apparent. These include the change in her level of physical activity and its effect on her social life and the weight gain that is worrying her. The falls themselves are significant, along with Alice's knowledge of the medications she takes for her arthritis. Fear of falling and loss of confidence in her physical capabilities may be significant, as well as the daughter's concern. Nutrition may also be an issue here.

Most older people have considerable skill in overcoming problems and can maintain and regain a high level of autonomy, quality of life and satisfaction with life if given appropriate support (Iliffe and Drennan, 2000). For Alice, this support might include a visit to her health centre for falls risk assessment as well as a medication review, including pain relief. Here, health professionals could assess just how she feels about the health issues affecting her and explore the options open to her. However, the decisions would need to be hers; much of the information she needs may be available within her own home, through use of the internet or appropriate reading. The daughter might also be able to obtain this information in a similar way.

The priorities for Alice would be about rebuilding confidence, making her feel safe to walk and engage in activity (Accalai, 2007). The type of health education she needs is questionable: she may already understand the impact of weight gain on arthritic joints and be similarly informed about the effects of exercise and diet. Nevertheless, information on local services such as exercise groups or diet clubs might be appreciated and information about healthy eating might be needed. Possibly the greatest support Alice can be given is the opportunity to discuss the options open to her, including what she would like to do and the support she believes she needs to be able to achieve this. Indeed, it is only by demonstrating respect, a partnership approach and a willingness to listen and learn ourselves that health promotion can be effective and achieve its goals.

CONCLUSION

Society is ageing and the evidence is all around us: people are living longer. While this represents a triumph, it also represents a challenge (Hunt, 2005). Maintaining and improving the health and wellbeing of older people is a vast undertaking, possibly the greatest charge the health and welfare services face. The starting point is essentially a philosophical one: the reshaping of attitudes and beliefs so the value of later life and the potential for a healthy, fulfilling old age are more widely accepted.

On a practical level, maintaining and enhancing physical health in later life can involve many activities and initiatives such as those identified within this chapter. Clearly, health promotion for older people is not always a highly technical or specialised area of professional practice, although it involves many types of knowledge, skills and personal qualities, and should never be underestimated.

For the future, it is evident that much needs to be done to address the needs of those sections of the older population who are frail, vulnerable and have limited access to health-promoting facilities and services. It is only with commitment, insight and determination that all people, regardless of age, will be given the opportunity to be actively involved in life and the realisation of their full potential.

FURTHER READING

Green, S. and McDougall, T. (2002) 'Screening and assessing the nutritional status of older people'. *Nursing Older People*, 14 (6): 31–2
An article exploring how a good diet can help older people enjoy many years of active life. It discusses risk assessment for malnutrition and provision of access to advice and support.

Tutton, E. and Ager, L. (2003) 'Frail older people: Participation in care'. *Nursing Older People*, 15 (8): 18–22
This article describes a research project designed to explore views of frail older people and their nurses on participation in care. From the research, a framework for participation in care has been developed. The article presents this framework and a consideration of questions that people can use to reflect on the extent to which they promote participation.

Watts, M. (2007) 'Incidences of excess alcohol consumption in the older person'. *Nursing Older People*, 18 (12): 27–30
This article explores the causes of excess alcohol consumption in older people, its consequences and treatment.

Useful websites

www.ageconcern.org.uk
Age Concern

www.fons.org/healthy_ageing
Healthy Ageing Projects

www.hpe.org.uk
Health Promotion England

www.arc.org.uk
The Arthritis Research Campaign

REFERENCES

Accalai, P. (2007) 'The effect of exercise in osteoarthritis'. *Practice Nurse*, 33 (4): 30–1

Andrews, G. (2001) 'Promoting health and function in an ageing population'. *British Medical Journal*, 332: 728–9

Antonovsky, A. (1996) 'The Salutogenic Model as a theory to guide health promotion'. *Health Promotion International*, 11 (1): 11–18

Archibald, C. (2003) *People with Dementia in Acute Hospitals: A Practice Guide For Registered Nurses*. Stirling: University of Stirling

Baltes, P.B. and Baltes, M.M. (1990) 'Psychological perspectives on successful aging: The model of selective optimization with compensation' in Baltes, P.B. and Baltes, M.M. (eds) *Successful Aging: Perspectives from the Behavioral Sciences*. New York: Cambridge University Press

Bernard, M. (2000) *Promoting Health in Old Age*. Buckingham: Open University Press

Bowker, L.K., Price, J.D. and Smith, S.C. (2006) *Oxford Handbook of Geriatric Medicine*. Oxford: Oxford University Press

Bourne, A. (2003) 'Promoting continence in nursing homes: responding to government guidelines'. *Nursing Older People*, 15 (8): 14–16

Brooker, C. (ed.) (2003) *Pocket Medical Dictionary*. Edinburgh: Churchill Livingstone/Elsevier

Cavanagh, S. and McLafferty, E. (2007) 'The recognition and use of patient expertise on a unit for older people'. *Nursing Older People*, 19 (8): 31–6

Chandler, J. (1986) 'Attitudes of nursing personnel towards the elderly'. *Gerontologist*, 26 (4): 551–5

Denby, N. (2006) 'The role of diet and lifestyle changes in the management of constipation'. *Journal of Community Nursing*, 20 (9): 20–4

Department of Health (2001) *National Service Framework for Older People*. London: TSO

Department of Health (2006) *A New Ambition for Old Age: Next Steps in Implementing the NSF for Older People*. London: TSO

Drennan, V. and Goodman, C. (2007) *Oxford Handbook of Primary Care and Community Nursing*. Oxford: Oxford University Press

Duffin, C. (2006) 'Pride and prejudice'. *Nursing Older People*, 18 (11): 12–13

Evans, G. (2000) 'Health promotion for older people' in Kerr, J. (ed.) *Community Health Promotion: Challenges for Practice*. Edinburgh: Bailliere Tindall

Ewles, L. and Simnett, I. (1999) *Promoting Health: A Practical Guide to Health Education* (4th edn). Edinburgh: Harcourt

Gott, M. (2006) 'Sexual health and the new ageing'. *Age and Ageing*, 35: 106–7

Grigg, E. (2000) 'Sexually transmitted infections and older people'. *Nursing Standard*, 14 (39): 48–53

Haggart, M. (2000) 'Promoting the health of communities' in Kerr, J. (ed.) *Community Health Promotion: Challenges for Practice*. Edinburgh: Bailliere Tindall

Hanlon, P. (1990) 'Health promotion under the new contract'. *British Journal of General Practice*, 349

Hargie, O. and Dickson, D. (2004) *Skilled Interpersonal Communication: Research, Theory and Practice* (4th edn). Abingdon: Routledge

Harris, G. (2004) 'Male sexual dysfunction'. *Practice Nurse*, 28 (8): 74–83

Harris, G. (2005) 'Osteoporosis in primary care'. *Practice Nurse*, 30 (6): 72–7

Haughey, A. (1995) 'Contemporary district nursing practice', in Sines, D. (ed.) *Community Health Care Nursing*. Oxford: Blackwell

Health Care Alliance (2003) *The National Service Framework for Older People in Wales*. **www.healthcarealliances.co.uk/Public/documents** (Accessed May 2008)

Heath, T. and Watson, R. (2002) 'The causes of urinary incontinence in men'. *Nursing Older People*, 14 (6): 15–19

Hunt, A. (2005) 'Keeping well: a local approach to delivering health advice and information'. *Nursing Older People*, 17 (9): 16–19

Iliffe, S. and Drennan, V. (2000) *Primary Care for Older People*. Oxford: Oxford University Press

Job, S. (2005) 'What older people want'. *Nursing Older People*, 17 (5): 10–12

Lane, N.E. (1999) *The Osteoporosis Book*. Oxford: Oxford University Press

Laverack, G. (2007) *Health Promotion Practice: Building Empowered Communities*. Maidenhead: Open University Press/McGraw-Hill

Luxton, T. and Riglin, J. (2003) 'Preventing falls in older people: A multi-agency approach'. *Nursing Older People*, 15 (2): 18–21

Marmot, M. (2001) 'A social view of health and disease' in Heller, T., Muston, R., Sidell, M. and Lloyd, C. (eds) *Working for Health*. London: Sage Publications

Marshall, T. (1997) 'Infected and affected: HIV, Aids and the older adult'. *Journal of the British Society of Gerontology*, 7 (4): 8–11

McCabe, C. and Timmins, F. (2006) *Communication Skills for Nursing Practice*. Basingstoke: Palgrave MacMillan

Midwinter, E. (2004) 'Never too late to learn'. *Nursing Older People*, 16 (1): 10–12

Mitchell, E. (2006) 'Evaluation of an integrated falls – education group programme'. *Nursing Older People*, 18 (1): 21–4

Naidoo J. and Wills J. (2000) *Health Promotion: Foundations for Practice* (2nd edn). Edinburgh: Bailliere Tindall

Neno, R. (2007) 'Feet for purpose'. *Nursing Older People*, 19 (8): 5–6

Nettleton, S. (1995) *The Sociology of Health & Illness*. Cambridge: Polity Press

NICE (2004) *Assessment and Prevention of Falls in Older People*. London: National Institute for Health and Clinical Excellence

O'Connell, N. and Sutcliffe, A. (2007) 'Improving adherence in osteoporosis'. *Practice Nurse*, 33 (4): 49–50

Penzer, R. and Finch, M. (2001) 'Promoting healthy skin in older people'. *Nursing Older People*, 13 (8): 22–8

Phillipson, C. (1985) *Health Education and Old People: Developing Positive Approaches in District Nursing and Health Visiting. Evidence to the Community Review*. Keele: University of Keele, Department of Adult Education

RCN (2005) *Clinical Practice Guidelines for the Assessment and Prevention of Falls in Older People*. London: Royal College of Nursing

Runciman, P. and Sander, R. (2006) 'Journal scan'. *Nursing Older People*, 18 (5): 36–7

Sanders, K. (2006) 'Developing practice for healthy ageing'. *Nursing Older People*, 18 (3): 18–21

Short, R. (2006) 'Falls'. *Nursing Older People*, 18 (18): 16–18

Sidell, M. (2003) 'Older people's health: Applying Antonovsky's Salutogenic Paradigm' in Sidell, M., Jones, L., Katz, J., Peberdy, A. and Douglas, J. (eds) *Debates and Dilemmas in Promoting Health: A Reader* (2nd edn). Basingstoke: Palgrave Macmillan

Siegrist, J., Von Dem Knesebeck, O. and Pollock, C. (2004) 'Social productivity and well being of older people: A sociological exploration'. *Social Theory and Health*, 2 (1): 1–17

Slater, R. (1995) *The Psychology of Growing Old*. Buckingham, Open University Press

Squire, A. (2002) *Health and Well-being for Older People: Foundations for Practice*. Edinburgh: Bailliere-Tindall

Suffolk Acre (Undated) *Vigour – 50+*. Ipswich: Suffolk Acre

Tannahill, A. (1985) 'What is health promotion?' *Health Education Journal*, 44: 167–8

The Stationery Office (2003) *Let's Make Scotland More Active: A Strategy for Physical Activity*. Edinburgh: The Stationery Office

Toofany, S. (2007) 'Empowering older people'. *Nursing Older People*, 19 (2): 12–14

Trueland, J. (2007) 'Stubbing it out'. *Nursing Older People*, 18 (12): 16–17

TSO (2007) *The Official Highway Code – 2007 Edition*. London, TSO

Tutton, E. and Ager, L. (2003) 'Frail older people: Participation in care'. *Nursing Older People*, 15 (8): 18–22

Uglow, J. and Dewing, J. (2004) 'Introducing a physical activity group on an intermediate care ward'. *Nursing Older People*, 16 (6): 19–22

Uitenbroek, D.G. (1996) 'A new public health model and ageing: The example of primary prevention by way of exercise and physical activity'. *Health Care in Later Life*, 1 (1): 15–27

Watson, H., McIntosh, J. and Tolson, D. (2006) 'Community nurses' health promotion work with older people'. *Journal of Advanced Nursing*, 55 (1): 46–57

Woodrow, P. (2002) *Ageing: Issues for Physical, Psychological and Social Health*. London: Whurr Publishing

Young, S. (2006) 'Taking a break'. *Nursing Older People*, 18 (3): 14–17

Chapter 15

Transitions

Angela Kydd

Learning outcomes

Reading this chapter will enable you to:

- explain what is meant by a life transition;

- examine the factors involved in making minor and pivotal life transitions;

- explore the concepts of coping and uncertainty during pivotal transitions;

- discuss how personal circumstances and attitudes might affect the way in which an older person adapts to life in a care home.

INTRODUCTION

Transitions occur throughout life and, with each transition, comes change. The change will affect the individual's normal social and emotional networks and this may result in growth or deterioration (Goodman *et al.*, 2006). These changes can be biological, social, psychological or spiritual in nature. All are inextricably linked as they react and interact not only with each other, but with the individual characteristics, coping mechanisms and support systems of the person undergoing the transition (Evans *et al.*, 1998).

Some life transitions are perceived to be positive and others as negative, some occur at a good time in the individual's life and some do not, some transitions are expected, while others may be unexpected. The context and timing of a transition in an individual's life will ultimately affect their interpretation of the transition. The life event may be the same for everyone, for example, pregnancy, divorce, retirement or moving into care, but the meaning of the transition to the person concerned and how they cope with it will be unique to that individual.

Should perceived negative transitions occur with frequency, the deleterious effect on the individual may be damaging. This is especially pertinent to those classed as the 'oldest old', those aged 85 and over. It is well-documented that people in this age group are more likely to have compromised health than their younger counterparts (Ketcham and Stelmach, 2001). In addition, this group are also more likely to undergo negative transitions (Woods, 2000b), such as bereavement, poor health, disability, increasing dependence, loss of independence or loss of one's home with a move into long-term care. It is therefore important that health and social care professionals are aware of the possible effects of life transitions on the oldest old, those over 85 (Office for National Statistics, 2003).

In this chapter the concept of coping (an essential part of transition) is explored. Then the ways in which transitions can be both defined and viewed are discussed with reference to the literature. Also examined are the ways in which personal attitudes and individual circumstances can colour the way in which a person interprets and copes with life changes in later life. Finally, the transition from home into long-term care is discussed, with a focus on the oldest old moving into a care home.

COPING

One major coping resource identified in the literature is a sense of 'mastery' or being in control. A study by MaloneBeach et al., (1992) proposes that feeling in control tends to lead to proactive behaviours, such as seeking help when required. Work by Zarit and Edwards (2000) reports that feeling in control is an effective buffer against stressors in a variety of situations. A sense of mastery in one's life is an internal resource and may result in better adaptation following major life transitions, such as moving into a care home (Aneshensel et al., 1995).

Coping can be described as reactions to stressors and is considered to be effective when the threat or problem has been reduced (Ekwall et al., 2007). Zarit and Edwards (2000) outline three different types of coping strategies:

- emotion-focussed;
- cognitive coping;
- problem-focussed.

Emotion-focussed coping will not change the threat, but involves management of the symptoms of stress. Cognitive coping does not change the threat, but changes the way an individual views the threat and problem-focussed coping centres on defining the threat with an attempt to alter it.

How individuals cope depends on the nature of the threat or stressor and the meaning it has to the individual. It also depends on the nature of coping, because, interestingly, stressors and coping have been found to have a reciprocal relationship. Zarit and Edwards (2000: 173) explain:

> Stressors evoke coping responses, but effective efforts at management may lower the rate at which stressors occur. Ineffective coping, in turn, can lead to exacerbations of behavioural and emotional problems.

They give the following example to illustrate this point:

> . . . confronting a dementia patient who asks to see her long-deceased mother is likely to make her more agitated and increase the frequency of her request. By contrast, comforting her and reminiscing about her mother can be calming and lead to a reduction in the frequency of this behaviour.

Control is an essential resource to coping and, according to Schulz and Heckhausen (1998), an essential part of human development. Magai (2001), summarising Schulz and Heckhausen's control theory, states that two types of control are apparent over the lifespan; primary and secondary.

> Primary control involves attempts to achieve effects change in the immediate environment through direct influence on the external world, whereas secondary control targets the self and attempts to achieve changes from within the individual.
>
> (Magai, 2001: 403)

Primary control peaks at the age of 40–50 and then declines. Secondary control, however, has a late onset development and increases well into old age. According to Schultz and Heckhausen (1998) this developmental change in control may compensate for the physical and social losses that come with age and lead to greater self reliance.

How do people cope?

Understanding how people cope, or do not cope, is an essential requirement for health care professionals (for further reading on coping in later life see Woods, 2000b). Coping mechanisms are unique to the individual. For example, some people like to take a walk when they are stressed, others may like to talk about their stressors. Such coping mechanisms are not always possible in an institution and health care professionals need to be sensitive to the fact that people do not always have their usual coping resources available to them. Careful care plans to assess the effect of a stressor on an older person can help identify symptoms and address emotion-focussed coping and the negative effects of poor coping (for example, insomnia) as described above.

One example is for health professionals to assess sleep patterns. Rodehn Fox (1999) suggests sleep plans to identify factors that may be keeping an individual awake. These may be external, such as noise, or internal, such as pain, worry or anxiety. Sleep has been highlighted as an integral part of recovery for older people (Ersser, 1999), yet sleep is rarely monitored in older people. Sleep deprivation can lead to confusion, irritability and apathy (Beck-Little and Weinrich, 1998). Such a state will not address the original anxiety caused by transition and may lead to inappropriate pharmacological interventions.

TRANSITIONS

There is now a growing body of literature on helping people to cope with transition and the concept of caring for patients in transition has been addressed in policy documents. Key examples include *Adding Life to Years* (Scottish Executive, 2001), *Moving On* (Audit Scotland, 2005), *Designed to Care* (Scottish Office, 1997), *A National Service Framework for Older People* (Department of Health, 2001), *The Strategy for Older People in Wales – Living Longer, Living Better 2008–2013* (Welsh Assembly, 2003) and *Healthcare Services used by Older People in NHS Scotland* (NHS Quality Improvement Scotland, 2004).

Defining transitions

Transitions are a natural part of life. In one's early years, biological transitions are ongoing and are usually seen as positive. Expected transitions would appear to be part of everyday life; a baby becomes a toddler, a school child, an adolescent and an adult. However, every transition is unique as each individual grows in a unique way within a unique environment and cultural context.

Biological or developmental transitions are determined by an indefinite number of factors that include:

- hereditary factors and genes;
- economic status;
- physical and mental health status;
- lifestyle and lifestyle choices;
- environmental status;
- accidents and chances;
- social, psychological and spiritual transitions.

Within the framework of biological transitions, social, psychological and spiritual transitions take place. Some occur as a direct result of biological transitions, others occur and react and interact with differing types of transitions. Brammer (1992: 1) defines transition as:

> . . . a short-term life change characterised by a sharp discontinuity with the past. Thus transitions have identifiable beginnings and usually definite endings.

He cites examples such as a holiday or bereavement and highlights the fact that transitions can be positive or negative, expected or unexpected and welcome or unwelcome. Transitions may also be minor, or pivotal and life changing. Pivotal periods of transition may result in one's past social histories being discarded and replaced with a new set of relationships and circumstances (Sampson and Laub, 1993). The effect of this can be to change the way an individual feels about themselves and their new roles. This is illustrated by Reich *et al.* (2007) who highlight recent work on seeing individuals as 'multiple selves' rather than unitary beings. They suggest that when an individual undergoes transition, this has the potential to create disturbances that often compel a person to query their social roles, relationships, status and core identities.

Bridges (1980) suggests that transitions have three stages and these always start with an ending. The stages he identifies are:

- an ending;
- a period of confusion and distress;
- a new beginning, in the cases that have come that far.

(Bridges, 1980: 9)

When the endings experienced are perceived as losses, and the resolutions are not desired, the individual is vulnerable to feelings of sadness and sometimes despair. Similarly, when the period of confusion and distress is protracted, the individual will undergo anxiety and uncertainty.

Uncertainty, anxiety and worry

Uncertainty is a dynamic state in which an individual is in a situation but does not know what the outcome will be and how it will impact on their life. This prompts a discomforting, uneasy sensation that may be affected (reduced or escalated) through cognitive, emotive or behavioural reactions or by the passage of time and changes in the perception of circumstances (Penrod, 2001).

Uncertainty is closely linked to anxiety, which is, in turn, linked to worry. Worry and anxiety are related but different concepts. Worry has been defined as the cognitive, or thinking, component of anxiety. Emotionality, the physical component of anxiety, describes a broad range of reactions that are related to bodily reactions such as an increased heart rate, raised blood pressure and/or gastrointestinal upsets. Worry, the cognitive component of anxiety, is characterised by negative thoughts and images about the outcome of events. These impact upon an individual's ability to think clearly and take in information (Turner and Beidel, 1986).

The cycle of anxiety and worry, caused by a negative transition affecting an older person's perceived mental and physical health status, can lead to a further worrying transition into dependence caused by ill-health. An extreme example would be a person having a stroke because their blood pressure was high (due to anxiety) for a sustained period. A less extreme but equally harmful example would be malnutrition brought about by an individual's feeling of nausea for any length of time.

Transition models

Brammer (1992) suggests three ways to view transitions from a counselling perspective:

- As metaphors from classical literature:
  Brammer states that Bridges (1980) used metaphors from classical literature to describe transitions over the lifetime. The journey through life is a common image and is embedded in many pieces of classical literature. The counsellor would encourage individuals to see their individual and serial transitions, and the meanings of these, as part of their personal life journey.

- As a social interaction model:
  This model is described by Schlossberg (1984) who categorises transition in terms of type, context and impact. She suggests transition must be explored with regard to:
  - the way a person appraises their transition;
  - the nature of the transition;
  - the coping resources present at that time;
  - the characteristics of the individual and the environment they are in.

Schlossberg developed this transition theory, which is typically seen as a theory of adult development. It examines an individual's personal and interpersonal life and sees the environment as an influential variable (Schlossberg, 1981; Goodman *et al.*, 2006):

- As predictable overlapping stages;
  Much of the work on psychological and spiritual transitions has its roots in the work on bereavement. The stages of bereavement, as identified by Parkes (1972) for example, speak of the tasks or stages of grief. Hopson (1981) adapted the bereavement model to transitions in general and identified the stages as:
  - confusion and emotional discomfort;
  - shock, if the loss is severe;
  - sadness and despair, sometimes alternating with relief and positive feelings;
  - a short period of stabilisation when defence mechanisms such as denial and rationalisation are mobilised;
  - previously learned coping skills being tapped;
  - stabilisation replaced with fears for the future;
  - self-esteem plummeting and sadness, dread and depression possibly occurring.

These models provide a useful framework in which to view transitions. They endeavour to describe how individuals may respond to change, but transitions are individual and personal. The aim of this literature is to provide transition awareness.

Transitions in later life

Erikson's (1963) stages of psychosocial development refer to later life as the period of 'integrity versus despair'. Integrity implies an acceptance of the traumas and disappointments in life. According to Yalom (1987) the developmental tasks in this period centre on abandoning ambitions and coming to terms with one's limitations and the finite nature of life. Vergere (1997) points out that an individual does not reach old age without mastering many life transitions and losses. He goes on to state that with repeated change comes learning and the norm is for older people to experience loss, but not become paralysed by it. He states:

> Conscious acceptance of limitations, along with the need for assistance in daily living, is indeed a progression and not a regression in a psychological sense.
>
> (Vergere, 1997: 243)

However, despair is on the other end of the continuum. Older people who do not feel in control of their lives or cannot adapt to new life events are vulnerable to the deleterious effects of worry and anxiety. Worry is closely related to fear, particularly with concern about the future (Borkovec *et al.*, 1986). More recently, Metzger *et al.* (1990) demonstrated that daily worry levels adversely affected an older person's cognitive processing difficulties, this affected memory, decision making and led to negative thoughts. Although worry is a common human experience, chronic and excessive worry can lead to constant discomfort, a loss of joy in living and may result in a diagnostic condition known as 'generalised anxiety disorder' (GAD) (Borkovec *et al.*, 1998).

Worry and anxiety also affect sleep patterns. Jensen and Herr (1993) state that sleep is an essential component of health. Lack of sleep negatively impacts on the quality of life and wellbeing of an individual and this in turn will affect the way an individual copes with his or her circumstances.

Transition to a care home

Several studies have focussed on the transition into long-term care but most report on the situation after the event. A study by Reed *et al.* (1998) found that many people described the experience as a profound change in their lives. Some had found the move distressing, while others reported that it was a relief from the anxiety and that life in the home was unexpectedly pleasant. One consistent theme found throughout their study was the passivity of older people in the process of moving. The findings suggested that the stoicism exhibited by the individuals might mask feelings of loss and anxiety (Reed and Stanley, 2000). However, it may also be a form of resignation or acceptance. Early studies relating to the circumstances leading up to the transition to long-term care include the works of Chenitz (1983) who developed a set of basic conditions seen to shape the adjustment to the new environment. These are:

- **centrality**: the perceived importance of the move in maintaining one's independence and autonomy;
- **legitimation**: knowing the reason for the move into care;
- **time and duration**: if the move is to be permanent, fixed or temporary.

Later work by Nolan and Grant (1992) has criticised this theory for the lack of positive response, stating that some people want to move into care. They suggest the addition of 'anticipation' and 'embracing' to reflect this.

Work by Challis and Bartlett (1988) suggests that transition is eased if the individual has choice. This choice operates on:

- when to enter care;
- the locality of the home;
- whether to stay in that particular home.

Biedman and Normoyle (1991) suggest that the possibility of entry to care is one of the most pervasive sources of anxiety marking later life. Research by Nolan *et al.* (1996) stated that not all transitions are like this and they suggest that four types of transition into care emerged from their work. These are:

- the positive choice;
- the rationalised alternative;
- the discredited option;
- the *fait accompli*.

Early work on how people adjust to being in care was carried out by Brooke (1987 cited in Patterson, 1995). Brooke interviewed 41 newly-admitted residents and followed them over a ten-month period. Four major phases were identified, which are similar to stages of bereavement identified by Parkes (1972):

- Disorganisation: the individual feels displaced and abandoned. Lasts for approximately 6–8 weeks.
- Reorganisation: begins to ask questions, explain needs, solve problems and justify being in a home. Occurs in the 2nd–3rd months.
- Relationship building: emotional links formed, engages in conflict, makes friends. Occurs in the 3rd month.
- Stabilisation: settling in process complete. Has sense of belonging. Begins to reach out to new residents. Occurs in the 3rd–6th months.

Patterson (1995) built on this work. Using the four phases identified by Brooke (1987), she studied the lives of 12 residents. Six had been newly admitted and six had been in the home for over a year. Patterson's small study found that emotional support and practical assistance by staff and other residents was the most valued and helpful supportive behaviour. The lack of it was identified as the most non-supportive behaviour, especially by nursing staff. Patterson recommends that support interventions by staff are required to help people adapt to life in care. A further study by Wilson (1997) found that the transition to care was made easier if a designated member of staff spoke at regular intervals to older people who had moved into a care home setting. Wilson stated that this person should have good listening skills, be empathetic and supportive.

A study by Nolan and Dellasega (1999) takes this recommendation further. They state that once a carer has placed a relative in long-term care, it is assumed that the initial stress of this transition for both parties will abate over time. They point out the literature that suggests this is not the case and recommend that staff have to work with residents and their carers to ease the stress caused by the transition to care.

Researchers have commented that work is needed on the actual experiences of older people as they adjust on a day-to-day basis to life in care (Lee et al., 2002) and how older people cope with being transferred from one institution to another (Coleman, 2003). There is a growing body of literature on older people's experience of being in care and examples include Reed et al., 2003; McCormack et al., 2008 and Kydd, 2008.

CASE STUDIES

The following interviews are between a researcher and two older people (Kydd, 2006). Read the two extracts and then complete the exercise below.

Case study

Interview one

Mrs A had been in hospital for ten weeks and was too frail to be discharged home. She was waiting until a care home bed could be found for her. She had no idea why she was originally admitted to hospital other than she had fallen at home and had recently lost her sight due to glaucoma.

AK – How have you coped with being in hospital?

Mrs A – Not very well at all. I had no idea anything was wrong. Now they [medical staff] have told me I can't go home because I can't see. Yet they say I can't stay here [the hospital], I'm not allowed to stay here.

AK – So where are you going?

Mrs A – I couldn't tell you, I've no idea. My son says I have to go to a nursing home but I don't want to go.

AK – How do you feel about that?

Mrs A – I can't cope with it . . . I'll never get used to not going home. I miss my friends, my neighbours and my home. I have a flat in [names town]. I was born in that town.

AK – What do you see is your future?

Mrs A – I have no future . . . I don't want to talk any more.

Interview two

Mrs B is also in hospital. She is to be moved to a care home, but she is unsure as to the details. She has been in hospital for over a year.

AK – What brought you into hospital?

Mrs B – I couldn't walk…it was so upsetting but thanks to that [zimmer] I can get around . . . I've got bad eyes, I can't see . . . I never had bother with my eyes before . . . losing my sight has been worse than anything. [Cries] . . . I've lost all my friends they've all gone, I'm just lonely but this is a good place. [Cries] The staff are very good, you get attended to and looked after you don't need to worry about anything. They give you a laugh . . . I used to laugh a lot up until I lost all my family; I had three brothers and three sisters – gone. My mother and father they're all gone. [Cries]

AK – You've had a lot to put up with, how do you get by?

Mrs B – I get by alright, you have to get used to it, the way of living here, it's a different way . . . It's not what you would like or think about, but you get what life throws you and you have to live that life.

AK – How do you feel about not being at home?

Mrs B – Well it's a terrible period isn't it, but you can't go back [cries] because I know I couldn't look after myself . . . I loved my house, I loved cleaning it, I liked to keep it nice, I went out with my sister every day . . . we went up the town to shop and visit friends, but our friends have all gone now. My sister died before I came here and then her husband . . . they all went away one after the other.

AK – Will you go into a care home?

Mrs B – Well if I got the chance . . . when you think away back long ago there was never anything like these homes. It's great. I'm 90 odd and there didn't used to be places for people at that age . . . I don't know where I will end up . . .

AK – That must be quite hard.

Mrs B – Well you don't know, you are just living from day to day. You know you are getting looked after here, but you just have to accept that, you don't know where you are going or what is going to happen to you, but I'm 92 and I can't be going on much longer.

Activity 1

The two women above are both going through a transitional phase. They have similar health problems but Mrs B appears to be more accepting of her fate than Mrs A. Read the interviews again and suggest reasons why you think the two women might be reacting as they are.

- Now look at some of the changes you have been through in your own life. Concentrate on one very positive event that has led to a change and one very negative event that has led to a change.
- What made the positive event so good? It may have been something you have been working hard towards, like an exam, or training for a race. It may have been something you planned for and had saved for, like a holiday. Or it may have happened unexpectedly like a prize, a new brother or sister, or release from a commitment that was onerous.

- Now look at the negative event. Why was it negative for you? What changes did it make to your life? How did you handle the disappointment/loss/failure? Do you think you coped well? Did you have adequate and relevant resources to help you cope such as friends, family, money, etc.?
- Finally, think about your life as it is now. Now imagine that you were going through what Mrs A and Mrs B were going through. Both women were suddenly unable to go back to their homes. Both were unable to walk and unable to see. Mrs B had been bereaved of her family and many of her friends. Both were moving to a new environment.
- How do you think you would cope?
- Do you think health care professionals recognise an older person's transition into care as a major life event?
- Do you think more could be done to help older people make a transition into care?

THE USER'S PERSPECTIVE

In the two case studies above, Mrs A has undergone a series of sudden, traumatic losses in a short space of time. She is horrified at the thought of going into care and has difficulty talking about it. Mrs B has undergone similar losses, which are still very upsetting to her, but she has had time to come to the realisation that she can no longer cope at home. Neither women can plan for the transition they still have to make as both are in a transitional environment and have no idea which care home they will be admitted to or when. They are in the stage of 'confusion and distress' as identified by Bridges (1980).

Case studies on adapting to life in care homes illustrate that many older people adapt well to life in a care home. Vergare (1997) states that strategies, such as personalising a person's room with items from their homes, can make a person's transition to care much easier.

IMPLICATIONS FOR JOINT WORKING

Penrod (2007) highlights the need for health care professionals to understand the effects of uncertainty on individuals. This is because they work routinely with clients and caregivers who are in the midst of health-related times of uncertainty. She goes on to state that more research is needed in this area to build on the existing theories of transition and uncertainty.

> Foundational theory building is critical to the development and testing of research-based interventions to enable accurate assessment and intervention to facilitate the transition from discomforting states of uncertainty towards more comfortable states marked by a sense of personal growth.
>
> (Penrod, 2007: 666)

An essential part of helping older people to cope with the transition into care is to include support workers in helping older people settle into life in care. Team working between professionals and unqualified staff within the care home is essential. Baldwin (2003) highlights the fact that direct care is now mostly carried out by support workers, yet little attention is given to training and supporting unqualified staff in specific areas. The relationship between support workers and care home residents is usually closer than the relationships professionals have with them. The knowledge support workers have about the daily lives, hopes and fears of the residents is frequently ignored, to the detriment of the residents' care. This is especially true of information on managing transition, with training focussing on health and safety and physical care.

Another major area of concern is the lack of team work between the statutory and private sector. Reed and Stanley (2003) suggest that better communication between hospitals and the care home sector is needed in order to facilitate a smoother transition from one institution to another. They suggest that a daily living plan of an individual's preferences should be designed by the hospital staff, in conjunction with the older person. This plan would then be passed on to the care home when the individual is admitted. Coleman and Fox (2004) substantiate such work by stating that older people in transition require skilled practitioners who will work with the individual and their relatives.

The complex needs of older people require a multi-agency approach to care (Easterbrook, 1999) and in the last decade there has been a policy drive to provide 'joined up' services for older people in health and social care (Department of Health, 2001). The statutory services are working towards providing links to care homes and, in some areas, communication has been excellent. National projects such as *My Home Life* (National Care Homes Research and Development Forum, 2006) have done much to raise the profile of care homes and the management of the transition into care.

CONCLUSION

Transitions are part of the life course and the experience of each transition is a unique occurrence. Individuals differ in their vulnerability to transitions and how they cope will depend on the meaning the transition has to them, as well as the resources they have available to them.

Multiple transitions can produce a cumulative deterioration, especially if the individual has not had time to recover from one event before another one occurs. The anxiety and worry that accompanies an uncertain future can lead to a physical deterioration, especially in those whose health is already compromised. The physical effects may lead to a transition to further dependence for some frail older people, or may adversely affect their quality of life, which in turn will adversely affect their coping abilities.

This chapter has identified the anxiety and worry experienced by some older people moving into long-term care. It has also outlined several strategies from research studies that have made a positive difference to the way individuals move from one institution to another, or adapt to a life in care.

Transition awareness is every health care worker's business. Recognising the nature of transition, being aware of the possible effects of transition and knowing some strategies that may facilitate a smoother transitional period for a resident is essential knowledge for both health care professionals and their support workers.

REFERENCES

Aneshensel, C., Pearlin, L., Mullan, J., Zarit, S. and Whitlach, C. (1995) *Profiles of Caregiving: The Unexpected Career*. New York: Academic Press

Audit Scotland (2005). *Moving On: An Overview of Delayed Discharges in Scotland*. Edinburgh: Audit Scotland

Baldwin, R. (2003) 'National Framework for Older People (editorial)'. *Psychiatric Bulletin*, 27: 121–2

Beck-Little, R. and Weinrich, S. (1998) 'Assessment and management of sleep disorders in the elderly'. *Journal of Gerontological Nursing*, April, 21–9

Beidel, D., Turner, S. and Dancu, C. (1985) 'Physiological, cognitive, and behavioral aspects of social anxiety'. *Behavioral Research and Therapy*, 23: 109–17

Biedman, P. and Normoyle, J. (1991) 'Elderly community residents' reactions to the nursing home: an analysis of nursing home related beliefs'. *The Gerontologist*, 31: 107–15

Borkovec, T. (1979) 'Pseudo (experiential) insomnia and ideopathic (objective) insomnia: Theoretical and therapeutic issues'. *Advances in Behaviour Research and Therapy*, 2: 27–55

Borkovec, T., Metzger, R. and Pruzinsky, T. (1986) 'Anxiety, worry and the self' in L.Hartman, L. and Blackenship, K. (eds) *Perception of Self in Emotional Disorders and Psychotherapy*. New York: Plenum Press

Borkovec, T., Ray, W. and Stöber, J. (1998) 'Worry: a cognitive phenomenon intimately linked to affective, physiological, and interpersonal behavioral processes'. *Cognitive Therapy and Research*, 22: 561–76

Brammer, L. (1992) *Coping with Life Transitions*. Eric Digest. Identifier ED350527 www.ericdigests.org/1992-1/life.htm (Accessed 24 March 2008)

Bridges, W. (1980) *Transitions: Making Sense of Life's Changes*. Harlow: Addison-Wesley Publishing Company

Brooke, V. (1987) 'Adjusting to living in a nursing home: toward a nursing intervention.' Unpublished dissertation in Patterson, B. (1995) 'The process of social support: adjusting to life in a nursing home'. *Journal of Advanced Nursing* 21: 682–9

Challis, L. and Bartlett, H. (1988) *Old and Ill: Private Nursing Homes for Elderly People*. London: ACE Books

Chenitz, W. (1983) 'Entry to a nursing home as a status passage: a theory to guide nursing practice'. *Geriatric Nursing*, March/April: 92–7

Coleman, E. and Fox, P. (2004) 'One patient, many places: managing health care transitions, Part II: Practitioner skills and patient and caregiver preparation'. *Annals of Long-Term Care*, 12 (10): 34–48

Coleman, P. (2003) 'Falling through the cracks: challenges and opportunities for improving transitional care for persons with continuous complex needs'. *Journal of the American Geriatrics Society*, 51: 549–55

Department of Health (2001) *National Service Framework for Older People*. London: HMSO

Easterbrook, L. (1999) *When We Are Very Old: Treatment, Care and Support for Older People*. London: King's Fund

Eckwall, A., Sivberg, B. and Hallberg, I. (2007) 'Older caregivers' coping strategies and sense of coherence in relation to quality of life'. *Journal of Advanced Nursing* 57 (6): 584–604

Erikson, E. (1963) *Childhood and Society* (2nd edn). New York: Norton

Ersser, S. (1999) 'Measuring the sleep patterns of older people'. *Nursing Times*, 6: 46–9

Evans, N., Forney, D. and Guido-DiBrito, F. (1998) *Student Development in College: Theory, Research and Practice*. San Fransisco, CA: Jossey-Bass Publishers.

Goodman, J., Schlossberg, N. and Anderson, M. (2006) *Counseling Adults in Transition: Linking Practice with Theory* (3rd edn). New York: Springer Publishing

Hopson, B. (1981) 'Response to papers by Schlossberg, Brammer and Abrego'. *The Counseling Psychologist*, 9: 36–40

Jensen, D. and Herr, K. (1993) 'Sleeplessness: advances in clinical research'. *Nursing Clinics of North America*, 28: 385–405

Ketcham, C. and Stelmach, G. (2001) 'Age-related declines in motor control' in Birren, J. and Schaie, K. (eds) *Handbook of the Psychology of Aging* (5th edn). London: Academic Press

Kydd, A. (2006) 'Life in Limbo: Delayed discharge from a patient and policy perspective' (unpublished dissertation). Aberdeen: Aberdeen University Press

Kydd, A. (2008) 'The patient experience of being a delayed discharge'. *Journal of Nursing Management*, 16: 104–14

Lee, D., Woo, J. and MacKenzie, A. (2002) 'A review of older people's experiences with residential care placement'. *Journal of Advanced Nursing*, 37: 19–27

Magai, C. (2001) 'Emotions over the life span' in Woods, R. (ed.) *Psychological Problems of Ageing: Assessment Treatment and Care*. Chichester: John Wiley and Sons Ltd

MaloneBeach, E., Zarit, S. and Spore, D. (1992) 'Caregivers' perceptions of case management and community based services: barriers to service use'. *Journal of Applied Gerontology*, 11: 146–59

McCormack, B., Mitchell, E., Cook, G., Reed, J. and Childs, S. (2008) 'Older persons' experiences of whole systems: the impact of health and social care organisation'. *Journal of Nursing Management* 16: 104–14

Metzger, R., Miller, M., Cohen, M., Sofka, M. and Borkovec, T. (1990) 'Worry changes decision making: The effect of negative thoughts on cognitive processing'. *Journal of Clinical Psychology*, 46: 78–88

Moxon, S., Lyne, K., Sinclair, I., Young, P. and Kirk, C. (2001) 'Mental health in residential homes: a role for care staff'. *Ageing and Society*, 21: 71–93

National Care Homes Research and Development Forum (2006) '*My Home Life*': *Quality of Life in Care Homes*. London: Help the Aged

NHS Quality Improvement Scotland (2004) *Healthcare Services Used by Older people in NHS Scotland. Draft Standards May 2004*. Edinburgh: NHS Quality Improvement Scotland

Nolan, M. and Dellasega, C. (1999) '"It's not the same as him being at home": creating caring parnerships following nursing home placement'. *Journal of Clinical Nursing*, 8 (10): 723–30

Nolan, M. and Grant G. (1992) 'Mid-ranging theory building and the nursing-theory practice gap'. *Journal of Advanced Nursing*, 17: 217–13

Nolan, M., Walker, G., Nolan, J., Williams, S., Poland, F., Curran, N. *et al.* (1996) 'Entry to care: Positive choice or fait accompli?'. *Journal of Advanced Nursing*, 24: 265–74

Office for National Statistics (2003) 'People Aged 65 and Over: Results of a Study Carried out on Behalf of the Department of Health as Part of the 2001 General Household Survey. TSO: London

Parkes, C. (1972) *Bereavement: Studies of Grief in Adult Life*. New York: International Universities Press

Patterson, B. (1995) 'The process of social support: adjusting to life in a nursing home', *Journal of Advanced Nursing*, 21 (4): 682–89

Penrod, J. (2001) 'Refinement of the concept of uncertainty'. *Journal of Advanced Nursing*, 34: 238–45

Penrod, J. (2007) 'Living with uncertainty: concept advancement'. *Journal of Advanced Nursing*, 57 (6): 658–67

Reed, J., Cook, G., Sullivan A. and Burridge, C. (2003) 'Making a move: care home residents' experience of re-location'. *Ageing and Society*, 23 (2): 225–42

Reed, D., Morgan, D. and Palmer, A. (1998). *Discharging Older People from Hospital to Care Homes: Implications for Nursing.* Newcastle-upon-Tyne: Faculty of Health, Social Work and Education, University of Northumbria

Reed, J. and Stanley, D. (2000) 'Discharge from hospital to care home: Professional boundaries and interfaces' in Warnes, A., Warren, L. and Nolan, M. (eds.) *Care Services for Later Life.* London: Jessica Kingsley Publishers

Reed, J. and Stanley, D. (2003) 'Improving communication between hospitals and care homes: the development of a daily living plan for older people'. *Health and Social Care in the Community*, 11 (4): 356–63

Rodehn Fox, M. (1999) 'The importance of sleep'. *Nursing Standard*, 3: 44–7

Sampson, R. and Laub. J. (1993) *Crime in the Making: Pathways and Turning Points Through Life.* Cambridge, MA: Harvard University Press

Schlossberg, N. (1981) 'A model for analyzing human adaptation to transition'. *Counseling Psychologist*, 9 (2): 2–18

Schlossberg, N. (1984) *Counseling Adults in Transition.* New York: Springer

Scottish Executive (2001) *Expert Group on Healthcare of Older People: Adding Life to Years.* Edinburgh: Scottish Executive

Scottish Office (1997) *Designed to Care.* Edinburgh: The Stationery Office

Schultz, R. and Heckhausen, J. (1998) 'Emotion and control: A life span perspective' in Magai, C. (2001) 'Emotions over the life span', in Woods, R. (ed.) *Psychological Problems of Ageing: Assessment Treatment and Care.* Chichester: John Wiley and Sons Ltd

Turner, S. and Beidel, D. (1986) 'Empirically derived subtypes of social anxiety'. *Behavior Therapy*, 16: 38

Vergare, M. (1997) 'Depression in the context of late-life transitions'. *Bulletin of the Menninger Clinic*, 6 (2): 240–5

Reich, W., Harber, K. and Siegel, I. (2007) 'Self-structure and well-being in life transitions'. *Self and Identity*, 7 (2): 129–50

Welsh Assembly (2003) *The Strategy for Older People in Wales – Living Longer, Living Better 2008–2013.* **www.new.wales.gov.uk** (Accessed 29 April 2008)

Wilson, S. (1997) 'Transition to nursing home life: A comparison of planned and unplanned admissions'. *Journal of Advanced Nursing*, 26 (5): 864–71

Woods, R. (2000a) 'Mental health problems in later life' in Woods, R. (ed.) *Psychological Problems of Ageing: Assessment Treatment and Care.* Chichester: John Wiley and Sons Ltd

Woods, R. (2000b) (ed.) *Psychological Problems of Ageing: Assessment Treatment and Care.* Chichester: John Wiley and Sons Ltd

Yalom, I. (1987) 'Forward', in Sadavoy, J. and Leszcz, M. (eds) *Treating the Elderly with Psychotherapy.* Madison, CT: International University Press.

Zarit, S. and Edwards, A. (2000) 'Family caregiving: Research and clinical Intervention' in Woods, R. (ed.) *Psychological Problems of Ageing: Assessment Treatment and Care.* Chichester: John Wiley and Sons Ltd

Chapter 16

Palliative Care, Death and Bereavement

Stuart Milligan and Elaine Stevens

This chapter will examine the principles of palliative care and discuss the relevance of palliative care to older people and the evidence that access to palliative care for this group is currently poor. It will go on to examine a number of issues relevant to older people, including pain assessment and management, palliative care in care homes, palliative care for people with dementia and palliative care at the end of life. The chapter will conclude with three case studies that highlight some of the major issues around loss, grief and bereavement and their relevance to older people.

Learning outcomes

Reading this chapter will enable you to:

- give a definition of palliative care;
- describe the benefits to older people of appropriate palliative care;
- discuss the principal challenges in providing appropriate palliative care for older people;
- identify the major issues around loss, grief and bereavement;
- discuss loss, grief and bereavement as they relate to older people.

INTRODUCTION

The term 'palliative care' was coined as recently as 1974, and the speciality of Palliative Medicine was only recognised by the Royal College of Physicians in 1987. However, in the intervening decades, palliative care has grown to become a significant theme in health care provision in the UK and around the world.

Palliative care seeks, first and foremost, to relieve suffering and improve quality of life. For this reason, palliative care approaches have traditionally been offered to those for whom cure is impossible. However, palliative care is increasingly being recognised not as an alternative to curative interventions but as an approach that is compatible with active disease management and appropriate at various points in the individual's disease journey (Sepulveda *et al.*, 2002). As a result, older people, by virtue of their higher rates of life-limiting illness and associated high levels of morbidity and mortality, might be expected to be prime users of palliative care services. The potential benefits of appropriate palliative care for older people, particularly in the areas of symptom relief, psychosocial comfort and carer support are considerable (World Health Organisation Europe, 2004a).

WHAT IS PALLIATIVE CARE?

Palliative care has its modern origins in the hospice movement and, particularly, in the work of Dame Cicely Saunders and her contemporaries at St Christopher's Hospice (opened in 1967) and elsewhere (Clark *et al.*, 2005). However, the roots of a concern for the welfare of those suffering from the effects of life-limiting illness can be traced back a century earlier to the work of the Sisters of Charity among the dying poor (particularly in Dublin and London) and to Mme Jeanne Garnier's *Dames de Calvaire* who first used the term 'hospice' in 1840s France. In truth, the origins of the practice of providing comfort, care and healing for people nearing the end of life lie well before recorded history.

According to the World Health Organisation (Sepulveda *et al.*, 2002: 92), palliative care is:

> . . . an approach that improves the quality of life of patients and their families facing the problems associated with life-threatening illness, through the prevention and relief of suffering by means of early identification and impeccable assessment and treatment of pain and other problems, physical, psychosocial and spiritual.

Palliative care:

- provides relief from pain and other distressing symptoms;
- affirms life and regards dying as a normal process;
- intends neither to hasten or postpone death;
- integrates the psychological and spiritual aspects of patient care;
- offers a support system to help patients live as actively as possible until death;
- offers a support system to help the family cope during the patient's illness and in their own bereavement;
- uses a team approach to address the needs of patients and their families, including bereavement counselling, if indicated;
- will enhance quality of life, and may also positively influence the course of illness;
- is applicable early in the course of illness, in conjunction with other therapies that are intended to prolong life, such as chemotherapy or radiation therapy, and includes those investigations needed to better understand and manage distressing clinical complications.

It should be apparent from the above that palliative care is an active approach to patient care with a focus on the individual and emphasis on support, symptom management and quality of life. It is applicable in many different settings and the older person with a life-threatening illness may receive palliative care not just in hospices but in acute hospitals, primary care, community hospitals and care homes (National Council for Palliative Care, 2006).

THE PROVISION OF PALLIATIVE CARE

The growing recognition of the benefits of palliative care to patients has led to the proliferation of dedicated palliative care services throughout the UK and Ireland (and increasingly around the world). By 2008, the Hospice and Palliative Care Directory (produced annually by the Hospice Information Service (HIS) at St Christopher's Hospice, London) was listing 223 In-patient Units, 304 Hospital Support Teams and 316 Home Care (community) Services (HIS, 2008). In addition to these dedicated units and services, many other health and social care providers incorporate elements of palliative care into the services they provide. In 1995, the National Council for Hospice and Specialist Palliative Care Services (NCHSPCS) identified three levels of palliative care provision: specialist palliative care (provided by specialist teams such as hospital palliative care teams and hospices), palliative interventions (short-term care provided by surgeons, anaesthetists and other specialists), and a palliative approach to care (provided by a range of health and social care professionals across all care settings) (NCHSPC, 1995).

Traditionally, palliative care has primarily been offered to people with cancer (Scottish Partnership for Palliative Care, 2006a). However, this situation has long been recognised as inequitable and current trends are towards ensuring that palliative care is provided on the basis of need, not diagnosis. Consequently older people with a range of disease processes (including cancer, progressive neurological conditions, heart failure, advanced respiratory disease, Parkinson's Disease and dementia-causing illnesses) may find themselves the recipients of palliative care provision and services (NCHSPCS, 2005; Scottish Partnership for Palliative Care, 2006a).

THE NEEDS OF OLDER PEOPLE FOR PALLIATIVE CARE

The potential benefits of incorporating a palliative approach into the care of the older adult include improved symptom control, psychosocial and spiritual support (for both patient and carer), open and effective communication, appropriate care at the end of life and support for the bereaved (World Health Organisation Europe, 2004a). Research has consistently shown that older people, particularly at the end of life, suffer worse symptoms, experience more isolation and receive poorer communication than their younger counterparts (Hockley and Clark, 2002). Calls from the NCHSPCS and other bodies for government policy to address this issue have resulted in successive health policy documents acknowledging the role of palliative care in the care of older people (for example, World Health Organisation Europe, 2004b; Department of Health, 2006; Scottish Executive Range and Capacity Review Group, 2006).

Evidence of underassessment and undertreatment in older people requiring palliative care

In spite of increasing attention to the palliative care needs of older people, a recent review of provision across Europe concluded that 'older people suffer unnecessarily because of widespread underassessment and undertreatment of their problems' (World Health Organisation Europe, 2004a). The main areas of concern highlighted by this report were underassessment of pain, lack of information and involvement in decision-making, lack of home care, lack of access to specialist services and lack of palliative care within nursing and residential homes. Taken together, these concerns point to a significant failure to meet the palliative care needs of older people, a situation referred to by Help the Aged as a 'national disgrace' (Help the Aged, 2008).

In the UK there is evidence that older people are less well represented among users of specialist palliative care services than might be expected (Eve and Higginson, 2000; Koffman and Higginson, 2004). There is also evidence that care homes have yet to fully respond to the challenge of incorporating palliative care into already established models of care (Department of Health, 2006). Also, in spite of UK government investments in care of the dying in recent years, it appears that many health care staff consider themselves unprepared to deliver effective end of life care for older people (Help the Aged, 2006).

Pain assessment and management

One of the ways in which palliative care might have most to contribute to the care of older people is in the area of the assessment and management of pain. The early work of Cicely Saunders helped to form current views of 'total pain' and the need for holistic assessment and management of the symptom (Saunders, 1978). Furthermore, the degree of expertise in pain control that has undoubtedly built up within specialist palliative care has important implications for the considerable amount of unrelieved pain known to be experienced by older people (Gagliese and Melzack, 1997).

The importance of adopting a holistic, person-centred approach to the management of pain in older people cannot be overstated. Research has shown that pain in older people is affected not only by a complex array of pathophysiological factors but also by the attitudes of older people themselves, the attitudes of their professional carers, ritual and routine, concerns about side effects of medication and communication difficulties (for example, Duggleby, 2000; Mitchell, 2001). Clearly a consistent and logical approach based on partnership working between the multi-professional team, the older person and his or her carers is called for (Twycross, 1997).

Frequently, however, pain management in older people falls at the first hurdle because assessment is inaccurate or incomplete. This is particularly the case when communication is restricted by cognitive impairment (Scherder et al., 2005; Regnard et al., 2006). Ideally, the primary assessor of any pain should be the sufferer him or herself (NHS Quality Improvement Scotland, 2006). To this end, Mitchell (2001) has listed useful suggestions for the design of self-assessment tools for older people. However, when communication problems are severe, for instance in profound cognitive impairment, even the simplest self-assessment tools are unsuitable. In such circumstances, health care professionals have tended to employ a complex combination of observation, familiarity with 'the normal' and seeking out corroborative evidence to arrive at workable pain assessments (Parke, 1998). In recent years, however, several dedicated tools have been devised to measure pain in the cognitively impaired older person including the Abbey Pain Scale and the DOLOPLUS 2 Scale (Lefebvre-Chapiro and the DOLOPLUS Group, 2001; Abbey *et al.*, 2004). Particularly when used within a framework of holistic management of pain and other causes of distress, these tools offer real opportunities to reduce levels of pain in this vulnerable group.

Palliative care in care homes

In the United Kingdom as many as one in five people die in residential or nursing care homes and, with the changing demography of society, care homes will become increasingly important providers of end of life care for older people (Philp, 2002). Given the range of diagnoses represented within the care home population, the multiple pathologies often suffered and the imperative to optimise quality of life, the case for introducing palliative care into care homes is readily made (Scottish Partnership for Palliative Care, 2006b).

There is little doubt that there is considerable interest from care home practitioners in expanding palliative care into that sector (Froggatt and Payne, 2006). However, evidence suggests that uptake of end of life care initiatives, while good in hospitals and hospices, has been poorer in care homes (Department of Health, 2006). Some of the barriers to the introduction of palliative care into care homes include variations in perceptions of concepts around end of life care among care home managers, the lack of stability in some care home workforces and well-intentioned but sometimes inappropriate staff training (Froggatt, 2002; Goodman, Woolley and Knight, 2003; Froggatt and Payne, 2006). The drafting of standards for palliative care in care homes has been a welcome development and provides a framework within which the considerable progress already made can be consolidated (for example, Scottish Partnership in Palliative Care, 2006b). Several education initiatives are enabling some of the expertise that is located in specialist palliative care to be shared with the care home sector. Providers of this education include the Royal College of Nursing, Macmillan Cancer Relief, Marie Curie Cancer Care and many specialist palliative care units and teams. Other initiatives aimed at sharing expertise between specialist palliative care and care homes have included domiciliary visits by specialist clinicians and the appointment of link nurses (Froggatt, 2002). Finally, integrated care pathways including the Liverpool Care Pathway offer tremendous scope for end of life care practice in care homes to harmonise with the very best of evidence-based care (Duffy and Woodland, 2006).

Palliative care for people with a dementia

Much interest has been directed towards the extension of palliative care from its traditional base of advanced cancer to include other progressive, life-threatening conditions including cardiac failure and chronic obstructive pulmonary disease (for example, Scottish Partnership for Palliative Care, 2006a). Increasingly this interest has also been directed at the complex of progressive disorders referred to as the dementias. Until relatively recently, the management of dementia was dominated by a biomedical model that focussed primarily on the medical needs of sufferers (Cox and Cook, 2002). This approach had the effect of restricting the scope of supportive care given to people dying of the condition and a recent report of The House of Commons Committee of Public Accounts (2008) has drawn parallels between recent attitudes towards dementia and those towards cancer in the 1950s.

Modern models of dementia care are firmly person-centred and are entirely compatible with the integrated, supportive approach that is central to palliative care. Indeed, there is growing evidence that end of life care for the person with dementia can be enhanced by a merging of dementia-focussed approaches with elements of palliative care (NHS Lothian, 2007). Some of the areas where an approach based on palliative care principles may be beneficial include communication, support for carers, openness about prognosis and end of life care.

Another important area of dementia care that could benefit from cross-fertilisation with palliative care is spirituality (Smith, 2005). The progressive and cumulative losses associated with dementia can disconnect the person from the people, places and things which gave his or her life meaning. Moving to a deeper knowledge of the person and instituting practices that acknowledge and express their unique personhood can be powerfully affirming for all concerned (Milligan, 2004).

Palliative care at the end of life

A consistent barrier to the improvement of care at the end of life for people of all ages has been reluctance to speak about issues around death and dying. A report from Help the Aged (2005) entitled *Dying in Older Age* called for the taboo surrounding death to be lifted so that standards of dying in older people could be addressed. Indeed there is evidence that some older people welcome and might even enjoy, discussing end of life issues (Catt *et al.*, 2005).

One of the legacies of palliative care has been to support a greater openness about death and dying. This openness means that older people can more freely engage with care providers to discuss how they wish to be cared for at the end of life (Help the Aged Peer Education Project Group, 2006). In 1999, Age Concern commissioned the Debate of the Age Health and Care Study Group to question older people about what, for them, constituted a good death. The result was the following principles of a good death:

1. To know when death is coming and to understand what can be expected.
2. To be able to retain control of what happens.
3. To be afforded dignity and privacy.
4. To have control over pain relief and other symptom control.
5. To have choice and control over where death occurs (at home or elsewhere).
6. To have access to information and expertise of whatever kind is necessary.
7. To have access to any spiritual or emotional support required.
8. To have access to hospice care in any location, not only in hospital.
9. To have control over who is present and who shares the end.
10. To be able to issue advance directives which ensure wishes are respected.
11. To have time to say goodbye, and control over other aspects of timing.
12. To be able to leave when it is time to go, and not have life prolonged pointlessly.

(Debate of the Age Health and Care Study Group, 1999)

It is clear from the above that older people want to have choices about how and where they die, and who provides the care they receive. They may be less likely than younger people to want help to end their own lives, but this should not be interpreted as implying acceptance of the current status quo (Catt *et al.*, 2005). There is a pressing need for older people in all care settings to have more control over their end of life care. The Department of Health's *End of Life Care Programme* is a positive development but it urgently requires the assurance of long-term funding and replication in other parts of the UK (Department of Health 2006; Scottish Partnership for Palliative Care, 2007).

LOSS, GRIEF AND BEREAVEMENT IN OLDER PEOPLE

Using the three case studies in this section, focus on how you, the professional carer, can provide support for the older person who is dying and their family and friends and also when an older person experiences the death of a family member or friend.

From research we know that when a person has a life-limiting illness it stretches their coping mechanisms and also the coping mechanisms of their family and friends (Reed and Rousseau, 2007). Indeed, we recognise that there is a strong link between the ability to cope with loss and an individual's quality of life (Payne, Horn and Relf, 2000). From this it is logical to assume that if better support is provided to the dying person and their families and friends the better their quality of life will be.

Loss and the person who is dying

Case study 1

Let's begin by looking at the case of George who is 79 and has been diagnosed with motor neurone disease. He has been advised not to drive because of his increasing muscle weakness. This is a huge issue for George as he lives alone in a rural community. He wonders how he will collect his pension, how he will get to church and how he will get to the doctors.

As each individual will experience their own unique losses we cannot cover every loss that George may experience. This example discusses those losses that are experienced by many older adults who have a life-limiting illness.

The enforced loss of a driving licence is one of the common causes of low mood and depression in older adults and is related to loss of independence and control (Windsor et al., 2007). This is especially true if the person is also experiencing the loss of physical health (Covinsky et al., 2003). In addition, the ensuing loss of social contacts and support such as, for example, church groups, compounds feelings of isolation leading to lower mood and depression, which may also have an impact on the person's motivation to get up, washed and dressed (Lochler *et al.*, 2004). Indeed, it has been noted that suicide rates in older adults, especially those with multiple co-morbid conditions and who are socially isolated, are above average in relation to the general population (Coon, DeVries and Gallacher-Thompson, 2007). The loss of health, independence and motivation to care for oneself may also mean a person requires admission to care. That, in itself, may result in depression. In fact, we know that depression in care home residents is more common than in older people living at home and although the reasons for this are multifaceted it causes added distress for residents (Choi *et al.*, 2008). Unfortunately the incidence of depression can increase as death nears (Lloyd-Williams, Spiller and Ward, 2003) and this can also have a negative impact on the quality of a person's death.

Loss and the death of a family member

Case study 2

Let's now look at our second case where we will focus on the quality of dying and possible reactions of specific family members to the loss of an older adult.

Jean is a widow of 76 who has advanced dementia. She lives in a care home where she is now confined to bed and sleeps most of the time. Her GP feels her prognosis is weeks rather than months. Jean has two very attentive daughters and a son who is estranged from his sisters due to alcohol addiction. He visits his mother once a month.

Society usually expects a lesser reaction from adults to the death of a parent who is old and indeed often thinks that the death of an older person who has been ill is a relief for the family left behind (Taylor and Norris, 1995). This may have implications for Jean's children as they may feel unable to show their grief and believe they have to get on with life as if nothing has happened. In reality the death of a parent is the most common reason for adults to request help with their bereavement (Cruse Bereavement Care, 2004).

We also know that the quality of death can affect the grief of those left behind. For example, many people can identify a 'good' death and indeed Bradbury's (2000) research identifies three main types of good death:

- a sacred good death – dying within one's religious and cultural framework;
- a medicalised good death – dying with good symptom management and a strong medical presence;
- a natural good death – dying with little medical intervention or dying doing something that the person loved to do, for example motor racing.

In addition, we also understand that if a death is anticipated or expected it may help family members to cope with the death of a loved one when it happens. Although a protracted death such as in dementia can have a negative effect on bereavement outcomes (Open University, 2004) as families may have witnessed their loved one struggle with illness for a long time. The quality of death can also be affected by the place of care and we know that in an ageing society many older adults die in care homes. However, it is recognised that their palliative care needs may not be addressed as many have a limited budget to train staff and therefore skills are lower (Hirst, 2004). This may, in turn, lead to a poorer quality of death and bereavement for those left behind.

Jean's daughters may have experienced many losses as her illness has progressed such as the loss of a friend, confidant and their family home as well as witnessing the progressive decline of their mother's health. We also have to remember that even though the two daughters are sisters their reactions may differ. For example, if one daughter had relied on their mother more for advice and support it may be more difficult for her to cope with both the illness and impending death as she has lost her main support mechanism (Parkes, Relf and Couldrick, 1997). This may result in one daughter seeming to be less interested in her mother's condition as she is unable to cope with 'bad news' and, as such, avoids asking about her mother's condition. We also know that when middle-aged women lose their mothers there may be significant changes in self identity and role that can have a negative effect on their grieving (Taylor and Norris, 1995) and, indeed, on marital relationships (Parkes, 2006). In addition accumulated important losses, including the loss of the head of a family and the lack of support in bereavement, can lead to both depression and suicidal thoughts (Parkes, 2006).

Jean's son, being an estranged family member, may find it difficult to cope with illness and death in the family as he may not get enough information about what is happening (Smith, 2004). This can lead to feelings of isolation and anxiety being displayed as anger and/or aggression (Worden, 2000). We also know that people's personalities affect the way they cope and that alcohol can be used as a coping measure (Parkes, 2006). However, alcohol used as a long-term coping mechanism can have a devastating effect on interpersonal relationships (Humphreys, Moos and Cohen, 1997), meaning that Jean's son may have no support in his bereavement, which will affect his quality of life. This is important for the care home team to be aware of as they may have to provide extra support to Jean's son themselves. Another avenue open to the care home team would be to, with his permission, advise Jean's son's GP of the current family situation and to request that the primary care team make contact with him so help is at hand if required. Indeed, many GP practices now have a counsellor as part of their team who could support Jean's son through this difficult time.

Experiencing the loss of a family member in old age

Case study 3

Our final case is Beryl who is 88 and has been in hospital for five months following a stroke that has left her physically frail and with expressive dysphasia. Her only son lives in Australia and her only sister visits the hospital once a week. Beryl's husband died of lung cancer 30 years ago. Beryl's sister has learned that Beryl's son has lung cancer and will die very soon. However she does not want Beryl to know this.

Families often want to protect their loved ones from harm. However, there is good evidence to suggest that deceit between family members can have far reaching effects on how they trust each other in the future (Open University, 2004). This will then affect the amount of support Beryl may receive as she may no longer feel she can rely on her sister. The notion that Beryl may not be able to understand the implications of her son's illness may be compounded by her inability to communicate and, as such, care staff may agree with Beryl's sister. Indeed, current opinion shows that care professionals may not always wish to communicate bad news to patients as they are afraid of the emotions it may cause (Buckman, 2000). However, we do know that, in fact, older adults are often more resilient than is thought and this, combined with the fact that Beryl has a right to be told the truth, leads us to believe that 'the truth may hurt but deceit hurts more' (Fallowfield, Jenkins and Beveridge, 2002: 297). However, what we do not want is to assault people with information they do not want or that harms their quality of life.

So, before opting to tell Beryl about her son's illness, preparatory work on how this may affect Beryl should be considered. This is especially true as Beryl may not be able to express her feelings due to her dysphasia. Parkes (2006) suggests that the loss of an adult child should not cause as much disruption as that of a younger child. However Stroebe and Schut (2001) suggest that the loss of an adult child results in a more severe grief reaction, especially if it is an only child, as the death is seen as both unnatural and as the loss of one's future heritage. Another issue that may affect Beryl is that of survivor guilt, feeling that she should be the one to die not her son (Worden, 2000). Beryl's fear for her son may also be increased by memories of the loss of her husband as both have the same diagnosis. Indeed we know that the experience of a past loss can have either a positive or negative effect on the ability to cope with further losses (Worden, 2000). Therefore, if Beryl's husband did not have the 'good death' previously defined, then this will colour her ideas of the type of death her son may have. As Beryl cannot communicate distress it is useful to consider how she has previously displayed distress so she can be well supported. This can be achieved by asking Beryl's day-to-day carers as Parke (1998) explains that they will have a good knowledge of Beryl's behaviours that indicate distress.

Support for those experiencing loss, grief and bereavement

This final section will discuss how to support people who are experiencing loss, grief and bereavement. Remember that grief is a natural response that we will all experience at some point in our lives and that each grief experience is unique and as such different emotions and behaviours will be displayed (Walter, 1999).

Dying people and their families need continuity of care so, consequently, a therapeutic relationship needs to be built based on openness and trust (Jarrett and Maslin-Prothero, 2004). This means that professional carers require good communication skills including the ability to actively listen

(Parkes, Relf and Couldrick, 1997). These skills also allow professional carers to accurately assess issues as they arise, including situations that can be changed to reduce losses being incurred. For example, in the case study about George, finding alternative means of transport may alleviate some of his issues or, in the case study about Jean, ensuring she has a good death will help all concerned. Indeed Loftus (2000) suggests a key nurse can ensure that services can be accessed in a timely manner. In reality this key worker can keep the rest of the care team informed so an individualised, holistic plan is developed in conjunction with the patient's or the family member's values and belief systems. Other ways of helping may be to sensitively approach spiritual or religious issues (Peberdy, 2000) either during the illness journey or in the bereavement phase. This can encourage people, like Jean's children in Case Study 2, to talk about their concerns thus reducing feelings of loss and isolation. Or, in Beryl's case, exploring the meaning of the loss of her son, should this occur.

Unfortunately, when people are experiencing loss there are times when nothing can be changed and the role of the helper is simply to be there. This can be difficult for professional carers as their main role is to reduce distress and the inability to do this may lead to embarrassment and difficulties in engaging with those experiencing loss (Parkes, Relf and Couldrick, 1997). However, Walter (1999) suggests that bereavement is part of a reflexive, ongoing dialogue with oneself and others in which the bereaved try and make sense of their world. Therefore being there for the bereaved is an important way of helping. Remember, however, that some individuals may experience an abnormal reaction to a loss no matter how good the support is and this requires formal psychological/psychiatric expertise (Parkes, 2006). Examples are those who totally withdraw from society, who abuse alcohol, like Jean's son in Case study 2, or who are fixated with the death of a loved one for a long period of time (Worden, 2000).

So, in conclusion, the older adult will experience their own unique losses either during their own illness or during the illness and/or death of a family member or friend and it befalls the professional team to support them as best they can to maintain their quality of life.

Activity

Does your organisation have any information available for the care team to help the care team support people who are experiencing loss, grief and bereavement? Find out from your line manager if there is any information available to give dying people or their family members, to show where they may find bereavement support. You could also visit the CRUSE Bereavement Care website at **www. crusebereavementcare.org.uk** to see what they suggest could be done to support the bereaved.

Commentary

If your organisation does have such information available then it is one of the few that has taken a holistic view of patients' care. It is more likely that outcomes of care are defined in terms of physical wellbeing with little or no real focus on the other areas of holistic care (Pearce and Duffy, 2005). It may be helpful to develop an information file along with other care team members so you are able to provide support to dying people and their families even if this is only being able to direct them to the most suitable professional or organisation who is able to do this.

CONCLUSION

This chapter has discussed the principles of palliative care and touched on some of the issues affecting older people living with life-threatening disease or approaching the end of life. It has also explored the often-hidden problem of grief and bereavement in this age group. It has demonstrated that many older people would benefit from the inclusion of some elements of palliation into their care. However, relatively few will receive specialist palliative care services. It is therefore incumbent upon the many other health care providers and settings, aided by specialist palliative care if necessary, to incorporate a palliative approach into the range of options they provide for older people.

FURTHER READING

Davies, E. and Higginson, I.J. (2004) *Better Palliative Care for Older People*. http://www.euro.who.int/document/E82933.pdf

Stevens, E. and Edwards, J. (eds) (2008) *Palliative Care: Learning in Practice*. Exeter: Reflect Press.

Walter, T. (1999) *On Bereavement: The Culture of Grief*. Buckingham: Open University Press.

Useful websites

www.eapcnet.org
European Association for Palliative Care

www.ncpc.org.uk
National Council for Palliative Care

www.palliativecarescotland.org.uk
Scottish Partnership for Palliative Care

www.who.int/cancer/palliative/en
World Health Organisation

REFERENCES

Abbey, J., De Bellis, A., Piller, N., Esterman, A., Parker, D., Giles, L. and Lowcay, B. (2004) 'The Abbey pain scale: a 1-minute numerical indicator for people with end stage dementia'. *International Journal of Palliative Nursing*, 10 (1): 6–13

Bradbury, M. (2000) 'The good death?' in Dickenson, D., Johnson, M. and Katz, J.S. (eds). *Death, Dying and Bereavement* (2nd edn). London: Sage/Open University Press

Buckman, R. (2000) 'Communication in palliative care: A practical guide' in Dickenson, D., Johnson, M. and Katz, J.S. (eds). *Death, Dying and Bereavement* (2nd edn). London: Sage/Open University Press

Catt, S., Blanchard, M., Addington-Hall, J., Zis, M., Blizard, R. and King, M. (2005) 'Older adults' attitudes to death, palliative treatment and hospice care'. *Palliative Medicine*, 19 (5): 402–10

Choi, N.G., Ransom, S. and Wylie, R.J. (2008) 'Depression in older nursing home residents: The influence of nursing home environmental stressors, coping, and acceptance of group and individual therapy'. *Aging & Mental Health*, 12 (5): 536–47

Clark, D., Small, N., Wright, M., Winslow, M. and Hughes, N. (2005) *A Bit of Heaven for the Few? An Oral History of the Hospice Movement in the United Kingdom*. Lancaster: Observatory Publications

Coon, D.W., DeVries, H.M. and Gallacher-Thompson, D. (2007) 'Cognitive behavioural therapy with suicidal older adults'. *Behavioural and Cognitive Psychotherapy*, 32: 481–93

Covinsky, K.E., Palmer, R.M., Fortinsky, R.H., Counsell, S.R., Stewart, A.L., Kresevic, D., Burant, C.J. and Landefeld, C.S. (2003) 'Loss of independence in activities of daily living in older adults hospitalised with medical illness: Increased vulnerability with age'. *American Journal of the American Geriatric Society*, 51 (4): 451–8

Cox, S. and Cook, A. (2002) 'Caring for people with dementia at the end of life' in Hockley, J. and Clark, D. (eds) *Palliative Care for Older People in Care Homes*. Buckingham: Open University Press

Cruse Bereavement Care (2004) *Cruse Annual Report*. Richmond: Cruse Bereavement Care

Debate of the Age Health and Care Study Group (1999) *The Future of Health and Care of Older People – The Best is Yet to Come*. London: Age Concern

Department of Health (2006) *NHS End of Life Care Programme: Progress Report March 2006*. London: Department of Health

Duffy, A. and Woodland, C. (2006) Introducing the Liverpool Care Pathway into nursing homes. *Nursing Older People*, 18 (9): 33–6

Duggleby, W. (2000) 'Enduring suffering: a grounded theory analysis of the pain experience of elderly hospice patients with cancer'. *Oncology Nursing Forum*, 27 (5): 825–31

Eve, A. and Higginson, I.J. (2000) 'Minimum dataset activity for hospice and hospital palliative care services in the UK 1997/98'. *Palliative Medicine*, 14 (5): 395–404

Fallowfield, L.J., Jenkins, V.A. and Beveridge, H.A. (2002) 'Truth may hurt but deceit hurts more'. *Palliative Medicine*, 16: (4): 297–303

Froggatt, K. (2002) 'Changing care practices: beyond education and training to practice development' in Hockley, J. and Clark, D. (eds) *Palliative Care for Older People in Care Homes*. Buckingham: Open University Press

Froggatt, K. and Payne, S. (2006) 'A survey of end of life care in care homes: issues of definition and practice'. *Health and Social Care in the Community*, 14 (4): 341–8

Gagliese, L. and Melzack, R. (1997) 'Chronic pain in elderly people'. *Pain*, 70: 3–14

Goodman, C., Woolley, R. and Knight, D. (2003) 'District nurse involvement in providing palliative care to older people in residential care homes'. *International Journal of Palliative Nursing*, 9 (12): 521–7

Help the Aged Peer Education Project Group (2006) *Planning for Choice in End of Life Care*. London: Help the Aged

Help the Aged (2005) *Dying in Older Age*. London: Help the Aged

Help the Aged (2006) 'Older people denied a "good death" as hospital staff face too many pressures to cope'. **http://press.helptheaged.org.uk/_press/Releases/_items/_endoflife.htm** (Accessed 9 September 2008)

Help the Aged (2008) 'Health and social care: end of life care'. **www.helptheaged.org.uk/engb/Campaigns/HealthandSocialCare/EndOfLifeCare/** (Accessed 9 September 2008)

Hirst, P. (2004) 'Establishing specialist palliative care provision for care homes'. *Cancer Nursing Practice*, 3 (2): 29–32

Hockley, J. and Clark, D. (Eds) (2002) *Palliative Care for Older People in Care Homes*. Buckingham: Open University Press

Hospice Information Service (2008) *Hospice and Palliative Care Directory United Kingdom and Ireland 2008*. London: HIS

Humphreys, K., Moos, R.H. and Cohen, C. (1997) 'Social and community resources in long term recovery for treated and untreated alcoholism'. *Journal of Studies on Alcohol*, 58 (3): 231–8

Jarrett, N. and Maslin-Prothero, S. (2004) in Payne, S., Seymour, J. and Inlgeton, C. (eds). *Palliative Care Nursing: Principles and Evidence for Practice*. Maidenhead: McGraw-Hill/Open University Press

Kinghorn, S. and Duncan, F. (2005) 'Living with Loss' in Lugton, J. and McIntyre, R. (eds) *Palliative Care the Nursing Role* (2nd edn). Edinburgh: Churchill Livingstone/Elsevier

Koffman, J. and Higginson, I.J. (2004) 'Equal access in palliative care' in Sykes, N., Edmonds, P. and Wiles, J. (eds) *Management of Advanced Disease*. London: Arnold

Lefebvre-Chapiro, S. and the DOLOPLUS group (2001) 'The DOLOPLUS 2 scale – evaluating pain in the elderly'. *European Journal of Palliative Care*, 8 (5): 191–4

Lloyd-Williams, M., Spiller, J. and Ward, J. (2003) 'Which depression screening tool should be used in palliative care?'. *Palliative Medicine*, 17: 40–3

Lochler, J.L., Ritchie, C.S., Roth, D.L., Baker, P.S., Bodner, E.V. and Allman, R.M. (2004) 'Social isolation, support and capital and nutritional risk in an older sample: Ethnic and gender differences'. *Social Science and Medicine*, 60 (4): 747–61

Loftus, L. (2000) 'A collaborative nursing model for advanced non-malignant disease'. *International Journal of Palliative Nursing*. 6: 454–8

Milligan, S. (2004) 'Perceptions of spirituality among nurses undertaking post-registration education'. *International Journal of Palliative Nursing*, 10 (4): 162–71

Mitchell, C. (2001) 'Assessment and management of chronic pain in elderly people'. *British Journal of Nursing*, 10 (5): 296–304

National Council for Hospice and Specialist Palliative Care Services (1995) *Specialist Palliative Care: A Statement of Definitions*. London: NCHSPCS

National Council for Hospice and Specialist Palliative Care Services (1998) *Reaching Out: Specialist Palliative Care for Adults With Non-malignant Diseases*. London: NCHSPCS

National Council for Palliative Care (2006) *Briefing Bulletin 14: Palliative Care Needs of Older People*. London: NCPC

NHS Lothian (2007) *West Lothian Dementia Palliative Care Project*. Edinburgh: NHS Lothian

NHS Quality Improvement Scotland (2006) *Management of Chronic Pain in Adults – Best Practice Statement*. Edinburgh: NHSQIS

Open University (2004) *Death and Dying: Workbook 2: Caring for Dying People*. Buckingham: Open University

Open University (2004) *Death and Dying: Workbook 4: Bereavement, Private Grief and Collective Responsibility*. Buckingham: Open University

Parke, B. (1998) 'Gerontological nurses' way of knowing: Realising the presence of pain in the cognitively impaired'. *Journal of Gerontological Nursing*, 24 (6): 21–8

Parkes, C.M. (2006) *Love and Loss: The Roots of Grief and its Complications*. Abingdon: Routledge

Parkes, C.M. (1998) *Studies of Grief in Adult Life* (3rd edn). London: Penguin

Parkes, C.M., Relf, M. and Couldrick, A. (1997) *Counselling in Terminal Care and Bereavement*. Exeter: British Psychological Society

Payne, S., Horn, S. and Relf, M. (2000) *Loss and Bereavement*. Buckingham: Open University Press

Pearce, C.M. and Duffy, A. (2005) 'Holistic Care' in Lugton, J. and McIntyre, R. (eds) *Palliative Care the Nursing role* (2nd edn). Edinburgh: Churchill Livingstone/Elsevier

Peberdy, A. (2000) 'Spiritual care' in Dickenson, D., Johnson, M. and Katz, J.S. (eds). *Death, Dying and Bereavement* (2nd edn). London: Sage/Open University Press

Philp, I. (2002) 'Introduction' in Hockley, J. and Clark, D. (eds) *Palliative Care for Older People in Care Homes*. Buckingham: Open University Press

Reed, P.G. and Rousseau, E. (2007) 'Spiritual enquiry and well being in life limiting illness'. *Journal of Religion, Spirituality and Aging*, 19 (4): 81–98

Regnard, C., Reynolds, J., Watson, B., Matthews, D., Gibson, L. and Clarke, C. (2006) 'Understanding distress in people with severe communication difficulties: developing and assessing the Disability Distress Assessment Tool (DisDAT)'. *Journal of Intellectual Disability Research*, 51 (4): 277–92

Saunders, C. (1978) *The Management of Terminal Disease*. London: Arnold

Scherder, E., Oosterman, J., Swaab, D., Herr, K., Ooms, M., Ribbe, M., Sargeant, J., Pickering, G. and Benedetti, F. (2005) 'Recent developments in pain in dementia'. *British Medical Journal*, 330 (7489): 461–4

Scottish Executive Range and Capacity Review Group (2006) *Second Report: The Future Care of Older People in Scotland*. Edinburgh: Scottish Executive

Scottish Partnership for Palliative Care (2006a) *Joined Up Thinking, Joined Up Care: Report of the Scottish Partnership for Palliative Care Big Lottery Fund Project: 'Increasing access to palliative care for people with life-limiting conditions other than cancer'*. Edinburgh: Scottish Partnership for Palliative Care

Scottish Partnership for Palliative Care (2006b) *Making Good Care Better: National Practice Statements for General Palliative Care in Adult Care Homes in Scotland*. Edinburgh: Scottish Partnership for Palliative Care

Scottish Partnership for Palliative Care (2007) *Palliative and End of Life Care in Scotland: The Case for a Cohesive Approach* (a report and recommendations submitted to the Scottish Executive). Edinburgh: Scottish Partnership for Palliative Care

Sepulveda, C., Marlin, A., Yoshida, T. and Ullrich, A. (2002) 'Palliative care: the World Health Organisation's global perspective'. *Journal of Pain and Symptom Management*, 24 (2): 91–6

Smith, P. (2004) 'Working with family caregivers in a palliative care setting' in Payne, S., Seymour, J. and Inlgeton, C. (eds) *Palliative Care Nursing: Principles and Evidence for Practice*. Maidenhead: McGraw-Hill/Open University Press

Smith, S.D.M. (2005) 'Dementia palliative care needs assessment: a focus on spiritual care'. *Scottish Journal of Healthcare Chaplaincy*, 8 (1): 13–19

Stroebe, W. and Schut, H. (2001) 'Risk factors in coping with bereavement: a methodological and empirical review' in Stroebe, M.S., Stroebe, W. and Hansson, R.O. (eds) *Handbook of Bereavement*. Cambridge: Cambridge University Press

Taylor, J.E. and Norris, J.E. (1995) 'Difficulties with inevitable loss: Middle-aged women and maternal death'. *Bereavement Care* Winter, 30–3

The House of Commons Committee of Public Accounts (2008) *Improving Services for People with Dementia*. London: The Stationery Office

Twycross, R. (1997) *Symptom Management in Advanced Cancer*. Oxford: Radcliffe

Walter, T. (1999) *On Bereavement: The Culture of Grief*. Buckingham: Open University Press

Windsor, T.D., Anstey, K.J., Butterworth, P., Luszcz, M.A. and Andrews, G.R. (2007) 'The role of perceived control in explaining depressive symptoms associated with driving cessation in a longitudinal study'. *Gerontologist*, 47 (2): 215–23

Worden, J.W. (2000) *Grief Counselling and Grief Therapy: A Handbook for the Mental Health Professional*. Abingdon: BrunnerRoutledge

World Health Organisation Europe (2004a) *Better Palliative Care for Older People*. Copenhagen: World Health Organisation Regional Office for Europe

World Health Organisation Europe (2004b) *What Are the Palliative Care needs of Older People and How Might They Be Met?* Health Evidence Network Evidence Reports. Copenhagen: World Health Organisation Regional Office for Europe

Chapter 17

Medication Management

Austyn Snowden

INTRODUCTION

Learning outcomes

Reading this chapter will enable you to:

- critically analyse the differences between compliance, concordance and adherence;

- understand risk factors in medication management in older adults;

- describe effective interventions in improving medication management for older adults.

This chapter looks at medication management in older adult care. It starts off by examining the concept of concordance and looks at the reasons why this concept has emerged. While agreeing with the principles behind this development, the chapter goes on to criticise concordance as being impossible to achieve. That is, concordance is a worthy but meaningless concept for the purpose of medication management in practice.

The chapter subsequently focusses on aspects of medication management specifically demonstrated to benefit older adults in particular. That is, examples are given from the literature of demonstrable risks and effective interventions. These risks and benefits are then discussed with a group of older adults in a Greenock community centre to see if they have any relevance to this group.

THE PROBLEM WITH CONCORDANCE

Definitions of key concepts in medication management	
Concept	*Summary Definition*
Compliance	The paternalistic view that the patient is a passive party who has their prescribed treatment enforced.
Adherence	The (still paternalistic) view that the informed (but still passive) patient will stick to taking their recommended treatment.
Concordance	The process of enlightened communication between the patient and their health care professional leading to an agreed treatment and ongoing assessment of this as the optimal course.

Figure 1 Definitions of key concepts in medication management (abridged from Treharne *et al.*, 2006)

Compliance with prescribed medication is about 50 per cent according to the National Prescribing Centre (Clyne *et al.*, 2007). Given that 15 per cent of the total NHS budget is spent on medication (Clyne *et al.*, 2007: 5) and the total NHS budget for 2007–2008 was £90.8 billion (Department of Health, 2007: 131) then non-compliance could cost about £6.8 billion in 2008. As older people take more medication than younger people the majority of this amount is attributable to people over 65 years of age (Lenaghan *et al.*, 2007). Reasons for non-compliance range from the unintentional and practical, such as an inability to open the bottle, to the intentional and attitudinal, such as the belief that the medicine does not work or does more harm than good. There is no evidence to suggest that these latter reasons differ across the life span; older people are just as unlikely to take a medicine that interferes with their lifestyle or beliefs as younger people (Carter *et al.*, 2003).

The concept of concordance has emerged as a principle underpinning suggested solutions to these problems (Medicines Partnership, 2003). This chapter first briefly examines the concept of concordance and concludes that, while useful as a principle, it is difficult to translate into practice. This is implicit in practical attempts to do so where concordance is either not found (Latter *et al.*, 2007) or is quickly substituted for something more meaningful, such as 'shared decision making' (Clyne *et al.*, 2007: 4), 'adherence' (Cribb and Barber, 2005) or even 'compliance' (van Eijken *et al.*, 2003).

In more detail, concordance is seen as the best way of managing medication (Medicines Partnership, 2003; Weiss and Britten, 2003; Latter *et al.*, 2007). The term means 'together-heart' and infers complete agreement on a contract. If a patient does not adhere to a regimen that arose from a concordant discussion then it is the discussion that was at fault, not the 'non-adherer'. This is a worthy ideal, but operationally problematic. For example, what if the medication prescribed is the best available option for someone? This knowledge can be based on high-quality evidence, yet the person can remain equally unconvinced (Jessop and Rutter, 2003). How can concordance be approached here?

This simplistic example suggests that the practice of concordance may be problematic if negotiations do not result in what the prescriber thinks is best. To give an example, Latter *et al.* (2000) found that when people with mental health problems had beliefs that facilitated medicine-taking, nurses worked with these beliefs and did not try to change them, even when the beliefs were related to the person's hallucinations. However, when people had beliefs that stopped them from adhering to their medicine regimen, nurses tried to modify these beliefs. In other words, the principle of concordance is fine as long as it does not compromise what the nurse sees as the duty of care.

A further problem is that to assume concordance should be the goal of medication management is to assume that everybody wants enlightened communication with the prescriber. There is evidence to suggest this is not so, particularly in an older adult population. For example, Neame *et al.* (2005) showed that 78 per cent of older adults felt they should be free to make 'everyday' decisions about medical problems, meaning more than one in five did not. When it came to 'important' medical decisions three out of four wanted to defer these decisions to the doctor and 50 per cent would comply even if they didn't agree. However, it has been argued that this acknowledgement of the person's wishes is within the spirit of concordance. That is, the person's view still takes precedence because their wish is to delegate decision-making authority to the prescriber (Pollock *et al.*, 2002).

This justification highlights the major difficulty with the concept: if concordance can be made to encompass any type of agreeable person-centred discussion then it becomes meaningless – it cannot be tested empirically if it simply subsumes all good practice in medication management. If it is beyond testing it is beyond criticism. A further complication is that concordance, in the context of medication management, contains a prescription and the recipient of a prescription. A prescription is an instruction that surely alludes to an unequal (non-concordant) relationship. A patient has to be told about the script and given directions. It could certainly be argued in the spirit of Pollock *et al.* (2002) that implicitly, if not explicitly, the patient and the prescriber therefore come to an agreement, a concord. It is clear, however, that this justification suffers from the same **tautological** problems as above. If concordance can be made into an all encompassing good it loses coherence as a testable concept.

What concordance seems to imply in the literature is an overarching statement of principle that includes respect for individual care through better communication. If this is the case then there is no justification for this principle to automatically exclude compliance or adherence. For example, van Eijken *et al.* (2003) make a strong case for compliance being compatible with a person-centred approach. The words concordance, compliance and adherence are, therefore, interchangeable in the literature – not because they are misunderstood but because they often seek the same end. For example, it can be seen that the principle of concordance runs through Cribb and Barber's (2005) model of measurable aspects of medication management (see Figure 2) but elements of compliance and adherence also persist. This is probably more realistic than simply abandoning terms because they are no longer politically correct.

There is also a more pragmatic reason to keep all the terms in mind. Since the term concordance is relatively new, much of the research on medication management is filed under the key terms 'compliance' and 'adherence'. The terms therefore need to stay alive if only for a comprehensive search of the literature. So, for the purpose of discussing the literature on medication management, all terms were searched. The assumption underpinning Cribb and Barber's pragmatic position is that effective interventions designed to specifically address aspects of concordance, compliance or adherence are likely to improve medication management generally. This is a worthy aim. For example, the finding that a medicine organiser reduced drug wastage from 18.1 per cent to 1 per cent in a study of frail elderly patients (Ryan, Woolley and Rees, 2005) would be of practical use to any patient–prescriber relationship, however this relationship is viewed. The secondary finding that there was also a significant decrease in the number of prescribed drugs and dosages in the intervention group alludes to the benefit of increased attention to medication management in general.

A. Following through decisions over time
Including:
- o The following through of professional recommendations about treatments/action; and/or
- o The following through of patient informed choices about treatments/action. (Following through here means carrying out and/or appropriately reviewing.)

B. Good quality decision making
Including:
- o The supporting of informed patient choice (patient education, understanding, decision-making involvement, responsibility); and/or
- o The supporting of informed professional choice (knowledge of patient specificities, perspectives and preferences).

C. Good quality health care relationships
Including:
- o Broader and deeper communication; and/or
- o Mutual respect; and/or
- o (Elements of) partnership working.

D. Good outcomes
Including:
- o Patient satisfaction with medicine taking and/or
- o Optimal health gain for individuals; and/or
- o Promoting cost-effective use of treatments; and/or
- o Stewardship – avoiding the waste of (often collective) resources (e.g. medicines, consultation time); and/or
- o Public health.

(Adapted from Cribb and Barber, 2005)

Figure 2 Measurable aspects of medication management

LITERATURE ON MEDICATION MANAGEMENT

Prevalence of chronic disease increases with age (Scottish Executive, 2005) and older adults receive the majority of prescriptions (Lenaghan *et al.*, 2007). Most prescriptions are for chronic disease, which infers that older adults use and waste the most medication. Within 10 days of filling a prescription, 30 per cent of patients with chronic disease have missed at least one dose, half unintentionally and half not (DiMatteo, 2004).

Four in five people over age 75 years are prescribed at least one medicine and 36 per cent are prescribed four or more medicines (Department of Health, 2001a).

It does not necessarily follow that too much medication is being prescribed. More than 10 per cent of older adult admissions to hospital are thought to be a direct result of not taking prescribed medication (Chia et al., 2006). As a further complication some suggest that older adults are not being prescribed medication when they should be. Rudd et al. (2004) found that whereas 71 per cent of patients under 65 years receive lipid-lowering drugs following admission for stroke, only 54 per cent of patients over 75 years received the drug. Competing concerns such as these were the impetus for the *National Service Framework for Older People* (Department of Health, 2001a), which proposed a regular review of care home residents' medicine as specified in the accompanying publication, *Medicines and Older People* (Department of Health, 2001b) (see Figure 3).

Effective interventions in medication management for older people

Appropriate prescribing for older people, and monitoring of their conditions, are key objectives. However, it is not only prescribing but how medicines are used by patients that is important. Patients and their carers need more support for medicine taking. There are five main types of intervention:

- prescribing advice/support;
- active monitoring of treatment;
- review of repeat prescribing systems;
- medication review (with individual clients and their carers);
- education and training.

(adapted from Department of Health, 2001b: 4)

Figure 3 Effective interventions in medication management for older people

Zermanski et al. (2006) tested these recommendations (Figure 3) by reviewing the medication of older adults living in care homes in Leeds. They reviewed 315 people in 65 care homes over six months. They found no change in hospital admission, mortality, cognitive function or activities of daily living as a result of their intervention. However, they found a reduction in falls and a change in medication regimens; more drugs were stopped than started, but there was no cost benefit as the drugs started were newer and more expensive. Lenaghan *et al.* (2007) found much the same in their study of a home-based medication review in people over 80 years. They demonstrated no positive outcomes in relation to clinical outcome or quality of life. Like Zermanski *et al.* (2006), Lenaghan *et al.* (2007) noted a change in overall prescribing but here there was also decreased cost associated with the change. They noted this was probably offset by the cost of the reviewing, but there may well be secondary benefits as yet unseen. Longitudinal studies are required. What is notable in both studies is that outcomes are measured in terms of measurable 'goods', mainly relating to cost. However, Leneghan *et al.* (2007) make the point that reducing falls and taking more appropriate or less overall medication may well correlate with longer term benefits.

There is no evidence that shows that older people are more or less likely to be non-adherent than members of other age groups (Carter *et al.*, 2003). Ho *et al.* (2004) found good compliance with prescribed inhalers in their study of 500 people over age 70 years with chronic obstructive pulmonary disease. However, the researchers found that people were not as compliant as they thought themselves to be. This is a common finding and suggests studies that rely on self-reported medication-taking data might be over-estimating compliance rates. However, there is also more objective evidence that older people are competent at managing complex medication regimens (Bytheway *et al.*, 2000). Given that these studies show that older adults can manage their medication then one conclusion must be that a proportion of older people fail to take their medications as prescribed because they do not want to take it, just like the rest of the population (Carter *et al.*, 2003). One opinion (Crome and Pollock, 2005) suggests this may be to do with issues of control. That is, autonomous people want to exert control over their illnesses, even to the extent of suffering pain rather than taking medication they don't believe in.

However, at least 10 per cent of hospital admissions are thought to be a direct result of non-adherence to medication (Chia *et al.*, 2006). Therefore, it is important to explore all potential factors relating to the causes of non-adherence; that is, hospital admission must surely be seen as undesirable by the vast majority, and especially by people who view themselves as autonomous agents. George *et al.*'s (2006) study of residents in sheltered housing complexes in Aberdeen found non-adherence in 28 per cent of people. Factors correlated with non-adherence included younger age, confusion about drugs, lack of drug supply and administration, perceived view of risks outweighing benefits, and the fact that treatment recommendations interfered with lifestyle. Lowe *et al.* (2000) found that factors of non-adherence included experience of the medicines in terms of side effects and the perceived inefficacy of treatments prescribed.

It is clear that side effects and inefficacy encompass a broad range of issues from the practical to the rational and emotional. As such it is no surprise to find they are difficult to address with a single strategy. Each person is different to the degree that they appear to have their own unique set of circumstances and beliefs about medication management. Interventions should ideally reflect this; however, there is common sense in looking for broader commonalities and targeting demonstrably effective interventions at those most in need. In other words, we should avoid those factors that demonstrably make matters worse in general and focus on interventions that likewise improve medication management. These will be discussed in turn.

WHAT MAKES MEDICATION MANAGEMENT WORSE? WHAT ARE THE RISK FACTORS?

Many different risk factors have been identified such as decreasing manual dexterity, cognitive dysfunction and personal beliefs. It is argued that these factors are a function of one or both of the following findings. Namely, older people are:

- more likely to take multiple medicines with high dose frequencies (Department of Health, 2001b), and
- just as likely as younger adults to not take medication as prescribed (Chia et al. 2006; Carter et al., 2003).

These factors will be considered in turn.

Taking multiple medications

Polypharmacy is a known risk factor for non-adherence and, more importantly, adverse events. When two drugs are given together it becomes very difficult to know how exactly they and the body will interact and react. Some of the more common interactions are shown in Figure 4. Reasons for these interactions differ but, for example, if both drugs are metabolised by the same enzyme then that enzyme may not be able to effectively metabolise both. This is increasingly the case with advancing age where kidney and liver function are known to decrease in most people (Durrance, 2003). The net effect may be an accumulation in the body of one or both drugs/metabolites. The cascade effect of that becomes difficult to predict. It is easier to predict that there will be an increase in falls, mental health problems, car accidents and hospital admission as a result (Loftipour and Vaca, 2007). Adverse reactions to medicines in older adults are implicated in between 5 per cent and 17 per cent of hospital admissions (Clyne *et al.*, 2007).

First Drug	Second Drug	Effect
ACE inhibitors	Potassium sparing diuretics	Increased risk of hyperkalaemia
Aminoglycosides	Diuretics	Increased risk of ototoxicity
Carbamazepine	Many antidepressants	Anticonvulsant effect reduced
Digoxin	St John's Wort	Plasma concentrations of digoxin reduced
Griseofulvin	Warfarin	Anticoagulant effect reduced
Lithium	Many analgesics	Lithium excretion reduced
Nitrates	Sildenafil	Hypotensive effect increased
Simvastatin	Itraconazole or ketoconazole	Increased risk of myopathy
Sulphonylureas	Antifungals	Increased risk of hypoglycaemia
Warfarin	Many antibiotics	Anticoagulation may be increased

Figure 4 Common Interactions (Reid and Chrome, 2005)

A reasonable question to ask is, therefore, why is polypharmacy so common in older adults? A simple answer is that older people have more chronic disease (Scottish Executive, 2005) and subsequently need more treatment. However, even this simplistic view belies the finding that many older adults are prescribed unnecessary drugs. There is also the 'Catch 22' of the prescribing cascade. This is where drugs are added to counter the side effects of the last drug, and so on. Constipation, nausea, headache and confusion are frequently consequences of prescribed medication as opposed to new disease. Treatment should therefore be through medication review rather than extra aperients, emetics, etc. Hirst (2003) gives a moving account of how stopping haloperidol as part of a medication review drastically improved one woman's wellbeing. The symptoms the woman was showing could easily have been mistaken for the side effects of haloperidol and another drug been added instead. Unnecessary prescribing of neuroleptics to older adults has been a long-term problem, particularly in nursing homes (McGrath and Jackson, 1996).

Not taking medication as prescribed

Chia *et al.* (2006) conducted a systematic review to explore the effects of beliefs on medication adherence in older adults. They found a number of factors were implicated in adherence. The researchers found the most potent predictor of adherence was self-efficacy; the belief that one can perform a specific behaviour under differing conditions, i.e. confidence in one's ability to maintain control over a medication regimen. Medication efficacy was also a factor. That is, if a medication was perceived to be of great benefit or necessity then it was more likely to be taken. This belief was found to be tempered by the perceived likelihood and severity of adverse events (Horne and Weinman, 2000) or the presence of alternatives (Brown and Segal, 1996). For example, major barriers to effective pain relief in older adults with cancer have been shown to be related to fears about tolerance and addiction (Thomason *et al.*, 1998). Illness perception is also a factor. For example, better adherence to asthma medication was found in older women who believed they had asthma and that it could be controlled. Also factorial were the beliefs that it was not caused by external factors, such as pollution or chance. Long-term adherence was also predicted by these beliefs (Jessop and Rutter, 2003). In other words, if older adults:

- don't believe they can take the medication as prescribed,
- don't see the necessity of it, or
- don't believe in the effectiveness of it, or
- feel concerned that adverse events outweigh perceived benefit . . .

. . . they are less likely to take medication as prescribed. Not all of these beliefs are necessarily groundless. In an extremely candid letter to the BMJ, Masters (2003) admitted to reading the BNF on 'quite a few occasions' in order to discover the clinical indication of some of the medicines he was responsible for prescribing. Given that this admission may be more commonplace than generally assumed, older adults may be right to suspend belief in some cases. Findings such as this should be borne in mind when examining figures about prescriptions not being dispensed or not taken as prescribed.

HOW IS MEDICATION MANAGEMENT IMPROVED? WHAT WORKS?

One of the most widely-used practical medication aids is the dosette box or medicines organiser (Ryan, Woolley and Rees, 2005). This is a compartmentalised device filled under supervision of a pharmacist and designed to simplify complex oral medication regimens. Dosette boxes/ pill organisers are widely believed to be effective and practical for people with difficulties remembering or with other sensory deficits. These devices seem intuitively helpful but are they? I know from personal experience that they are not necessarily as straightforward as they seem and that if they don't fit with someone's lifestyle they may not work as planned. For example, I once visited a lady at home who appeared to be confused about her medication regime. We discussed a dosette box as an option and she thought it sounded good. When I went round to see how she was getting on a few days later I found she had received the box and then carefully removed all the tablets from it and put them in separate containers that she then labelled by date and time. I never fully understood her rationale for this. The most likely rationale is a lack of guidance on my part. Perhaps it may be correlated with Crome and Pollock's (2005) earlier suggestion that issues of control and autonomy are major factors in successful medication management. The fact is she remained much less confused with her medication and grateful for the box.

However, Moisan et al. (2002) found pill organisers to have no effect on compliance in their study of older adults who had difficulty reading. McGraw (2004) found them to be beneficial for people trying to control diabetes but ineffective for people with hypertension. The reasons for this were not absolutely clear but thought to be attributable to participants' views of the severity of their illness and the need for medication. The populations studied were not exclusively older though, and the review had very strict exclusion criteria.

In a very small study Higgins et al. (2004) found that 'concordance therapy' enhanced antidepressant medication compliance in older adults, but not by much. Higgins et al. (2004) described concordance therapy as an amended version of Kemp et al.'s (1996) 'compliance therapy' with increased focus on the negotiation element of medication management. Compliance therapy has proved successful outside the clinical trial context according to Surguladze *et al.* (2002) and could therefore offer real benefit in practice. It can be broken down into the following three areas:

1. Eliciting the patient's stance towards treatment.
2. Exploration of ambivalence.
3. Working towards treatment maintenance.

It was difficult to see how concordance therapy as described by Higgins *et al.* (2004) differed from compliance therapy, as they followed the same three-stage process. The intervention was based on a model of cognitive behaviour therapy and outcome measures were related to adherence. Nevertheless, it had a marginal effect and it was interesting to note that the control group in this study also improved their medication adherence. This would suggest some other factor might be involved. For example, the **Hawthorne effect** is an enduring, if flawed, theory of the beneficial consequences of increased observation and attention (Mayo, 1933). Certainly secondary benefits often appear to emerge as a result of medication review (Ryan Woolley and Rees, 2005).

In reviewing the evidence on the efficacy of written instructions for medication management, Raynor *et al.* (2007) reviewed over 50 000 citations and concluded that written information alone was not valued by patients. This would add weight to the theme that simplistic generic or non-individualised approaches appear broadly ineffective in enhancing medication management. For example, Roter *et al.* (1998) conducted a systematic review of interventions designed to improve compliance in people taking antipsychotic medication. They found individualised tailored approaches most effective. In a Cochrane review of interventions targeted at enhancing compliance in the general population, Haynes *et al.* (2005) also concluded that the best interventions were complex and individually tailored. However, even they did not lead to large improvements in treatment outcomes.

One of the more innovative studies was that of Dow *et al.* (1991). Their study differed in that it focussed on educating patients about how to ask questions regarding their medication instead of attempting to educate patients about their medication. This method had the added benefit of improving patient confidence when talking to prescribers, which in turn enabled prescribers to elicit more pertinent and relevant information, which subsequently enhanced compliance. In many ways this should be no surprise as this patient-centred intervention aligns with the most effective methods of learning. This was the only study found that sought to systematically empower patients rather than teach them.

Cox *et al.* (2004) attempted to explore this further and conducted a systematic review of communication between patients and professionals in regard to medicine management. They found that nurses speak about concordance and pharmacists and doctors speak about information and evidence. Arguably the most pertinent comment in the report comes from Alison Lawrence, the 'lay' member of the team, who summarises her view as 'remember, it's as important to listen as to speak!' This quote maybe needs to be borne in mind when considering the evidence that nurses weren't as good at practising concordance as they thought they were (Latter *et al.*, 2007) and that GPs overestimated the amount of time they spend giving people information about their medicines (Nolan *et al.*, 2004).

Nolan *et al.* (2004) concluded that the best predictor of good medication management is the extent to which people feel able to discuss their treatment options with the prescriber. This makes sense as it allows for a more thorough investigation of beliefs and related actions that may or may not align. That is, if a person is acting in a certain way because she believes she should, yet her actions contradict this or her information is incomplete, then discussing this may improve the chances of her actions being congruent with her fully informed beliefs.

THE USER VIEW

In order to discuss some of the issues raised in this chapter with the relevant group I went to a community centre in Greenock to talk with a group of eight women over the age of 65. This evidence should therefore be considered as no more than anecdotal. However, I think it contrasts with the literature nicely, and presents a 'real' voice of experience.

I began by asking general questions about medication management and found they all took medication. All but one took more than one medicine a day, and two took more than ten. One lady gave an accurate breakdown of her regime and then said: 'you get used to it'. This sentiment appeared to be echoed around the group. I asked if others knew what all the medicines did and another lady said sometimes she had to look up the indications by reading the enclosed leaflets. Most people concurred with this but some said they didn't read these leaflets at all. Those that did wanted information on adverse effects of the prescribed medication.

I asked what benefit they got from their medication: 'If I didn't take them I wouldn't be walking about.' The lady who said this clarified the statement by asserting her faith in antibiotics. This faith in 'physical' medication recurred throughout the session. That is, there was more willingness to accept drugs for infection, stroke prevention and blood **dyscrasia** than mood-altering drugs for example. Likewise the medications that the ladies were most keen to stop tended to be the psychotropics. One lady tried to come off an antidepressant she was taking but:

> '. . . had bad symptoms and had to go back on them. So I think I'm on them for good'.
>
> I asked: 'How do you feel about that?'
>
> 'I just take them along with the rest' (laughs).

There was further evidence that most wanted to stop some of the medicines they were taking and some had approached their doctors in this regard. However, without exception, the doctor had just told them to carry on. This didn't appear to be problematic however, and the consensus was that they would do what they were told quite willingly and there was no expressed desire to contradict medical directions. The desire to stop medication didn't have a single origin. That is, one woman wanted to stop due to a fear of addiction, another was worried about the amount of medication she was taking and another was concerned about the timing of the regime. They all appeared quite reassured by the doctor restating the necessity for the regime in question.

As far as knowledge was concerned one woman had a very clear idea of what she could and couldn't take with her prescribed medication, possibly as a result of the regime she was on and the importance of subsequent avoidance of certain other medicines. The others were less clear.

All agreed that if their doctor prescribed them something they would take it without question. They would stop only if they got side effects. Some of the women had regular medication reviews whereas some claimed never to have had one. There was some confusion over whether they could ask for a review or not, although some had clearly done so. Again this was related to dissatisfaction with psychotropic medication:

> It makes you awful tired. I think they slow you down. I was on five milligrams, then 10, then 20. That's the highest you can go. He said that'll get you up and going but they didn't (laughs).

However, where a reason was seen for taking the tablets there was no question of not taking it.

Most people forgot to take their medicine on occasions. One woman who took multiple medications would often forget to take the afternoon doses. She stated she would prefer to remember as she had a great deal of faith in the preventative power of the medication:

> The blood pressure tablets keep the blood pressure down and the cholesterol tablets keep cholesterol down . . . I'd be terrified I had another stroke.

None used the internet to research medicines or asked their doctor for a specific medicine as recommended by a friend. They denied discussing medication with each other and generally appeared content to leave these issues to the doctor:

> 'We just take them, that's all.'

> 'You just take it and hope for the best.'

> 'That's it, you hope for the best.'

I asked if they felt they were listened to and one said 'sometimes' with a shrug of the shoulders. This action seemed best to represent the general stoicism of the group.

Reflection

How does this account compare with the literature? Was anything a surprise? What do you think is the most important principle here: concordance, compliance or adherence?

CONCLUSION

There are no simple strategies for improving medication management in older adults. Concordance is a useful concept only to the degree that it engenders individual approaches and encourages deeper communication to elicit medication-taking beliefs. Success is still measured and discussed in terms of compliance and adherence in the literature. There are useful frameworks to guide the nurse in supporting these discussions (for example, the National Prescribing Centre, (Clyne *et al.*, 2007). Good outcome predictors include patient confidence to discuss medicines. Multiple medicines are a good predictor of non-compliance and should be reviewed. An older adult's view of the efficacy of medication and perception of illness are useful indicators of treatment adherence. Individually tailored approaches to medication management are undoubtedly best and should be explored as far as is practical.

Key points

- Positive medication management is currently discussed under the term concordance.
- However, concordance is a normative concept and therefore impossible to meaningfully evaluate.
- It is more clinically useful to focus on interventions that are demonstrably effective in addressing all aspects of medication management.
- Older people have similar reasons for non-adherence as younger people.
- Individually tailored approaches focussed on empowering people to discuss their views of illness and medicines appear most effective.
- This does not exclude discussions on compliance and adherence.

Useful websites

www.nmc-uk.org/aDisplayDocument.aspx?DocumentID=3251
All nurses should understand the professional and legal framework within which they operate. Here are the professional guidelines for administration of medicines, incorporated into 'Standards for medicine management' along with standards for dispensing, carrying, disposing of, storing and delegating by the Nursing and Midwifery Council in 2007.

http://en.wikipedia.org/wiki/Health_Belief_Model
Many of the points above consider the role of beliefs in decision making. A good place to start for further exploration of this topic in relation to health is the Health Belief Model. Type this phrase into a search engine for lots of information. Wikipedia has a good visual model.

www.sdo.lshtm.ac.uk/files/project/76-final-report.pdf
For a more in-depth analysis of the implications of confusing the terms compliance, concordance and adherence see the document 'Concordance, Compliance and Adherence in Medicine Taking' by the National Co-ordinating Centre for NHS Service Delivery and Organisation Research and Development. Among wider discussion of pertinent practical issues this has Cribb and Barber's excellent analysis in Chapter 5.

Acknowledgements

Part of this chapter appeared in: Snowden, A. (2008) 'Medication management in older adults: A critique of concordance'. *British Journal of Nursing*, 17 (2): 114–27

Thank you to Mark Allen Healthcare for permission to reproduce parts of this paper.

REFERENCES

Brown, C. M. and Segal, R. (1996) 'The effects of health and treatment perceptions on the use of prescribed medication and home remedies among African American and white American hypertensives'. *Social Science and Medicine*, 43 (6): 903–17

Bytheway, B., Johnson, J., Heller, T. and Muston, R. (2000) *The Management of Long-Term Medication by Older People. Final Report to the Department of Health.* Buckingham: Open University Press

Carter, S., Taylor, D. and Levenson, R. (2003) *A Question of Choice – Compliance in Medicine Taking. A Preliminary Review* **http://www.npc.co.uk/med_ partnership/assets/research-qoc-compliance.pdf** (Accessed 9 September 2008)

Chia, L., Schlenck, E.A. and Dunbar-Jacob, J. (2006) 'Effect of personal and cultural beliefs on medication adherence in the elderly'. *Drugs and Aging,* 23 (3): 191–202

Clyne, W., Granby, T. and Picton, C. (2007) *A Competency Framework for Shared Decisionmaking With Patients Achieving Concordance for Taking Medicines.* Keele: National Prescribing Centre. Available at: **www.npc.co.uk/ pdf/Concordant_Competency_Framework_2007.pdf** (Accessed 7 January 2008)

Cox, K., Stevenson, F., Britten, N. and Dundar, Y. (2004) *A Systematic Review of Communication Between Patients and Health Care Professionals About Medicine-taking and Prescribing.* London: Medicines Partnership

Cribb, A. and Barber, N. (2005) 'Unpicking the philosophical and ethical issues in medicines prescribing and taking' in National Co-ordinating Centre for NHS Service Delivery and Organisation Research and Development, *Concordance Adherence and Compliance in Medicine Taking.* **www.sdo.lshtm. ac.uk/files/project/76-final-report.pdf** (Accessed 20 February 2008)

Crome, P. and Pollock, K. (2005) 'Age discrimination in prescribing: accounting for concordance'. *Reviews in Clinical Gerontology,* 14: 1–4

Department of Health (2001a) *National Service Framework for Older People.* **www.dh.gov.uk/en/Publicationsandstatistics/Publications/ PublicationsPolicyAndGuidance/DH_4003066** (Accessed 19 October 2007)

Department of Health (2001b) *Medicines and Older People: Implementing Medicines-related Aspects of the NSF for Older People.* London: Department of Health. **www.dh.gov.uk/en/Publicationsandstatistics/Publications/**

PublicationsPolicyAndGuidance/DH_4008020 (Accessed 16 January 2008)

Department of Health (2007) *Departmental Report 2007*. London: Department of Health. **www.dh.gov.uk/en/Publicationsandstatistics/Publications/AnnualReports/DH_074767** (Accessed 16 January 2008)

DiMatteo, M.R. (2004) 'Variations in patients' adherence to medical recommendations: a quantitative review of 50 years of research'. *Medical Care*, 42: 200–9

Dow, M.G., Verdi, M.B. and Sacco, W.P. (1991) 'Training psychiatric patients to discuss medication issues. Effects on patient communication and knowledge of medications'. *Behaviour Modification*, 15 (1): 2–21

Durrance, S.A. (2003) 'Older adults and NSAIDS: avoiding adverse reactions'. *Geriatric Nursing*, 24 (6): 348–52

George, J., Munro, K., McCaig, D.J. and Stewart, D. (2006) 'Prescription medications: beliefs, experiences behaviour and adherence of sheltered housing residents'. *The Annals of Pharmacotherapy*, 40: 2123–9

Haynes, R.B., Yao, X., Degani, A., Kripalani, S., Garg, A. and McDonald, H.P. (2005) 'Interventions for enhancing medication adherence'. *Cochrane Database of Systematic Reviews*, 4 Article No.: CD000011

Higgins, N., Livingstone, G. and Katona, C. (2004) 'Concordance therapy: an intervention to help older people take antidepressants'. *Journal of Affective Disorders*, 81: 287–91

Hirst, B. (2003) 'A memorable patient: Polypharmacy remains an issue in elderly patients'. *BMJ*, 326: 1251

Ho, S.F., O'Mahoney, M.S., Steward, J.A., Breay, P. and Burr, M. L. (2004) 'Inhaler technique in older people in the community'. *Age and Ageing*, 33 (2): 185–8

Horne, R. and Weinman, J. (1999) 'Patients' beliefs about prescribed medicines and their role in adherence to treatment in chronic physical illness'. *Journal of Psychosomatic Research*, 47 (6): 555–67

Jessop, D.C. and Rutter, D.R. (2003) 'Adherence to asthma medication: the role of illness representations'. *Psychological Health*, 18 (5): 595–612

Kemp, R., Hayward, P., Applewhaite, G., Everitt, B. and David, A. (1996) 'Compliance therapy in psychotic patients: randomised controlled trial'. *British Medical Journal*, 312: 345–9

Latter, S., Yerrell, P., Rycroft-Malone, J. and Shaw, D. (2000) 'Nursing, medication education and the new policy agenda: the evidence base'. *International Journal of Nursing Studies*, 37 (6): 469–79

Latter, S., Maben, J., Myall, M. and Young, A. (2007) 'Perceptions and practice of concordance in nurses' prescribing consultations: findings from a national questionnaire survey and case studies of practice in England'. *International Journal of Nursing Studies*, 44 (1): 9–18

Lenaghan, E., Holland, R. and Brooks, A. (2007). 'Home-based medication review in a high risk elderly population in primary care – the POLYMED randomised controlled trial'. *Age and Ageing*, 36: 292–7

Loftipour, S. and Vaca, F. (2007) 'Commentary: Polypharmacy and older drivers: beyond the doors of the emergency department (ED) for patient safety'. *Annals of Emergency Medicine*, 49 (4): 535–7

Lowe, C.J., Raynor, D.K., Purvis, J., Farrin, A.J. and Hudson, J. (2000) 'Effects of a medicine review and education programme for older people in general practice'. *British Journal of Clinical Pharmacology.* 50: 172–5

Masters, N.J. (2003) 'Compliance enhanced by drug indication on every repeat script'. *BMJ,* 14 October 2003 **www.bmj.com/cgi/eletters/327/7419/819** (Accessed 28 November 2007)

Mayo, E. (1933) *The Human Problems of an Industrial Civilization.* New York: Macmillan

McGrath, A.M. and Jackson, G.A. (1996) 'Survey of neuroleptic prescribing in residents of nursing homes in Glasgow'. *BMJ,* 312: 611–12

McGraw, C. (2004) 'Multi-compartment medication devices and patient compliance'. *British Journal of Community Nursing,* 9 (7): 285–90

Medicines Partnership (2003) *Project Evaluation Toolkit.* London: Medicines Partnership

Moisan, J., Gaudet, M., Grégoire, J. and Bouchard, R. (2002) 'Non-compliance with drug treatment and reading difficulties with regard to prescription labelling among seniors'. *Gerontology,* 48 (1): 44–51

National Co-ordinating Centre for NHS Service Delivery and Organisation Research and Development (2005) *Concordance Adherence and Compliance in Medicine Taking.* **www.sdo.lshtm.ac.uk/files/project/76-final-report.pdf** (Accessed 20 February 2008)

Neame, R., Hammond, A. and Deighton, C. (2005) 'Need for information and involvement in decision making among patients with rheumatoid arthritis: a questionnaire survey'. *Arthritis Care and Research,* 53: 249–55

Nolan, P., Bradley, E. and Carr, N. (2004) 'Nurse prescribing and the enhancement of mental health services'. *Nurse Prescriber,* 1 (11): 1–9

Pollock, K., Blenkinsopp, A. and Grime, J. (2002) 'Concordance – a valuable contribution to make to debate'. *The Pharmaceutical Journal,* 268: 837–8

Raynor, D.K., Blenkinsopp, A., Knapp, P. R., Grime, J., Nicolson, D.J., Pollock, K., Dorer, G., Gilbody, S. M., Dickinson, D., Maule, A. J. and Spoor, P.A. (2007) 'A systematic review of quantitative and qualitative research on the role and effectiveness of written information available to patients about individual medicines'. *Health Technology Assessment,* 11: 1–177

Reid, J. and Crome, P. (2005) 'Polypharmacy: causes and effects in older people'. *Prescriber,* 19 October, 57–62

Roter, D. L., Hall, J.A., Mersica, R., Nordstrom, B., Cretin, D. and Svarstad, B. (1998) 'Effectiveness of interventions to improve patient compliance: a meta analysis'. *Medical Care,* 36 (8): 1138–61

Rudd, A.G., Lowe, D., Hoffman, A., Irwin, P. and Pearson, M. (2004) 'Secondary prevention for stroke in the United Kingdom: results from the National Sentinel Audit of stroke'. *Age and Ageing,* 33 (3): 280–6

Ryan, B.M., Woolley, M. and Rees, J.A. (2005) 'Initialising Concordance in Frail Elderly Patients via a Medicines Organiser'. *The Annals of Pharmacotherapy,* 39 (5): 834–9

Scottish Executive (2005) *Building a Health Service Fit for the Future* **www. scotland.gov.uk/Resource/Doc/924/0012112.pdf** (Accessed 19 October 2007)

Surguladze, S., Timms, P. and David, A. (2002) 'Teaching psychiatric trainees "compliance therapy"'. *Psychiatric Bulletin*, 26: 12–15

Thomason, T. E., McCune, J. S., Bernard, S.A., Winer, E. P., Tremont, S. and Lindley, C. M. (1998) 'Cancer pain survey: patient-centred issues in control'. *Journal of Pain Symptom Management*, 15 (5): 275–84

Treharne, G.J., Lyons, A.C., Hale, E.D., Douglas, K.M.J. and Kitas, G.D. (2006) 'Compliance is futile but is concordance between rheumatology patients and health professionals attainable?'. *Rheumatology*, 45 (1): 1–5

van Eijken, M., Tsang, S., Wensing, M., de Smet, P.A.G.M. and Grol, R.P.T.M. (2003) 'Interventions to improve medication compliance in older patients living in the community'. *Drugs and Aging*, 20 (3): 229–40

Weiss, M. and Britten, N. (2003) 'What is concordance?' *The Pharmaceutical Journal*, 271 (7270): 493

Zermanski, A. G., Alldred, D.P., Petty, D.R., Raynor, D.K., Freemantle, N., Eastaugh, J. and Bowie, P. (2006). 'Clinical medication review by a pharmacist of elderly people living in care homes – randomised controlled trial'. *Age and Ageing*, 35: 586–91

Chapter 18

Homelessness

Jennifer Stewart

Learning outcomes

Reading this chapter will enable you to:

- understand the possible causes of homelessness;

- recognise the particular health and social care needs of older homeless people and the role of professionals in supporting them appropriately;

- highlight examples of good practice in the field of health and social care;

- understand the existing barriers and limitations in the successful resettlement of older homeless people.

INTRODUCTION

This chapter is written in the context of a United Kingdom (UK) perspective through the use of largely Scottish experiences. Across the four nations of the UK, social care in each country is guided by a set of National Care Standards that exist to regulate and monitor the care of service users across all service providers. It is therefore advisable that as and when applicable you refer to the Care Standards relevant to your own country of residence (England – Commission for Social Care Inspection at **www.csci.org.uk**; Northern Ireland – Northern Ireland Social Care Council found at **www.niscc.info**; Wales – Care Standards Inspectorate for Wales found at **www.csiw.wales.gov.uk**).

The National Care Standards for Scotland base themselves upon the following principles; dignity, privacy, choice, safety, realising potential, equality and diversity (The Scottish Government, 2008). Homelessness should not exempt older people from these rights but the extent to which opportunities enable them to be exercised is indeed questionable. Despite the fact that older homelessness is not a recent or new phenomenon, it remains vastly under represented and misunderstood among researchers, policy makers and practitioners. Within the current climate the needs of our older homeless population remain unmet far too often. This chapter aims to highlight some of the key issues surrounding this vulnerable group and to explore the importance of health care and social work professionals working alongside other service providers in order to meet their needs appropriately. The discussion will raise awareness and understanding of the issues surrounding older homelessness and make suggestions for further reading at the end of the chapter.

The benchmark at which we define homeless people as older is open to debate. In line with the rest of the UK, The Scottish Government's Housing Statistics Branch currently uses a cut off age of 65 for men and 60 for women (The Scottish Government, 2007a). Nevertheless, there is a general consensus among researchers and social care practitioners that the ageing process among the homeless population often occurs prematurely (Warnes and Crane, 2000; Rich *et al.*, 1995; Help the Aged and the Older Homelessness Development Project, 2003). The following discussion will therefore apply to all homeless people aged 50 and over. Individuals will be referred to as homeless should they be **rough sleepers**, **hostel dwellers** or of **No Fixed Abode** (NFA). Those at risk of homelessness will encompass anyone vulnerable to any of these situations including individuals who are resettled after long periods of homelessness.

Although the discussion will largely explore the current situation and service provision across Scotland, various comprehensive UK studies exist that highlight issues relevant across borders which should not be overlooked, such as the causes and impact of homelessness on older people. Therefore, references will be made to a selection of these including Clapham and Evans (2000) 'Social exclusion: the case of homelessness', Crane (1998) 'The associations between mental illness and homelessness among older people: an exploratory study' and Crane (2001) *Our Forgotten Elders: Older People on the Streets and in Hostels*. Nevertheless, there are also slight differences across Social Policy which should be taken into consideration. One key difference is that unlike England, Scotland and Wales, where individual Local Authorities take responsibility for tackling homelessness, Northern Ireland has one regional housing authority established to do this called the Northern Ireland Housing Executive. Therefore, although the Scottish situation is in many ways representative of the UK as a whole it is advisable to make reference to individual government sites for specific policy details.

REVIEW OF THE CURRENT LITERATURE

The historical perspective

Throughout the first half of the twentieth century homelessness across the UK was considered to be a criminal act and responses were punitive rather than supportive (Warnes and Crane, 2000). Therefore, homelessness was perceived to be the result of individual behaviour rather than a social problem (Avramov, 1997). Some perceived such behaviour as a moral and spiritual weakness and, in response, set up services with salvation on the agenda (Warnes and Crane, 2000). This remained the case up until the late 1960s when the rediscovery of poverty led to a shift within UK social policy. This shift was reflected in public opinion with homelessness increasingly being perceived as a social problem (Jacobs *et al.*, 1999). It is now well accepted that homelessness is a **social construction**. Therefore the nature of, and attitudes towards, homelessness are ever-changing among society, policy makers, social care professionals as well as homeless people themselves. Often such changes are a reflection of the changing individual experiences of homelessness and the responses to it. This is largely driven by society's current social, economic and political agendas. Over the last decade more money has been invested in an attempt to tackle homelessness. One of the principal responses to increasing numbers of rough sleepers in Scotland came in 1997 when the Labour Government established the **Rough Sleepers Initiative** (RSI). Comprehensive reports reviewing the success of this can be found in the recommended websites section at the end of the chapter where an abundance of other publications can be sourced.

The extent of older homelessness

Across the UK the images attributed to older homelessness are often those that depict 'street drinkers' and 'bag ladies'. Despite Harman's (1989) view that homeless people look homeless, the reality, especially for older homeless people, is that the majority remain hidden and rarely engage with services. Crane (1999) supports such findings, stating that isolation and little or no contact with family is a common trait among this group. This results in a gap in service provision with many organisations needing to review policies and procedures that directly address the needs of this particular group. Indeed, Kalaga and Kingston (2007) highlight an increased risk of **discriminatory abuse** among older homeless people as a direct result of their exclusion from the wider community and services across health and social care. Such exclusion can make the rapport building process a tricky one. Care workers, in whatever capacity, should bear these factors in mind as well as the fact that the causes of homelessness are rarely unitary.

Taking into consideration hidden homelessness and double counting as a result of **transient** lifestyles, the extent of older homelessness remains unclear. Additionally, other factors such as the lack of homeless people on the electoral roll and those registered with a local general practitioner (GP) leads to further isolation (Crane, 2001). Therefore, deciphering the extent of older homelessness can be extremely problematic. The Scottish Government's (2007a) publication *Operation of the Homeless Persons Legislation in Scotland: National and Local Authority Analyses 2006–07* states that, to date, a total of 1,517 people over retirement age submitted Local Authority homeless applications. Of these, 651 were men and 866 were women. As is the situation across the UK, unofficial homelessness cannot be counted and so such figures only provide the smallest picture. Others over and above these statistics will include those who are NFA, rough sleepers and those who have been accommodated in temporary accommodation but remain at high risk of becoming homeless. In addition to this we cannot account for those who are banned from specific services and, in unique cases where risk assessments prove necessary, some may be banned from Local Authorities themselves.

Older homelessness is often a result of intertwining personal, social, economic and housing issues and the inability to cope with these. Crane's (1998) study of the links between mental illness and older homelessness found that common triggers preceding homelessness include major life changes such as bereavement and retirement. Additionally, relationship breakdown, eviction, discharge from the Armed Forces or indeed the end of any employment that included accommodation are other factors that can lead to older homelessness (Third and Yanetta, 2000; Allen, 2002). Such circumstances affect thousands every year. Although the majority of such groups do not end up homeless it is imperative to recognise that those who struggle to find adequate coping strategies, have pre-existing issues and/or lack any form of support network can make homelessness very much a reality. Working in the field of homelessness quickly highlights the fact that anyone can become homeless, irrespective of age, gender, ethnicity or socioeconomic class and this is something that all emerging professionals should bear in mind. For some homeless people, self-harm, alcohol and drug abuse can become coping mechanisms. Additionally, some individuals develop mental health problems which can, although not always, increase high risk behaviour patterns and coping strategies such as those noted previously (Crane, 1998). When any of these issues impede upon the ability to function throughout everyday life it is not uncommon for individuals to experience relationship breakdowns and become isolated from family and friends. Additionally, for those who have never experienced homelessness and who have perhaps lived lives many would consider 'normal' or, indeed, regimented for those in the forces, then this inability to cope is rarely addressed or picked up on. A lack of knowledge about where to go for support or advice can also fast track individuals on the road to homelessness, which may involve stays in hostels and periods of rough sleeping.

Health and social care needs

The support needs of older homeless people vary. Whereas issues such as **substance misuse**, mental ill-health and transience may prelude other, just as serious, needs it is crucial that professionals do not fail to address these. For instance, support needs surrounding nutrition, exploitation, budgeting and challenging behaviour are just as in need of appropriate response as the aforementioned. Indeed, 'complex' and 'multiple' needs are currently buzz words among policy makers, managerial and frontline staff. The majority of local councils have been working towards such a definition but Rankin and Regan (2004) summarise it clearly as:

> People with complex needs may have to negotiate a number of different issues in their life, for example learning disability, mental health problems, substance abuse. They may also be living in deprived circumstances and lack access to suitable housing or meaningful daily activity . . . there is no generic complex needs case. Each individual with complex needs has a unique interaction between their health and social care needs and requires a personalised response from services.
>
> (Rankin and Regan, 2004: 1)

Additionally, support packages often need to focus on areas such as employability alongside these other health and social care needs (Hawes, 1999; Scottish Government, 2004).

A common occurrence that lies uneasily among those supporting older homeless people is the lack of health care and social services provision invested in those who are affected by some form of **dual diagnosis**. Crane (1999) found that staff reported great difficulties and barriers to appropriate support for those service users who suffered ongoing mental health problems as well as substance misuse due to the fact that no one appeared willing or qualified to deal with such complex issues (Crane, 1999). In support of this a support worker who spoke at length to the author stated that:

> Often mental health professionals and nursing staff explain that they cannot address the mental health issues unless the individual stays off alcohol or drugs. This often isn't viable and so they are left unsupported. This can end up in a vicious cycle, often in and out of prison. Because some are incarcerated for petty crimes with short term sentences there is often no social work input and unfortunately, for both the individual and the public, their behaviour continuously becomes more risky.

With regards to the impact that mental illness has on older homelessness and vice versa, few studies exist that explore the true extent of this correlation. However, Crane's (1998) study, which interviewed 225 homeless people over the age of 55, found that 41 per cent of participants admitted to experiencing mental health problems prior to becoming homeless. As previously stated, mental health issues can lead to individuals withdrawing from others, and this often includes relevant healthcare services. The fact that older homeless people are continuing to remain hidden needs to be addressed and should not be taken lightly as this will only result in further social isolation and increased physical and mental health needs (Gorton and Borrill, 2007).

Accommodation

In Scotland the majority of hostel providers, both voluntary and statutory, strive towards the successful **resettlement** of homeless people into tenancies with appropriate support on a needs-led basis. Once, and if, a tenancy is allocated a referral can be made to Supporting People. Supporting People was established in Scotland in 2003 with the aim of promoting independent living in tenancies among vulnerable groups through a structured needs-led support package (The Scottish Government, 2007b), and whose commitment is to assist with the promotion of independence. Additionally, the government's focus on Community Care interventions principally strives to keep individuals in their homes (Means, 2007). Undisputedly such interventions meet the needs of older people each year. However, a gap that emerges is direct support that leads to a successful outcome for older people with a history of rough sleeping. Without ongoing supportive joint working between care providers, successful resettlement becomes problematic. Clapham and Evan's (2000) study of homelessness found that many older long-term hostel dwellers have a feeling of safety within hostel environments. It becomes a way of life within which they are accepted and supported. Indeed Gorton and Borrill's (2007) study into the resettlement of older people supports this. They advise that the promotion of unrealistic goals, such as sustaining independent tenancies, continues to fail older people for whom this will never work. If anything they found that it can result in ever increasing numbers of older homeless people residing in hostels where their complexity of needs supersede the support services available. So what is the answer? As the following case study will show, some older people will choose to seek independent resettlement. Quite simply, in today's society there is often not a suitable answer. Intensive care in the community packages are very expensive and budgets are simply too restricted to provide such comprehensive support to all those who would need it. Permanent wet houses have their place and can be incredibly successful in re-engaging older homeless people with health care, social and living skills while, at the same time, offering the individual a safe and secure home. However, unfortunately, as recognised by the UK Coalition on Older Homelessness (2007), there is a definite lack of such units as well as specialist care homes across the UK.

Day services

At present there are 214 Day Centres across the UK offering a range of support services to homeless people as well as those at high risk of homelessness (Watson, 2007). The majority (193) are in England, 55 of which are in London alone (Watson, 2007). In comparison to this, there are 14 in Scotland, four in Wales and three in Northern Ireland (Watson, 2007). Such centres often provide much needed **crisis intervention**, as well as **ongoing support**. One day centre support worker highlighted the importance of this ongoing support for the older resettled service users. He explained that many older people struggle to cope with the isolation and fear that having a tenancy often brings. Often older people are reluctant to have workers in their homes and, instead, continue to access day centres as a way of not only accessing support services, but also in order to maintain the social circles they have long since established. Both Anderson (2000) and Crane (1999), whose studies addressed the use of day centres, support this. Both found that social networks established in Day Centres continue to play a pivotal role in the individual's overall wellbeing following resettlement. Crane's (1999) publication, *Understanding Older Homeless People*, expands on this stating that those who move on to tenancies often continue to display homeless behaviour and access day centres for support. Yet the study also found that it is not uncommon for rough sleepers to avoid such services, including direct access hostels. Crane suggests that fears of violence or intimidation from other younger homeless people as well as a distrust of staff meant that it was not unusual for such **service users** to access for food services only, failing to actively seek help before leaving promptly. The role of active intervention by both support staff and **outreach services** is therefore essential. Once an initial rapport based on trust is established professionals can create opportunities by providing advice and information enabling the individual to make informed choices about their lifestyle.

So far the literature review has highlighted some of the key issues surrounding older homelessness, all of which should be understood, respected and addressed by health care and social work professionals. The following Case study takes us a step further, offering an insight into just one example of the impact that professionals can have on determining the lives of older homeless people.

Case study

Bruce is 66 years old and currently resides in a small voluntary sector hostel. He first became homeless aged 58 following a burglary in his home after which time he felt unable to cope and, with no support networks in place, he decided to leave his hometown. He moved to another city on the other side of Scotland where he slept rough for a while until a *Big Issue* vendor signposted him to a homeless day centre. Workers referred him to a local hostel where he stayed intermittently, sleeping rough when a bed was unavailable. By this time Bruce was drinking excessively and he had formed trusting friendships with other street drinkers. He continued to engage with homeless and outreach health care services but, due to his chaotic lifestyle, this support was crisis intervention, dealing with immediate needs only.

Since relocating to the East of Scotland Bruce has had three tenancies, all of which have failed due to antisocial behaviour by individuals who would access the tenancy for drinking purposes. Despite receiving tenancy support he struggled to stay away from those who threatened his tenancy and found it difficult saying no when they turned up at his door.

Following the loss of his last tenancy and two years residing in local hostels and rough sleeping, Bruce was accommodated in a fully supported accommodation unit. Unfortunately, Bruce struggled to control his levels of drinking, was failing to engage with staff and was involved with conflict among other residents. This led to the termination of this tenancy agreement and Bruce returned to the emergency bed hostel. Bruce's alcohol misuse has advanced his restricted mobility, leading to a number of falls, one of which resulted in hospital admission. Bruce remained there for five weeks because of problems finding suitable accommodation. Constraints upon the homeless hostel's environmental and professional capacity to deal with restricted mobility meant that readmitting Bruce would further jeopardise his wellbeing and health.

Joint working between the hostel and social services highlighted that Bruce had a social worker but that his case had been closed. Following lengthy advocacy meetings on behalf of Bruce, the hostel agreed to accommodate Bruce on the condition that a social worker would be allocated to support his additional needs as well as a physiotherapist. An assistant social worker was appointed and Bruce moved back into the hostel. A physiotherapist was also appointed but this ceased after two weeks when Bruce could show that he was able to climb one flight of stairs.

When reviewing options with Bruce, Social Services suggested **sheltered housing** where he could still maintain his independence but would have to refrain from alcohol. Bruce turned this down, explaining that alcohol was a part of his lifestyle and any suggestions that he refrain from it only made him feel devalued and disrespected. Bruce also explained that agreeing to such a commitment would result in failure as deep down it is not what he wants to do. Bruce has asked for a ground floor flat and has recently received a letter to say that his case is being presented at the **Varying Needs Panel** and a decision should be made shortly. He has not seen his social worker for six weeks as she said she would be in touch when she heard of the panel's decision.

Since returning to the hostel Bruce's drinking is controlled and he visits his GP regularly. At each appointment his alcohol intake is reviewed and health implications are discussed but the expectation that Bruce maintains sobriety is not enforced. Bruce is accepting of such **harm reduction** methods and feels that there is a balance between the role of the GP and an understanding of his lifestyle. He is currently prioritising his health needs and ensuring his medication is taken at regular intervals.

When Bruce is asked what he would like to happen he simply says, 'to settle down in a flat with some support, keep my independence, meet new friends and maybe find a nice woman friend to share life with me'.

Activity

Bruce's case is not unique. There are many older homeless people in this position and for whom the system seems to have limited answers. Read over Bruce's case a few times and review the following questions. Try to provide as full an answer as possible to each question. You should bear in mind the key principles of the National Care Standards specific to your own country. For example, the Scottish principles are dignity, privacy, choice, safety, realising potential, equality and diversity (The Scottish Government, 2008). It may also be useful to refer to Figure 1, Maslow's Hierarchy of Needs. This indicates that each developmental stage is only attainable if the lower needs are satisfied. Without this, individuals will lack the ability and motivation required to move on.

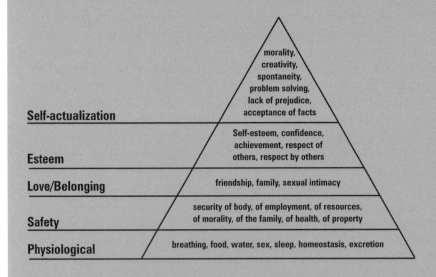

Figure 1 Maslow's Hierarchy of Needs

1. What do you think are Bruce's main issues that influence his lifestyle?
2. Who do you see as the core care provider for Bruce's care and why?
3. What do you think Bruce's immediate needs are?
4. What do you think Bruce's long-term needs are?
5. What support do you think needs to be put in place in order to address both his short-term and long-term needs?
6. What do you see as Bruce's own priorities?
7. What does Bruce appear to value from the professionals he engages with?
8. In what ways do Bruce's priorities conflict with the needs you have identified?
9. Were you surprised by Bruce's circumstances and why?
10. What type of support package do you think is needed for Bruce and who do you think should manage it?
11. Can you devise a care plan for Bruce? Doing so may highlight the difficulties that professionals have when faced with a conflict of interests between themselves and the individual.

THE USER'S PERSPECTIVE

The health needs of homeless people aged 50 are often comparable to those aged 60–70 living in secure accommodation. This is predominantly due to the chaotic nature of homelessness and the life choices made. Many do not prioritise health care, often living with ailments rather than addressing them. This is especially the case for those with mental health and/or substance misuse issues. Outreach services are pro-active in crisis intervention but longer-term preventative measures prove more challenging. Ad hoc support and transience means that establishing a rapport based on trust can be difficult. Additionally, workers are often unable to engage appropriately if individuals are under the influence of substances. Harm reduction therefore plays a key role in health promotion among the homeless population. Many older people with whom we have spoken discussed instances where pressure from workers to abstain from substances after years of reliance left them feeling misunderstood and devalued. Often this had resulted in them withdrawing from their support networks altogether.

Another trend that emerged through talks with older homeless people was a reluctance to access GP surgeries. Many individuals spoke about the importance of seeing a nurse within their own environment, whether that be a day centre, hostel or on the street. This was largely because they do not have to question the nurse's understanding of homelessness. Neither do they have to risk a potential hostile reaction from receptionists and others in the waiting area of general surgeries. Therefore, the establishment of specialised health care services across cities such as Glasgow, Perth and Edinburgh as well as many other cities across the UK certainly appear to have been successful in re-engaging the older homeless population. In contrast to this, Allen's (2002) study of health care among older homeless people found that negative experiences of Accident and Emergency departments were not uncommon, with individuals being on the receiving end of verbal insults and even on occasion being refused treatment. For those who have positive experiences of their GP, time, honesty and understanding were three key elements that individuals expressed as important in order to feel valued and respected. Indeed, older homeless people tend to value the attitudes of health care workers specialising in the field of homelessness because they have fewer experiences of feeling judged or undermined. The majority felt this was due to a better understanding of their lifestyle.

IMPLICATIONS FOR JOINT WORKING

Having reviewed some of the general users' perspectives, it is important to review some of the barriers to joint working experienced by workers. Multi-agency working sits at the heart of current best practice guidelines. In 2000 the Scottish Government stated that:

> Tackling and preventing homelessness is not just a matter for local authority housing departments. It requires concerted and co-ordinated efforts from a range of bodies, both public and voluntary, to make in-roads into the underlying problems and despair caused by drug abuse, mental and physical illness and household breakdown.
>
> (Scottish Government, 2000: 8)

Therefore a willingness to take on board the ideas and visions of others in related yet often politically diverse fields, such as the voluntary and statutory sectors, is crucial if such joint working is to be successful in practice (Kennedy, Lynch and Goodlad, 2001; Scottish Government, 2004). An example of when such partnerships break down was provided by a senior manager of a charitable organisation. He spoke about the regular withdrawal of social work support once a tenancy support worker had been allocated. On another occasion, a senior nurse discussed the breakdown of multi-agency forums due to poor attendance from other voluntary and statutory sector professionals. Both these examples led to a breakdown in communication, ill feeling among workers and inevitably jeopardised the support of this vulnerable group.

Help the Aged and the Older Homelessness Development Project (2003) also recognise the importance of such joint working throughout their evaluation of the discharge of older homeless people from hospital. They strongly recommend joint working between health and social care services and homelessness agencies in order to meet the needs of hospital patients. The report discusses the high rates of older homeless people discharging themselves from hospital, and the lack of intervention that takes place when they decide to leave prematurely (Help the Aged and the Older Homelessness Development Project, 2003). Although Bruce's situation highlighted areas of good practice, one hostel support worker I spoke to informed me that often they only found out about someone's stay in hospital after contacting their local hospital following raised concerns about the individual's whereabouts. The problem here is that by the time hostel workers make such contact it is not uncommon for the individual to have already self-discharged without secure accommodation or appropriate treatment.

One of the key barriers to successful joint working is the policies and procedures surrounding confidentiality (Kennedy, Lynch and Goodlad, 2001). As promoted within the Scottish Government's (2001) *Guidance on Single Shared Assessment of Community Care Needs*, all service users, or their representatives, should be given the opportunity to sign a consent form that indicates which agencies workers can liaise with should this be considered appropriate and in their best interests. (See Chapter 7 for further information on Single Shared Assessment in the UK.) However, across the different social work, health care, housing and other support agencies, the content within confidentiality and information-sharing policies differ. For example, it is not uncommon for specialist support services to share information, on a need-to-know basis, with health care and social work practitioners but such practice is not always a two-way process due to fear of breaching the rights of the individual (Support Worker, 2007). Again this potentially risks the successful resettlement of the individual and can leave the worker feeling under-valued and disrespected (Project Worker, 2007).

CONCLUSION

The emphasis on the resettlement of homeless people that has taken place over the last decade is a far cry from the decades of punitive responses and containment in mental institutions (Crane, 1999) yet, on many levels, the needs of the older population remain unmet. Examples of this have been highlighted throughout the chapter and it is clear to see that such complexity cannot be addressed through the establishment of one unitary response. The fact that many older homeless people as well as those at risk of becoming homeless remain hidden from mainstream services means that professionals need to possess an understanding and awareness of the issues and behaviour that this group can present with. Sensitivity is paramount, bearing in mind that some may have negative experiences or perceptions of mainstream services. Individuals themselves are not always averse to accessing health and social care services. They simply seek support from professionals who are respectful, honest and possess an understanding of their situations and life choices. Additionally, professionals should bear in mind the simple fact that anyone can become homeless. Individuals respond to and cope with life changing circumstances in a variety of ways. Often one does not know how they would cope until the situation arises. Therefore often preconceived ideas about the causes and nature of homelessness can be erased as it is a far more complex issue than generally understood. It is useful for workers entering the care sector to reflect upon such preconceived ideas. Through reflection professionals are able to challenge their own, as well as societal, attitudes which exist towards this vulnerable group.

Although increased provision of affordable housing would address the needs of some, the reality is that the successful resettlement of older people often exceeds the realms of housing issues and comprehensive support packages should be sought. Resettlement is not always the magic answer as many of their problems rarely end there. As Hawes states, homelessness is surrounded by a number of issues and factors including: 'low skills, poor education, drugs, alcohol, mental ill-health, disrupted family life, ejection from the cocooning effect of institutional life' (Hawes, 1999: 202). The importance of addressing multiple needs should not be overlooked as, without the required, often intensive, support, a cycle of homelessness can emerge. Therefore, continued support from homeless services can often continue to play a pivotal role in the success of any resettlement care package. The continued use of day centres has been discussed. This highlighted the importance of sustained support and socialisation for many who move on into secure tenancies but continue to display homeless behaviour. Additionally joint working is crucial if older homeless people are to receive the intense support they often require.

Only when services work together can we ensure that the varied needs of this vulnerable group are being addressed. Without such intervention individuals can remain homeless and hidden. For those who are resettled, a lack of joint working or miscommunication between professionals can lead to further isolation and a failure to cope with the responsibility involved in maintaining a roof over their heads.

Overall, all emerging professionals should remember that successful health and social care practice is about enabling informed choices while protecting the individual from further harm and exploitation. This can only be successful through a willingness to overcome the many barriers that may be in the way of the practitioner and the service user as well an enthusiasm for working together across all sectors.

FURTHER READING

Fitzpatrick, S., Pleace, N. and Bevan, N. (2005) *Final Evaluation of the Rough Sleepers Initiative*. Edinburgh: The Scottish Government. Found at **www. scotland.gov.uk/Publications/2005/03/20886/54982** (Accessed February 2008).
A comprehensive evaluation of the success and limitations of the *Rough Sleepers Initiative*, one of the biggest financial investments tackling homelessness over the last decade.

Lane, R. (2005) *The Road to Recovery – A Feasibility Study into Homeless Intermediate Care*. London: Homeless Intermediate Care Steering Group
An invaluable text evaluating the health needs of homeless people and the need for nurse-led intermediate care.

Lomax, D., Lancaster, S. and Gray, P. (2000) *Moving On: A Survey of Travellers' Views*, Edinburgh: Scottish Executive
A detailed analysis of Travellers' views and experiences of mainstream services. An excellent resource for anyone supporting this group.

Willcock, K. (2003) *Journeys out of Loneliness: The Views of Older Homeless People*. London: Help the Aged
A focussed piece of research that provides the reader with an increased awareness into the experiences of, and attitudes towards, health care among the homeless population.

Useful websites

www.scotland.gov.uk/Topics/Housing/homeless/H-M-G
A comprehensive guide to the Homelessness Monitoring Group, established in 2002 to review proposals put forward by the Homelessness Task Force.

www.crisis.org.uk
An excellent resource raising awareness about homelessness at a national level.

scotland.shelter.org.uk
A guide to housing issues across Scotland. The site includes details about current campaigns, policy, service providers and publications.

www.homeless.org.uk
A site devoted to homelessness that includes good practice guidelines, publications and current issues.

www.homelesspages.org.uk
A guide to resources, services and publications across the UK. An excellent resource for keeping up to date with national issues.

REFERENCES

Allen, D. (2002) 'A refuge for rough sleepers'. *Nursing Older People*, 13 (10): 10–13

Anderson, I. (2000) 'Social exclusion and housing: conclusions and challenges' in Anderson, I. and Sim, D. (eds) *Social Exclusion and Housing: Context and Challenges*. Coventry: Chartered Institute of Housing

Avramov, D. (1997) 'Social images of homelessness' in Parmentier, C. (ed) *Third International FEANTSA Congress – Where to Sleep Tonight? Where to Live Tomorrow?: Orientations for Future Action*. Brussels: FEANTSA

Bradley, T., Cooper, A. and Sycamore, R. (eds) (2004) *Homeless Link Day Centres Handbook: A Good Practice Guide*. London: Homeless Link

Clapham, D. and Evans, A. (2000) 'Social exclusion: the case of homelessness' in Anderson, I. and Sim, D. (eds) *Social Exclusion and Housing: Context and Challenges*. Coventry: Chartered Institute of Housing

Crane, M. (1998) 'The associations between mental illness and homelessness among older people: an exploratory study'. *Aging and Mental Health*, 2 (3): 171–80

Crane, M. (1999) *Understanding Older Homeless People*. Buckingham: Open University Press

Crane, M. (2001) *Our Forgotten Elders: Older People on the Streets and in Hostels*. London: St. Mungo's

Gorton, S. and Borrill, A. (2007) *Guide to Resettling Older Residents from Hostels*. London: UK Coalition of Older Homelessness

Harman, L. D. (1989) *When a Hostel Becomes a Home: Experiences of Women*. Ontario: Garamond Press

Hawes, D. (1999) 'Old and homeless: A double jeopardy' in Kennett, P. and Marsh, A. (eds) *Homelessness: Exploring the New Terrain*. Bristol: The Policy Press

Help the Aged and the Older Homelessness Development Project (2003) *The Discharge of Older Homeless People from Hospital*. London: Help the Aged

Jacobs, K., Kemeny, J. and Manzi, T. (1999) 'The struggle to define homelessness: a constructivist approach' in Hutson, S. and Clapham, D. (eds) *Homelessness: Public Policies and Private Troubles*. London: Cassell

Kalaga, H. and Kingston, P. (2007) *A Review of Literature on Effective Interventions that Prevent and Respond to Harm Against Adults*. Edinburgh: Scottish Government Social Research, found at **www.scotland.gov.uk/socialresearch** (Accessed February 2008)

Kennedy, C., Lynch, E., Goodlad, R. (2001) *Good Practice in Joint/Multi-Agency Working on Homelessness*. Edinburgh: Scottish Executive

Means, R. (2007) 'Safe as houses? Ageing in place and vulnerable older people in the UK'. *Social Policy & Administration*, 41 (1): 65–8

Project Worker (2007) *Personal Communications*, 21 December 2007

Rankin, J. and Regan, S. (2004) *Meeting Complex Needs: The Future of Social Care*. London: Turning Points/Institute of Public Policy Research

Rich, D., Rich, T. and Mullins, L. (eds) (1995) *Old and Homeless – Double Jeopardy: An Overview of Current Practice and Policies*. Westport, VA: Auburn House

The Scottish Government (2000) *Better Homes for Scotland's Communities: The Executive Proposals for the Housing Bill*. Edinburgh: The Stationery Office

The Scottish Government (2001) *Guidance on Single Shared Assessment of Community Care Need*. **www.sehd.scot.nhs.uk/publications/DC20011129CCD8single.pdf** (Accessed May 2008)

The Scottish Government (2004) *Code of Guidance on Homelessness*. Edinburgh: The Stationery Office

The Scottish Government (2007a) *Operation of the Homeless Persons Legislation in Scotland: National and Local Authority Analyses 2006–07*. Edinburgh: The Scottish Government. **www.scotland.gov.uk/Publications/2007/10/30092316/36** (Accessed February 2008)

The Scottish Government (2007b) *Supporting People*. **www.scotland.gov.uk/Topics/Housing/Housing/supportpeople** (Accessed February 2008)

The Scottish Government (2008) National Care Standards. **www.scotland.gov.uk/Topics/Health/care/17652/9325** (Accessed February 2008)

Third, H. and Yanetta, A. (2000) *Homelessness in Scotland: A Summary of Research Evidence*. Edinburgh: Scottish Homes

UK Coalition on Older Homelessness (2007) *Audit of Older Homeless People September 2007: Summary of Findings*. London: UK Coalition on Older Homelessness

Warnes, A. and Crane, M. (2000) *Meeting Homeless People's Needs: Service Provision and Practice for the Older Excluded*. London: King's Fund

Watson, P. (ed.) (2007) *Directory of Day Centres for Homeless People 2007*. London: Resource Information Service

Chapter 19

Life in Care

Angela Kydd and Eveline Kearney

Learning outcomes

Reading this chapter will enable you to:

- explain the term 'quality of life' and what this might mean to older people;

- describe the barriers to autonomous living for older people in a care home setting;

- explore how joint working might improve the experience of life in a care home;

- discuss the various perceptions of care home life, the reasons underlying these and what might be done to change them.

INTRODUCTION

The population of the Western world is ageing. Ageing is a very diverse concept and how an individual ages and copes with the deleterious effects of ageing is unique to that individual (Baltes and Baltes, 1990). Ageing encompasses not only the chronological years a person reaches, but how their biology has responded to their physical, psychological and social environment.

People are living longer and many older people enjoy a long, relatively independent and healthy life. Some older people will, however, become dependent on spouses, family members, neighbours or friends to support them. This can be a precarious position, as should support suddenly cease, a crisis move to long-term care may have to be made. The frail older person is extremely vulnerable at such a time. There is also a growing number of frail older people who will go into care because they can no longer cope alone or no longer wish to struggle on alone in their own homes.

For the sake of uniformity, any establishments offering institutionalised care with the remit of providing all aspects of accommodation, support and care, will be referred to within this chapter as care homes.

Once in a care home, most residents stay for the rest of their lives. What happens in that setting, the older person's new home, affects their quality of life. As these people represent one of the most powerless groups in society, it is essential that their voice is heard.

What life is like in care is a subject relevant to all professionals who work with adults, as some older people will be admitted to hospitals from care homes, or be discharged from hospital to a care home because they are no longer able to cope at home.

This chapter refers to the work in Chapter 2 on the demographic and welfare changes that have led to an increasingly frail and ill population of care home residents. It then goes on to explore the media, public and professional attitudes towards care homes and how these can negate some excellent work being done in the care home sector. Finally, entry to, and life in, care is discussed, with the aim of providing an insight into some of the issues involved in spending the remainder of one's life in an institution.

DEMOGRAPHICS

As mortality and fertility have declined, there has been a global increase in the proportion of older people (United Nations, 2002). The fastest growing age grouping is people aged 80 and over as is detailed in Chapter 2. Exact figures are difficult to estimate, but it is essential to look at demographic trends in order to plan services for the population. Given the rapidly increasing numbers of those people classed as the 'oldest old', it is inevitable that there will be increasing numbers of people requiring care services and long-term care.

WELFARE REFORMS

Since the late 1980s there has been a drive to keep older people in their own homes for as long as possible. An Audit Commission report (1986) *Making a Reality of Community Care* strongly criticised central government on organisational fragmentation, poor planning and the perverse incentive of supporting people in care homes and not at home. The government response was to set up a working party led by Sir Roy Griffiths, whose remit was to review the way in which public funds should be used to support people in the community. The Griffiths Report (1988) recommendations included providing people with greater consumer choice, setting up the social services to act as lead agencies and encouraging joint training and working between different professions. The White Paper, *Working for Patients* (Department of Health, 1989) was the government's response to the Griffiths Report and was one of three White Papers that underpinned the NHS and Community Care (1990) Act.

The NHS and Community Care Act (1990) brought a change in the provision of services in the National Health Service (NHS) as the emphasis was on reducing the cost of care and keeping people in the community. When the Act was fully implemented in 1993, indiscriminate state funding for residential and nursing home care ceased. Detailed accounts of the complexities of the reforms have been well documented elsewhere (Victor, 1997; Means and Smith, 1998; Glasby and Glasby, 1999; Malin *et al.*, 1999). Further welfare reforms following devolution in 1997 occurred within the four United Kingdom (UK) countries. With differing emphasis, all have worked towards enhancing the principles of the NHS and Community Care Act (1990) and are aiming to manage people with chronic conditions in the community, prevent hospital admissions, facilitate supported discharge, provide intermediate care and avert premature admission to a care home (Scottish Executive, 1998; Department of Health, 2001a; Welsh Assembly Government, 2002).

THE VULNERABILITY OF OLDER PEOPLE IN CARE HOMES

As admission to a care home is now intended for the frail old who cannot be supported at home, those admitted usually have either severe physical and/or cognitive problems and, as a result, have little voice with regard to the care they do or do not receive.

This group are also politically vulnerable. Until recently they have been overlooked by the government. *The Health Study for England 2000* (Falaschetti, Malbut and Primatesta, 2002) was the first to include data regarding people in institutional environments. Care home residents have no security of tenure as most fall outside the protection of the Human Rights Act (1998) if the home is privately owned, as is primarily the case with most UK care homes. An example of this is the case of an 84-year-old woman whose family challenged the decision of the care home that had given her notice to quit. The Law Lords ruled that, as the home was not a public authority, the Act did not apply. A private members bill is currently being brought in, in order to clarify the meaning of 'public function' in an attempt to afford protection to the residents of private care homes (House of Commons, 2007).

THE PERCEPTION OF LIFE IN CARE HOMES

The media invariably portrays negative stories regarding care homes and this is not confined to the tabloids. Broadsheet newspapers also focus on negative government reports that highlight sexual assaults, malnutrition and bullying (Joint Committee on Human Rights Enquiry, 2007). Although such allegations and proven cases are legitimate, the fact that good care is not reported means that little balance is offered to the public, therefore, the enduring public perception of life in care is negative.

Further negative images are plentiful regarding practices within care home settings when consultations are requested. For example, the Commission for Social Care Inspection sought the views on restraint from professionals and asked whether restraint should be banned (Commission for Social Care Inspection, 2007). The images conjured up by such an enquiry were not likely to be positive, although the fact that action was being taken on this controversial topic gives hope that life in poor care homes will improve.

The largely negative response to the concept of care home life is under review. A study is currently being carried out, collating the views of people in care homes and their relatives and friends, with a view to evidencing what value exists in such an environment (National Care Forum, 2008).

Older people's attitudes to life in care

Admission to a care home is not generally regarded as a positive option. Part of this attitude is historical, with the stigma of 'being put away in a home'. Many care homes were originally converted workhouses, described by Townsend (1964) as the old workhouse buildings, redeployed to house the decrepit older people who were 'too mad, too poor and too unloved' to be looked after at home.

The negative attitude towards admission to care is supported by recent welfare reforms. Recent government policies support the view that people should be kept at home for as long as possible, with admission to a care home as a last resort. The 'last resort' option is reminiscent of Townsend's *Last Refuge* (1964) and underlines the hopelessness of the situation for those who have to go into a care home.

A study by Boaz, Hayden and Taylor (1999) questioned older people in the community about their old age. The participants reported a fear of dependency and having to leave their homes and move into a care home. The desire of older people to remain independent is also highlighted in the Audit Commission report (2004).

Although independence is relative and subjective, the wish of older people to make choices and to exercise control over their lives is well reported (Audit Commission and Better Government for Older People, 2004; Age Concern and the Mental Health Foundation, 2006). This does not necessarily mean being totally independent as, in some areas of life, independence can be facilitated by accepting help. Older people value lower level assistance with shopping and cleaning, for example, as it helps them to maintain a degree of independence (Raynes *et al.*, 2001).

The National Service Framework for Older People (NSF) identified that older people preferred to remain at home and not to be in a care home or communal environment (Department of Health, 2004). Attitudes of older housebound people toward care home life tended to reflect that of the general public, perceiving care homes as places for people who are confused or without a caring family (Economic and Social Research Council (ESRC), 2003).

Nurses' perceptions of life in care

Murphy (2006) identified six factors that nurses perceived as facilitating quality in a care home. These were:

1. promoting independence;
2. a home-like environment;
3. person-centred care;
4. knowledgeable staff;
5. a knowledge of the person;
6. adequate resources.

Limiting factors identified by nurses were:

- lack of time;
- lack of resident choice;
- resistance to change;
- constraints of routine.

A study by Severance (2005) shows that the perceptions that nurses and carers have regarding quality of care differs from those of residents and their relatives. The staff have a more positive perception of the standard of care than those in receipt of care. The frames of reference differ for each role. For example, the carer may feel that they have done well to attend to a call from a resident within two minutes, given that they have to complete a care task for another resident beforehand but, for a resident with a urinary urgency, this may seem like a long time or may in fact be too late.

A study by Milke *et al.* (2006) collated responses from three groups of people, one group of family and friends and two groups of staff. Although many of the responses to the questionnaire items asked were similar across the groups, the responses of the family and friends group differed from the two groups of staff in responses relating to rights and freedoms, specifically, residents' rights to refuse medication, get up during the night, choice of dining area and flexibility of rising and bed times. In these areas the family and friends group were more critical of how well these aspects of care were delivered.

People in residential and care homes have inevitably been regarded as vulnerable and in need of protection and this attitude has resulted in a disinclination to allow risk. Care home staff have to judge between managing risk and duty of care. A common example is deciding whether to let an older person make the decision to walk without assistance, even though the staff know that this person is unsteady and at risk of falling. Such decisions result in a conflict of values for care staff and, as Suber (1992) points out, showing love can involve protecting individuals from harm, as opposed to respecting their freedom. This has resulted in regulations that, when applied in a blanket manner, can be constraining of personal autonomy. Risk can never be completely eliminated and risk decisions are a balancing act. Managing risk is a complex issue and, in order to enable individuals to remain as independent as possible, they must be permitted to take risks.

The user's perspective

Each individual's perceptions of life in care will be coloured by the life events that led them to admission, their state of mental and physical health and the way their expectations of the home are realised. This area is a growing area of interest to researchers.

Bergland and Kirkevold (2006) conducted a study, from a resident's perspective, to investigate factors that enabled people to thrive in a care home environment. One factor identified was the individual's own attitude to their circumstances. Interestingly, those who coped well had purposely reduced their expectations and reconceptualised their life in a care home. A further key issue identified was the quality of care delivered, which is discussed later in this chapter (see the section on 'Quality of life in care' on page 370).

Tester *et al.* (2003) found that the perceptions of people living in care homes identified four main themes. These are:

1. retaining a sense of self;
2. the care environment;
3. relationships;
4. activities.

Of these, retaining a sense of self by having the opportunity to 'be oneself' was a key determinant of their perceived quality of life.

Legislation, policies and procedures can be limiting to personal autonomy. An example of this is the health and safety issue surrounding personal items such as bedding and the need for them to be fire retardant. This can preclude personalisation of a resident's living space. McCormack (2001) identifies constraints such as 'routinised practices'. Communal dietary provision inevitably reduces real choice of menu. At home, people can eat what, when and where they choose. In a care home environment, residents mainly rely on staff to offer food and drink and though the menu will offer a choice, it may not be something that the resident feels like having at that particular time.

The Economic and Social Research Council (ESRC) Growing Older (GO) Project (2003) interviewed several groups of older people including care home residents and found that quality of life issues fell into three broad categories:

- diversity;
- social exclusion; and
- the value of formal and informal support.

Quality of life was determined by individual expectations and the ability to adapt; also by family, health and home. Emotional wellbeing, independence and mobility were also identified but functional capacity and health status were not identified as pre-requisites for good quality of life. Irrespective of health or disability status, those in residential homes reported a relatively poor quality of life. Although this group were older and had less cognitive capacity, neither these factors nor their greater health problems seemed to account for this result. The report concluded that the most important factor directly predicting individual quality of life for older people is the social environment.

ENTRY INTO CARE

Entry into long-term care has many different determinants; no two individuals experience the same circumstances. The reasons for going into care may be determined by personal choice, family choice, they may be directed by professionals or the availability of formal and/or informal care within the older person's geographical area.

The determining factors will be based not only on the needs of the individual, but on their current state of physical and mental health, their social circumstances and the resources available to them. These resources may include a package of community care services to enable them to stay at home with intensive support, financial resources to buy in necessary support, family and/or friends willing and able to take care of the individual at home and, of course, the internal resources of the individual. As frail older people become older and more frail, they also become more vulnerable on all counts. Their health status is delicate, making them susceptible to falls, infections and exacerbations of existing conditions; their support networks may be straining to cope with the extra work of caring for them, or their spouses – if they are the principal carer –may also be ageing and more susceptible to illnesses and may even die. Any sudden changes in a frail older person's condition or in their loved one's condition may precipitate admission to long-term care.

Studies relating to admission to long-term care include early works by Chenitz (1983), who developed a set of basic conditions seen to shape the adjustment to the new environment, Challis and Bartlett (1988) with respect to individuals selecting a care home and Nolan *et al.* (1996) on the types of entry to care. These are a few of the important studies carried out to investigate this phenomenon. However, Lee *et al.* (2002) point out that more work is needed on the actual experiences of older people as they adjust on a day-to-day basis to life in care. This criticism is being addressed in a growing body of literature, which includes the UK-wide initiative, *My Home Life* (Help the Aged, 2007).

QUALITY OF LIFE IN CARE

The term 'quality' has many definitions and connotations. One definition is that quality means 'fitness for purpose' (Juran and Gryna, 1988). In this definition 'fitness' is determined by the consumer or user. The quality of a care home and the quality of life in a care home is a very subjective topic and it should be measured by the individual's perception of their quality of care, not just by inspectors' reports.

The Commission for Social Care Inspection has introduced a star rating system for care homes with the intention of providing the public with information on which to base informed choices about the quality of their local care services (Commision for Social Care Inspection, 2005). The idea of this system is to offer providers an incentive to improve standards and also let residents and their relatives know what level of care they can expect, in comparison with similar establishments. Because potential clients will be able to see the quality rating at a glance, custom is expected to gravitate toward those with higher ratings. As inspectors will also report to commissioning bodies such as social services regarding homes with poor ratings, there will be an impact on referrals resulting in a virtual blacklisting of some homes, which will affect occupancy levels, reputation and the revenue of the home. In Scotland, the Scottish Commission for the Regulation of Care (the regulatory body covering residential care in Scotland) has set up a grading system (Scottish Commission for the Regulation of Care, 2007), which came into force on 1 April 2008. The grading system dictates that quality of care indicators must involve people who use the service.

If ratings are to be meaningful, then the qualitative aspects of care have to be judged and this is done best by asking the residents and taking account of their views. Concerns about the system of star ratings include providers 'chasing ratings', by focussing on some key areas at the expense of others. There is a danger that some important aspects of care will be overlooked. The report, *Bridging the Gap – Participation in Social Care*

Regulation (Better Regulation Task Force, 2004) points to the precedence that paperwork has taken over people and suggests that the emphasis has been placed on processes rather than on the outcomes for individuals.

Some of the major complaints about life in a care home are boredom, inactivity and pain. These are important areas to address as activity is linked to good mental health and activity is restricted if an individual is in pain (Age Concern and the Mental Health Foundation, 2006). Exercise and meaningful activity can lift the mood and ease the mind (Age Concern and the Scotland and Highland NHS Board, 2001). It is necessary for care staff to recognise that the support needed to take exercise is no less a priority than the support given with tasks such as washing and dressing. Those with access to physiotherapy clearly benefit in terms of improved mobility, confidence, mood and self esteem (Donaghy, 2007).

Recent research found, on observing activity levels in a residential care setting, that residents were sitting for 97 per cent of the time and engaged in no activity 61 per cent of the time. Only 2.5 per cent of observations identified residents interacting with staff and, of this observed contact, only 0.4 per cent was in a social context (Sackley *et al.*, 2006).

Positive events and wellbeing are linked and yet, to date, there has been little research into what residents perceive as positive events. Faulkner *et al.* (2006) have designed a tool called 'Combined Assessment of Residential Environments' (CARE) profile. This takes the form of three questionnaires, one each for residents, staff and relatives, taking account of the frequency of positive daily events. As positive events may not mean the same to everyone, events are described in different terms such as 'enjoyable' or 'satisfying'. The questionnaire is based on underpinning values such as having the sense of security, belonging, continuity, purpose, achievement and significance. Although early testing suggests that the tool is reliable, the views of cognitively impaired residents do not appear to be adequately represented. The use of such a tool might well enhance the quality of life of care home residents by identifying what is positive for them as individuals.

Pain

As the care home population in the UK is becoming increasingly dependent, and many residents suffer from conditions more prevalent in old age such as arthritis and osteoporosis, chronic pain is common in care home residents. Studies have, for some time now, identified that pain is not well controlled in older people in many settings but particularly so in those in care home environments. A study by Allcock, McGarry and

Elkin (2002) identified that 37 per cent of residents suffered chronic non-malignant pain that was not addressed.

The effects of chronic pain can include depression, irritability, disturbed sleep and poor mobility (Cairncross *et al.*, 2007). The same study suggests that both care home staff and older people come to accept pain as part of growing older, not helped by the stoical attitude to pain common in the older generation. Accepting and enduring the pain also impacts on their social activities, further reducing their quality of life.

Case study

The following is an extract from an interview with a woman who, for the purposes of anonymity, has been referred to as 'Miriam' (Kydd, 2006). Miriam had been waiting in hospital for a place in a care home. She knew she was no longer able to cope on her own at home and, although the home was not of her choice, it was in the area she wanted. The home is near where her nieces live. The month is November.

I was shown to Miriam's room by a pleasant member of staff. She knocked on Miriam's door and entered immediately. I followed. Miriam was clearly delighted to see me. I asked how she was and she told me she had not been too good. She said she had been breathless and had pains in her hands, arms and knees. She then laughed and said, 'Oh here I am moaning to you already and you've only just walked through the door.' She went on to tell me that her pains were so bad that she could not sit for any length of time. She said:

'It's [her osteoporosis] got worse since Christmas Day. I was in bed and I thought – I can't spend Christmas in bed – so I got up and went downstairs . . . we had a lovely Christmas lunch and I went into the lounge. Three girls had come to sing carols – it was a lovely treat. I sat and listened, but I must have sat too long, because when I started to get up I nearly fell over. I was so stiff. Luckily my niece had just arrived and so she helped me up to my room. Since then I've not been able to sit in a chair for long and tend to spend most of the time in my room just lying on my bed. I can get more comfort this way. If only I could get some periods of relief, it would be so nice.'

I asked Miriam about what pain-relieving tablets she was on and she told me that she was on stronger painkillers. She did not take the very strong ones because they caused her to have hallucinations and become very confused.

I asked if she was in pain now. She said that she was. She only got up today because the hairdresser was here. She had told the care assistant this morning that she felt unable to get washed and dressed in time to have her hair done. She was so pleased when the care assistant had offered to help her get ready and take her to have her hair done as she likes to look smart.

I asked about companionship. Miriam had one friend, Connie. Connie comes to Miriam's room for a chat. They have meals together in the upstairs lounge. Miriam told me:

> 'Connie's been in here for six months now and has never really settled – she didn't want to come in here at all, but had to when her husband died. I shouldn't really talk about her but I think she was having blackouts or something and one of her granddaughters arranged for her to come in here. I've got no complaints because for the last three years at home I had hardly been out of my nightclothes.'

I asked about the staff. She told me that the manager of the home was a young man. She went on: 'I think everyone's young in here.' She went on, 'There's a little girl called Rosy – only looks about 14. I found out that Rosy had been here for 16 years and has a little boy of five. She's pregnant; her baby is due in May.' Miriam doesn't like Rosy to bathe her as she is frightened that Rosy may lose the baby and she would not want to be the cause of such a dreadful thing.

I ask if Miriam if she is happy. She tells me that she couldn't have asked for more . . . many of the staff have been here for years, although they do have to get in agency nurses from time to time. She said that she was very happy, it was a shame that her friend Connie wasn't so happy – but she wouldn't be happy with anything because she just doesn't want to be here . . . Miriam likes the place, it is very peaceful. She tells me: 'There are some poor souls downstairs who don't know what they are doing – it's awful for them – makes you realise how lucky you are.'

Activity

Read the above Case study again then answer the following questions:

- Do you think Miriam had good quality care?
- What factors do you think contributed to Miriam's quality of life in the home?
- What factors do you think need to be addressed in Miriam's care?
- What are your thoughts on Connie's quality of life?
- What factors do you think need to be addressed in Connie's care?

Now answer the questions below as honestly as you can. What are your hopes for your old age?

- Do you plan to end your days in a care home?
- Have you ever thought about this before?
- What are the reasons for your answers?
- List the positives and negatives about your perception of care home life that have prompted you to respond in this way.

When you have completed this exercise, ask a friend or relative the same questions and compare the answers given. Many people will not have considered living in a care home. In fact, only a small percentage of older people are admitted to care homes and yet this seems to be something many older people still fear. Look at the responses you and your colleague gave to the above questions and then answer the following:

- On what information about care homes have you based your answers? For example, have your opinions been shaped by the press, personal experience, written materials?
- How many of your perceptions do you think are real and how many may be unfounded?

IMPLICATIONS FOR JOINT WORKING

Several studies show that the input from doctors, multiprofessionals and specialist gerontological nurses to care homes is inadequate (O'Dea, *et al.*, 2000; Barodawala *et al.*, 2001; Glendinning *et al.*, 2002; Jacobs, 2003). A recent report from the Alzheimer's Society (2007) identified that 33 per cent of care home managers questioned reported major challenges in accessing external services such as mental health services.

The need for collaborative working across the various disciplines involved in providing care for older people was highlighted in a report by Meyer *et al.* (2006). All care home residents are entitled to the same primary care services as people in the community and are dependent on GP support, but this is not always equitable. In some cases, for example, retainers are paid to GPs, which would not be the case if the person lived within the same community outwith the home (Glendinning *et al.*, 2002). Access to specialist services and therapists is often curtailed (Goodman *et al.*, 2003, 2005). Care homes without in-house nursing support are dependent on primary health care professionals such as district nurses for their residents' health care needs. This input is rarely recognised and their role and the services they provide to older people in care homes are generally ad hoc (Goodman *et al.*, 2003).

Essence of Care (Department of Health, 2001b) developed from a commitment to look at the benefits of benchmarking with a view to improving quality of life. Davies and Goodman (2008) suggest that this may be one way of improving health care for residents, through building closer working practices between health and social care staff, enabling the identification of shared objectives and improving communication between their agencies. Health and social care providers have been historically uncomfortable with joint working (Hiscock and Pearson, 1999). They suggest that benchmarking, encouraging negotiation, review and shared planning between health and social care staff will improve partnership working and so improve the quality of health care support available to care home residents.

Interprofessional education has been suggested as a way forward in collaborative working. A Cochrane Review (Reeves *et al.*, 2008) stated that evidence collected so far does not allow a conclusion to be reached about the key elements of interprofessional education and its effectiveness or impact on professional practice and health care outcomes.

Meyer *et al.* (2006) conclude that research undertaken from the viewpoint of a single discipline, as it currently tends to be, does not further the cause of interdisciplinary working; they also highlight the need for collaboration with care home residents in order to ensure that their voice is heard.

CONCLUSION

So how can we improve the actual and perceived experience of care home life for the older people that we care for? Government policy and media representation both play a part in the negative perception, as do the actual experiences of poor care within some care homes.

It has been shown that a positive adaptation to care home life is more likely if the resident is prepared and involved in the choice of placement (Davies and Nolan, 2003).

Recurrent themes in the research are the fear of loss of autonomy and independence. Managing risk sensitively is essential to maintaining this. Although there are inevitably legislative constraints, it is usually possible to look at issues from the resident's perspective and, in collaboration with them and their families, arrive at a workable solution. A life without risk is not much of a life and it cannot be right to deny an element of risk-taking behaviour to someone, just because they are old or living in a care home. To do so is to deny them the chance of reaching their potential.

Further themes identified by care home residents as important included retaining a sense of self, the care environment, relationships, activities and boredom. These are all areas where provision of good quality person-centred care can make a real difference. The use of tools such as CARE might help to identify specific needs of residents with regard to any deficiencies in the quality of care offered to them.

Staff in care homes tend to have a more positive perception of the standard of care on offer than do residents or relatives. This suggests that the standard that we as professionals are striving for does not necessarily equate to the quality that is expected. Bear in mind that quality is that which is perceived by the 'customer' or resident. We might do well to think of residents as 'customers' whose opinions are central to shaping our service provision if we are to seek more positive outcomes.

Access to pain relief is a fundamental human right, but pain in older people within the community and within a care home setting remains under-addressed. Raising awareness of this problem is essential. When the problem is identified it is then possible to liaise with specialists such as, for example, palliative care teams or rheumatology specialists, in order to seek solutions. In addition to providing appropriate analgesia in traditional ways, the pain-relieving effects of specialist equipment and appliances should not be overlooked. Pain is whatever the patient says it is, but in the case of older people we must be further aware that a stoical generation may not be complaining enough and we may have to be proactive in helping them to become comfortable and pain free.

Instances of poor practice must be challenged; often it is difficult to challenge established practice, even if is known to be wrong. Edmund Burke (1729–97) is attributed with saying that, 'It is necessary only for the good man to do nothing for evil to triumph' (*Little Oxford Dictionary of Quotations*, 2008). The code of practice for social workers states that the social care worker must use, 'established processes and procedures to challenge and report dangerous, abusive, discriminatory or exploitative behaviour and practice' (General Social Care Council, 2004: 15). Similarly, the Nursing and Midwifery Council (NMC) states that clients are entitled to safe and competent care and specifically that 'You are personally accountable for your practice. This means that you are answerable for your actions and omissions, regardless of advice or directions from another professional' (Nursing and Midwifery Council, 2004: 4). Provision of good care is everyone's business.

Current good practice, from whatever discipline it comes, should be shared and built upon. Joint working, not only across professional divides, but essentially including residents in planning care and services, will enhance quality and provide the quality service that eventually will allay the fears that many older people currently have regarding care home life.

FURTHER READING

Agich, G. J. (2003) *Dependence and Autonomy in Old Age: An Ethical Framework for Long-term Care* (2nd edn). Cambridge: Cambridge University Press
This is a revised version of the previously published *Autonomy and Long-term Care* by the same author. Although the book is written from a North American perspective, it is relevant to care in the UK and does not offer a purely philosophical and abstract discussion, but looks at the practical and cultural issues surrounding ethical caring and the barriers to this.

Perrin, T. (ed.) (2004) *The New Culture of Therapeutic Activity with Older People*. Bicester: Speechmark
Tessa Perrin is an occupational therapist in the UK. In this interesting and perceptive book, she merges the boundaries of occupational and

recreational therapy to describe a new culture, where activity is recognised as essential to wellbeing. This book is very readable and contains illustrative examples of real scenarios.

Schofield, P. (ed.) (2007) *The Management of Pain in Older People*. Chichester: John Wiley
Patricia Schofield edits this useful resource that looks not only at the anatomy and physiology of pain but the attitudes, perceptions and socioeconomic issues surrounding pain and older people. Also discussed is communication, pain assessment, interventions and specifically how pain is understood and managed within the care home setting.

Walker, A. (ed.) (2005) *Understanding Quality of Life in Old Age*. Maidenhead: Open University Press/McGraw-Hill
This book looks at the findings of the ESRC Growing Older (GO) Programme, referred to within this chapter, and considers what quality of life means to older people, how it can be measured and how it is affected by social policy.

Useful websites

http://new.wales.gov.uk/cssiwsubsite/cssiw/?lang=en
Care and Social Services Inspectorate Wales (CSSIW)

www.csci.org.uk
Commission for Social Care Inspection (CSCI)

www.alzheimers.co.uk
Home from Home

www.myhomelife.org.uk/Resources.htm
My Home Life Report

www.carecommission.com/index.php?option=com_content&task=view&id=16&Itemid=112
Scottish Commission for the Regulation of Care

REFERENCES

Age Concern and the Mental Health Foundation (2006) *Promoting Mental Health and Well-being in Later Life: A First Report from the UK Inquiry into Mental Health and Well-Being in Later Life*. London: Age Concern
Age Concern Scotland and Highland NHS Board (2001) *The Case for Promoting Physical Activity Among Frail and Older People*. Edinburgh: Age Concern
Allcock, N., McGarry, J. and Elkan, R. (2002) 'Management of pain in older people in the nursing home: a preliminary study'. *Health and Social Care in the Community*, 10: (6) 464–71

Alzheimer's Society (2007) *Home from Home: A Report Highlighting Opportunities for Improving Standards of Dementia Care in Care Homes.* **www.alzheimers.org.uk/downloads/home_from_home_full_report_2_.pdf** (Accessed 25 January 2008)

Audit Commission (1986) *Making a Reality of Community Care.* London: HMSO.

Audit Commission and Better Government for Older People (2004) *Older People – Independence and Well-being: The Challenge for Public Services.* London: Audit Commission

Baltes, P. and Baltes, M. (eds) (1990) *Successful Aging: Perspectives from the Behavioral Sciences.* Cambridge: Cambridge University Press

Barodawala, S., Kesavan, S. and Young. K. (2001) 'A survey of physiotherapy and occupational therapy provision in UK nursing homes'. *Clinical Rehabilitation,* 15: 607–10

Bergland, A. and Kirkevold, M. (2006) 'Thriving in nursing homes in Norway: contributing aspects described by residents'. *International Journal of Nursing Studies,* 43 (6): 681–91. **http://find.galegroup.com/itx/printdoc. do?contentSet=IAC-Documents&docType=IA** (Accessed 23 January 2008)

Better Regulation Task Force (2004) *Bridging the Gap – Participation in Social Care Regulation.* **http://archive.cabinetoffice.gov.uk/brc/upload/assets/ www.brc.gov.uk/bridgegap.doc** (Accessed 8 February 2008)

Boaz, A., Hayden, C and Bernard, M. (1999) *Attitudes and Aspirations of Older People: A Review of the Literature.* (DSS Research Report No. 101) Leeds: CDS

Cairncross, L., Magee, H. and Askham, J. (2007) *A Hidden Problem – Pain in Older People: A Qualitative Study.* London: Pickers Institute Europe

Challis, L. and Bartlett, H. (1988) *Old and Ill: Private Nursing Homes for Elderly People.* London: ACE Books

Chenitz, W. (1983). 'Entry to a nursing home as a status passage: A theory to guide nursing practice'. *Geriatric Nursing,* March/April, 92–7

Commission for Social Care Inspection (2007) *Rights, Risks and Restraints: An Exploration into the use of Restraint in the Care of Older People.* **www.csci. org.uk/PDF/restraint.pdf** (Accessed 06 May 2008)

Commission for Social Care Inspection (2008) *Quality Ratings for Care Services: Ratings Rules Available.* **www.csci.org.uk/professional/care_providers/all_ services/inspection/ratings_and_reports/quality_ratings_for_care_servi/ ratings_rules.aspx** (Accessed 25 March 2008)

Davies, N. and Nolan, M. (2003) 'Making the best of things: relatives' experiences of decisions about care home entry'. *Ageing & Society,* 23: 429–50

Davies, S. and Goodman, C. (2008) 'Supporting quality improvement in care homes for older people: the contribution of primary care nurses'. *Journal of Nursing Management,* 16 (2): 115–20

Department of Health (1989). *Working for Patients.* London: HMSO

Department of Health (1990). *Community Care in the Next Decade and Beyond: Policy Guidance.* London: HMSO

Department of Health (2001a) *National Service Framework for Older People.* London: HMSO

Department of Health (2001b) *Essence of Care. Patient-focused Benchmarking for Health Care Practitioners.* London: The Stationery Office

Department of Health (2004) *Better Health in Old Age.* London: Department of Health. **www.dh.gov.uk/en/Publicationsandstatistics/Publications/ PublicationsPolicyAnd Guidance/DH_4092957** (Accessed 22 January 2008)

Donaghy, M. (2007) 'Exercise can seriously improve your mental health: Fact or Fiction?'. *Advances in Physiotherapy,* 9 (2): 76–89

Economic and Social Research Council (2003) *Growing Older Programme – Project Summaries.* Swindon: ESRC. **www.imsersomayores.csic.es/ documentos/documentos/progsummaries-growingolder-01.pdf** (Accessed 6 May 2008)

Falaschetti, E., Malbut, K. and Primatesta, P. (2002) *Health Survey for England 2000: The General Health of Older People and their use of Health Services.* London: The Stationery Office

Faulkner, M., Davies, S., Nolan, M. and Brown-Wilson, C. (2006) 'Development of the combined assessment of residential environments (CARE) profiles'. *Journal of Advanced Nursing,* 55 (6): 664–77

General Social Care Council (2004) *Code of Practice for Social Care Workers and Code of Practice for Employers of Social Care Workers.* London: GSSC

Glasby, J. and Glasby, J. (1999) *Paying for Social Services: Social Services and Local Government Finance.* Birmingham: PEPAR Publications

Glendinning, C., Jacobs, S., Alborz, A. and Hann, M. (2002) 'A survey of access to medical services in nursing and residential homes in England'. *British Journal of General Practice,* 52: 545–8

Goodman, C., Woolley, R. and Knight, D. (2003) 'District nurses' experiences of providing care in residential care home settings'. *Journal of Clinical Nursing,* 12: 67–76

Goodman, C., Robb, N., Drennan, V. and Woolley, R. (2005) 'Partnership working by default, district nurses and care home staff providing care for older people'. *Health Social Care Community,* 13 (6): 553–62

Griffiths, R. (1988) *Community Care: An Agenda for Action.* London: HMSO

Grundy, E., Tomassini, C. and Festy, P. (2006) 'Demographic Change and the Care of Older People: Introduction'. *European Journal of Population,* 22: 215–18

Help the Aged (2007) *My Home Life: Quality of Life in Care Homes: A Review of the Literature.* **www.helptheaged.org.uk/NR/rdonlyres/26BF7E76- F7AB-41DF-AD99-9BF59AB78ECD/0/wd_myhomelife_lit_020307.pdf** (Accessed 16 February 2008)

Hiscock, J. and Pearson, M. (1999) 'Looking inwards, looking outwards: Dismantling the Berlin Wall between health and social services'. *Social Policy and Administration,* 33: 150–63

House of Commons (2007) *Human Rights Act 1998 (Meaning of Public Authority) Bill* (43). London: TSO. **www.publications.parliament.uk/pa/ cm200607/cmbills/043/2007043.pdf** (Accessed 14 March 2008)

Jacobs, S. (2003) 'Addressing the problems associated with general practitioners' workload in nursing and residential homes: findings from a qualitative study'. *British Journal of General Practice,* 53: 113–19

Joint Committee on Human Rights Enquiry (2007) *Eighteenth Report*. **www. publications.parliament.uk/pa/jt200607/jtselect/jtrights/156/15602.htm** (Accessed 13 March 2008)

Juran, J.M. and Gryna, F. (eds) (1988) *Juran's Quality Control Handbook* (4th edn). New York: McGraw-Hill

Kydd, A. (2006) *Life in Limbo: A Study of Delayed Discharge from a Patient and Policy Perspective*. Aberdeen: Aberdeen University Press

Lee, D., Woo, J. and MacKenzie, A. (2002) 'A review of older people's experiences with residential care placement'. *Journal of Advanced Nursing*, 37: 19–27

Little Oxford Dictionary of Quotations (2008). **www.askoxford.com/results/?view=quot&freesearch=edmund+burke&branch=14123648&textsearchtype=exact** (Accessed 16 May 2008)

Malin, N., Manthorpe, J., Race, D. and Wilmot, S. (1999) *Community Care for Nurses and the Caring Professions*. Buckingham: Open University Press

McCormack, B. (2001) *Negotiating Partnerships with Older People: A Person-Centred Approach*. Aldershot: Ashgate

Means, R. and Smith, R. (1998) *Community Care: Policy and Practice*. Basingstoke: Macmillan

Meyer, J., Heath, H., Holman, C. and Owen, T. (2006) 'Moving from victim blaming to an appreciative inquiry: Exploring quality of life in care homes'. *Quality in Ageing, Policy, Practice and Research*, 7 (4): 27–36

Milke, D.L., Beck, C.H.M. and Danes, S. (2006) 'Meeting the needs in Continuing Care of Facility-Based Residents Diagnosed with Dementia: Comparison of Ratings by Families, Direct Care Staff and Other Staff'. *Journal of Applied Gerontology*, 25: 103–119

Murphy, K. (2006) 'Nurses' perceptions of quality and the factors that affect quality care for older people living in long-term settings in Ireland'. *Journal of Clinical Nursing*, 16: 873–84

National Care Forum (2008) *Survey to Examine Attitudes to Life in Care for Older People*. **www.nationalcareforum.org.uk/forums/forum_posts.asp?TID=2061&PN=1** (Accessed 15 January 2008)

NHS and Community Care Act (1990) Office of Public Sector Information. **www.opsi.gov.uk/ACTS/acts1990/ukpga_19900019_en_1** (Accessed 6 May 2008)

Nolan, M., Walker, G., Nolan, J., Williams, S., Poland, F., Curran, N. *et al.* (1996) 'Entry to care: Positive choice or fait accompli?'. *Journal of Advanced Nursing*, 24: 265–74

Nursing and Midwifery Council (2004) *The NMC Code of Professional Conduct: standards for conduct, performance and ethics*. London: NMC

O'Dea, G., Kerrison, S.H. and Pollack, A.M. (2000) 'Access to health care in nursing homes: a survey in one English Health Authority'. *Health and Social Care in the Community*, 8 (3): 180–5

Office for National Statistics (2003) *People Aged 65 and over: Results of a Study Carried Out on Behalf of the Department of Health as Part of the 2001 General Household Survey*. London: TSO

Randers, I., Olson, T.H. and Mattiasson, A.C. (2002) 'Confirming older adults' views of who they would like to be'. *Nursing Ethics*, 9: 4

Raynes, N., Temple, B., Glenister, C. and Coulthard, L. (2001) *Quality at Home for Older People: Involving Service Users in Defining Home Care Specifications*. York: Joseph Rowntree Foundation/The Policy Press

Reeves, S., Zwarenstein, M., Goldman, J., Barr, H., Freeth, D., Hammick, M. and Koppel, I. (2008) 'Interprofessional education: effects on professional practice and health care outcomes'. *Cochrane Database of Systematic Reviews 2008*, Issue 1. Article No.: CD002213

Regulation of Care (Scotland) Act 2001 Statutory Instruments, Office of Public Service Information. **www.scotland-legislation.hmso.gov.uk/legislation/scotland/s-200201.htm** (Accessed 6 May 2008)

Report of the Joint Future Group (2000) *Scottish Executive Publications: Report of the Joint Future Group*. **www.scotland.gov.uk/library3/social/rjfg-00.asp** (Accessed 13 March 2008)

Sackley, C., Levin, S., Cardoso, K. and Hoppitt, T. (2006) 'Obervations of activity levels and social interaction in a residential care setting', *International Journal of Therapy and Rehabilitation*, 13 (8): 370–3

Scottish Commission for the Regulation of Care (2007) *Grading is Coming – 1 April 2008! What You Need to Know*. Dundee: SCRC Communication

Scottish Executive (1998) *Modernising Community Care – An Action Plan*. Edinburgh: Scottish Executive

Severance, J. S. (2005) *Divergent Perceptions of Nursing Home Care as a Barrier to Organizational Change*, Paper presented at the annual meeting of the American Sociological Association, Marriott Hotel, Loews Philadelphia Hotel, Philadelphia, PA. **www.allacademic.com/meta/p21455_index.html** (Accessed 23 January 2008)

Suber, P. (1992) *Self-Determination and Selfhood in Recent Legal Cases*. First delivered as the 1992 Emerson Lecture at Earlham College. **www.earlham.edu/~peters/writing/emerson.htm** (Accessed 25 January 2005)

Tester, S., Hubbard, G., Downs, M., McDonald, C. and Murphy, J. (2003) *Exploring Perceptions of Quality of Life of Frail Older People During and After Their Transition to Institutional Care*. Sheffield: ESRC Growing Older Research Programme, Department of Sociological Studies, University of Sheffield

The Commission for Social Care Inspection (2006) *Inspecting for Better Lives: A Quality Future*. **www.carestandards.org.uk/pdf/quality_ratings_tagged_v2.pdf** (Accessed 25 January 2008)

Townsend, P. (1964) *The Last Refuge: A Survey of Residential Institutions and Homes for the Aged in England and Wales*. Abingdon: Routlege and Kegan Paul.

United Nations (2002) *World Population Ageing, 1950–2050*. New York: United Nations

Victor, C. (1997) *Community Care and Older People*. Cheltenham: Stanley Thornes

Welsh Assembly Government (2002) *Intermediate Care Guidance*. WHC (2002) 108/NAWF 43/02. Cardiff: WAG

Chapter 20

Social Networks and Older People

Catherine Rae

Learning outcomes

Reading this chapter will enable you to:

- gain an understanding of the importance of social networking for older people;

- gain an understanding of what social isolation means for older people;

- gain an understanding of what can be done to combat social isolation and increase the social networks of older people in your care.

DEFINITIONS

Social networks

A **social network** can best be described as the circle of people you know through your family, interests, work or where you live. They are not necessarily all 'good friends' but can simply include people with whom you have contact. The reason(s) you have a relationship with them and the function of that relationship will be varied. It is well documented that our social networks not only change throughout our life but, as we grow older, they reduce in size due to retirement from work, death of a spouse, siblings and friends and failing or ill-health. Of course some of these situations such as retirement and ill-health will be the beginning of a new social network (Wenger, 1995). Typically, an individual's social network will consist of between 16 and 50 people, while the social network of an older person will consist of between five and seven people (Wenger, 1995). Heath and Schofield (1999) suggest 'that being embedded in a social network is vital for general wellbeing, and that involvement in a social network appears to play a critical role in enabling frail older people to remain in their own home' (p. 373–4).

Social inclusion

Social inclusion is when someone can access and benefit from the full range of opportunities available to members of society and older people often identify social inclusion as an important factor in their quality of life and independence (Wenger, 1995; Heath and Schofield, 1999). Although older people living alone are most at risk of becoming socially isolated, those who live in residential facilities are also at risk, especially if the opportunity to participate in activities outside the facility are few or non-existent (Squire, 2002). This can be overcome by encouraging links with local community centres, schools, churches and volunteer groups (Copel, 1998). A person-centred approach when planning activities should ensure older people feel valued members of their community. Most people would like good relationships with family, friends and work colleagues, to feel useful and have a role, as well as being treated with respect. To be given the opportunity to participate and make a positive contribution in their community are essential for autonomy and dignity (Heath and Schofield, 1999).

Social exclusion

Social exclusion occurs when certain groups of people are pushed to the margins of society and prevented from playing a full and active part in normal activities because of poverty, low education levels or inadequate life skills. This makes it difficult for them to access jobs, income and education opportunities, or to play a normal role in society and community networks. It means they have little access to power, little chance of influencing decisions or policies that affect them and little chance of bettering their standard of living (Combat Poverty Agency, 2004). A growing problem among older people is that of loneliness (Copel, 1998). It is a major contributory factor to many of the problems faced by older people in society (Lewis *et al.*, 1994). It can cause apathy and lack of interest and lead to problems such as malnutrition, hypothermia, depression and general self-neglect. The Scottish Government website reports: 'Of all suicides, 25 per cent happen in older people, although they account for only 15 per cent of the population. Ninety per cent of such cases had serious depression and had visited their doctor in the three months before they died. Even among frail and very old people trials show positive results for people who become more active' (**www. scotland.gov.uk**). In recent years there has been increased interest in the role social networks and support play in helping us cope with the stresses of life. However, as Heath and Schofield (1999) point out, it is imperative that we do not equate living alone or being alone with feeling lonely.

A REVIEW OF THE LITERATURE

Social inclusion features prominently in current government policy. The White Paper *Our Health, Our Care, Our Say* (Department of Health, 2006) sets out a vision to provide people with good quality social care and NHS services in the communities where they live. It acknowledges social exclusion, isolation and loneliness as significant contributory factors in the incidence of mental illness, particularly depression. The report emphasises the need for a universal approach to inclusion from services such as transport, health and housing.

In Scotland, *Better Outcomes for Older People: Framework for Joint Services* (Scottish Executive, 2005) promotes the development and mainstreaming of joint and integrated services, as part of the *Joint Future* drive for better outcomes for individuals and their carers. It also sets out requirements that the local partnerships of NHS Boards and local authorities should meet in developing and delivering joint and integrated services. The framework is a tool for developing joint and integrated services that assist older people to lead more independent lives and have more personal control over their lifestyles, care and environment (Scottish Executive, 2005).

Reaching Out: An Action Plan on Social Inclusion (Cabinet Office Social Exclusion Task Force, 2006) sets out the government's renewed approach to tackling the problem of social exclusion. It offers a series of opportunities for disadvantaged people that, if successful, will ease the lifelong effects of social exclusion and prevent them being passed down to future generations (Cabinet Office Social Exclusion Task Force, 2006).

A web only report entitled *Effective Social Work with Older People* (Kerr *et al.*, 2005) was commissioned by the Twenty-first Century Social Work Review Group to inform their work and includes a section on social isolation and older people. It reviews the evidence base for effective social work with older people. The aim was to explore 'what works' in terms of effective practice by qualified social workers and what leads to quality outcomes for older people and their carers.

Partnerships for Older People Projects [POPPs] (Care Services Improvement Partnership, 2006) is an initiative being led by the Department of Health. It is a project that aims to test and evaluate innovative approaches that sustain preventative approaches to care in order to improve the lives of older people, giving them greater personal control over their physical and emotional health, and helping them to remain independent wherever possible.

Living alone can equate to freedom and independence but, with increasing age, can be a risk factor for isolation. The benefits of promoting independent living for older people are enormous for individuals, public services and wider society. Extending years of active life will allow older people to play a full role in family life and in their local communities. *Home Alone: Combating Isolation with Older Housebound People* (McCarthy and Thomas, 2004) argues that users need to become 'co-producers' of personalised services.

Risk factors that can contribute to the social isolation of older people with a learning disability (as well as older people in general) can include poverty, bereavement, poor health, loss of work and age discrimination as well as other forms of discrimination. The Department of Health has established the Dignity Challenge as part of its *Dignity in Care* campaign. The challenge lays out what constitutes a service that respects dignity focussing on ten different aspects of dignity, including social isolation. In England, the practice guide, *Dignity in Care*, issued by the Social Care Institute for Excellence (SCIE, 2007), identifies factors that can cause social isolation and gives practical guidance to support service providers and practitioners in developing best practice.

A Sure Start to Later Life: Ending Inequalities for Older People (Cabinet Office, 2006) is a policy document from the Social Exclusion Unit that sets out a cross-government action plan to increase the quality of life for older people and ensure they are valued in families, the workplace and communities (Cabinet Office, 2006).

SOCIAL SUPPORT

In a study by Fisher *et al.* (2002) **social support** was generally agreed to be one of the most important components for older people when discussing quality of life. He also reported that, for many older people, practical and emotional support was most often provided by family and friends, although voluntary organisations did play a vital role in providing support in terms of information and advice. Older people who have a spouse, friends and family members who give psychological, emotional and material support tend to be healthier than those who do not have these relationships. Some studies report that having contact with a social network and social support is associated with longevity (Del Bono *et al.*, 2007). The influential work in this area was that of Berkman and Syme (1979) who carried out a large study in California and found that the mortality rates of people who had few social networks or contacts were two- to four-and-a-half times higher than those with strong social networks. The support we receive from our social networks can have a profound effect on the way we react and recuperate from illness and disease (Helgeson *et al.*, 1999, 2001). Social support has also been associated with improved recovery from serious illnesses such as cardiovascular disease and stroke (André-Peterson *et al.*, 2006). Support given through social attachments with family and friends has been shown to have a direct affect on us physically and psychologically as well as acting as a defence mechanism that helps us to control the damaging effects stress can have on our health and wellbeing. Peterson (2000) suggests this can be encouraged in a number of ways:

- By helping the older person and their families to identify strengths and weaknesses in their relationships. If relationships are difficult attempts should be made to promote effective communication and improve coping mechanisms within the older person's social network.
- By encouraging and assisting the person to value and maintain relationships with their friends as well as the relationships they have with their family.
- By encouraging the setting up of new relationships in all situations where older people are being cared for.
- By encouraging older people to use appropriate services, local support and self-help groups for any health problems they may be experiencing. In our techno-society there are many support groups available via the World Wide Web, which many older people could have access to either at home or with help via a local library or internet café. By seeking help themselves and interacting with others experiencing similar situations their social network and therefore possible sources of support will increase.
- Health care workers should compile a list of resources to which they can refer if they feel an older person is at risk of social isolation or in need of additional social support. People who would be in the at risk group would be those with little or no support from family, those with an illness which could lead to dysfunctional social interaction

such as those with dementia and/or learning disabilities or those who have depression.

- By using the existing professional support systems that have specific skills. This may range from professional counselling to home help services depending on the health care needs of the older person.
- By encouraging give and take within existing support relationships which will give recognition to the person's abilities and improve their self-esteem and sense of belonging.

Evaluation

The evaluation of social support can be determined by how the person feels they have been supported and the extent to which the support can be returned. There are a number of instruments available to evaluate social support such as the following three instruments designed by nurse researchers, which have been psychometrically tested for validity and reliability in social support measurement (Stewart and Tilden, 1995).

- The Norbeck Social Support Questionnaire [NSSQ] (Norbeck *et al.*, 1981) is widely used to measure perceived availability of types (affect, affirmation, and aid) and sources (network members) of social support.
- The Personal Resource Questionnaire (PRQ), which was developed to measure intimacy, social integration, nurturance, worth and assistance (Brandt and Weinert, 1981). This is a 25-item scale assessing perceived social support. All items are rated on a five-point Likert scale. Scaling for items ranges from 1 – 'strongly disagree' to 5 – 'strongly agree'.
- The Tilden Interpersonal Relationship Inventory (IPRI), which is derived from the social exchange theory and includes costs and benefits of supportive relationships (Tilden *et al.*, 1990), was developed in response to gaps in measurement of social relationships and contributed scales for reciprocity and conflict to a measure of social support (Tilden *et al.*, 1990).

Relationships

The social networks and relationships of older people over the course of their life will include family, friends, neighbours and co-workers who can potentially offer support over time. The membership of someone's social network is fluid and constantly changing as events such as the birth of a child, divorce or death of a spouse, the loss of work colleagues through retirement or the addition of new relationships will have a bearing on their lives. During significant life changes such as retirement, network members such as spouses, children and grandchildren can be strong sources of support. However, significant life changes can alter the relationship dynamics between the members of the older person's social network (Victor, 1989). The impact of a significant life event extends beyond the older person, and relationships and family dynamics will vary considerably and can be affected by other factors such as socioeconomic status, race and ethnicity. While relationships with friends, neighbours and former work colleagues are important to older people, the basis for most social support will be the family. Family as a social institution and network has a lifelong hold and influence on all of us (Victor, 1989, 1991).

For many older people the most supportive relationship and the major source of support will be the relationship the person has with his/her spouse. However, as we age, the probability of having the support of our spouse diminishes because of illness or death. This is arguably the most difficult life event older people will have to deal with. Earlier plans that were made for life together may have to be modified or even abandoned. The issues created by these difficulties can lead to an increased likelihood of depression and a potentially devastating reduction in social support. In Britain in 1990 it was estimated that the suicide rate for those aged 65 and older was 50 per cent higher than that in the population as a whole, with men being more vulnerable. According to Banerjee and MacDonald (1996) and Victor (1991), depression is the most common major mental health problem in older people yet very few older people will have active treatment compared to other age groups.

Retirement offers the opportunity to spend more time with children and grandchildren. It also provides an opportunity for the older person to feel useful. Many older people who enjoy relatively good health are able to offer support to their children in terms of childcare and financial help as well as emotional support with child-rearing, work and family issues. Because of the longevity of people and the opportunity to retire at a relatively young age most people with children will experience being a grandparent as well as being retired. What most grandparents want is companionship with their grandchildren and the opportunity to get to know them in a way they could not with their own children because of the constraints and obligations of parenthood. The strong desire to live near children and grandchildren can result in some older people living in their pre-retirement community rather than moving to a new location that may be more suited to their needs. The reverse may also be true where some older people could move many miles to live closer to their children and grandchildren, which could have a considerable impact on social networks (Banerjee and MacDonald, 1996; Victor, 1991).

Older people, once they have retired, may have the opportunity to have more contact with siblings and extended family members. These relationships can be very important due to shared experiences of same or similar life events within a similar time frame. They also have a long history of shared memories and understanding. When an older person has lost their spouse or when there are no children or grandchildren, siblings can be a vital source of support for an older person.

Activity 1

To illustrate the diversity and value we place on social networks, use the diagram below (see Figure 1) to represent your own social network. You may need to add more layers/circles. Place yourself in the centre layer/circle. In the next layer place those closest to you, the third next closest and so on.

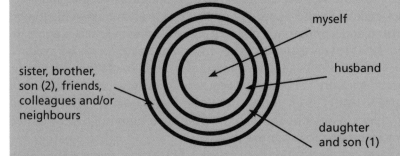

Figure 1 Personal social network

Compare this with the social network of an older person in your care or a grandparent.
1. What are the differences?
2. What are the similarities?
3. How could you increase the social network of the older person?

Discussion points based on above questions.
1. The people closest to you will probably be family, spouse, children and siblings. For the older person it could be a paid carer. How might this impact on the older person?
2. Even if the older person has children, they may, for example, live far away, therefore, they would be in an outer circle.
3. Networks could be developed through community resources, volunteer programmes or social activities.

IMPLICATIONS FOR JOINT WORKING

Policy makers must learn from voluntary and community sectors to help older people develop networks of social support. It is possible for health care workers to assist in increasing the size of an older person's social network, improve its structure and reinforce existing relationships. They can also strengthen links between the formal primary care system and informal lay care social systems which, in return, will impact on the older person's sources of social support. The encouragement of the use of self-help, neighbourhood and community groups, volunteers and community resources may improve social life as well as delivering important health messages to older people. It is important to point out that close friendships cannot be forced and attempts to put older people into situations where they are expected to establish friendships could result in embarrassment, depression, withdrawal and isolation. However, there are many opportunities for making use of existing social networks, especially if they are relevant to current concerns and interests and promote social roles that older people see as being meaningful and useful. Greater attention should be given by health care workers to strengthen existing relationships before attempting to create new ones (Wenger, 1995).

Since the 1970s, the ways social support and social networks impact on the lives of older people has been of considerable interest in all areas of society, not just nursing and health care. In order for a health professional to encourage the development of social support and improve an older person's social network, it is necessary to establish what is already in place. The requirement for social support and how satisfied that person is with the support will change over their life course depending on the different stresses put upon them and how the person copes with these stressors. Therefore, assessment of support must focus on the person's existing support, the timing and duration of that support, an awareness of the types of support available, evaluation of the cost and/or benefits of the support and the older person's perceived satisfaction with the support. Assessing social support accurately is not a straightforward task and can involve consultation with a number of significant others before achieving a complete picture (Heath and Schofield, 1999).

To demonstrate how varied and complex social networking can be, read the following Case study and answer the questions which follow it.

Case study

Ella is 63-years-old, living with her parents who are in their 80s, in a small village five miles from the nearest large town. Ella has Down's syndrome. Her mum had a stroke three years ago and now requires a walking stick to aid her mobility. Her dad is hard of hearing and uses a hearing aid and, because of a heart condition, is unable to lift heavy objects. Ella has a younger brother who has moved out the family home and lives over 500 miles away.

Ella has recently been diagnosed with dementia. Prompted by Ella's deterioration in behaviour, it took over 12 months with input from psychology, community nursing (learning disability) and social work for a diagnosis of dementia to be given.

Ella's support includes two days per week at a resource centre (she is collected and returned to her home by car) and 12 hours per week from a community service provider for respite for her parents. She also receives personal care for one hour each morning, seven days per week. Following the diagnosis of dementia, respite services were increased to 22 hours per week. She also has a two-day block every four months of residential respite. Due to her high level of disability she has a car (driven by support workers) through a mobility scheme.

There is now discussion taking place for Ella to be considered for residential placement due to her parents' failing health. Ella has a disturbed sleep pattern, erratic behaviour such as hitting out or sitting down in public places and refusing to move. She also requires someone to feed her. She has recently been put on a soft diet due to a choking risk identified by the speech and language therapist. Ella's mobility is very poor and she is at present being assessed for a wheel chair by a physiotherapist.

Despite her brother being interested, concerned and supportive, he lives too far away to be of any physical help to her parents, although they do value the emotional support he is able to give. Ella's parents have cared for her for 63 years and had intended to continue this care until she died, which at the time of her birth was estimated to be no longer than her late teens or early twenties. However, advances in modern medicine, technology, antibiotics and surgical techniques have increased her life expectancy. Because of their own failing health they are now faced with placing Ella into residential care. The implications of Ella being in residential care will have a devastating effect on both her and her parents.

For Ella, she will be taken from the social network of her family and, although this will be replaced by the social networks gained from staff, other residents, visitors and professionals connected with her care home, she will lose her existing social networks with all the support services she has received all her adult life. For someone who has dementia, it is beneficial to retain everything that is familiar around them. But, for Ella, at this particularly difficult time of her life, everyone who is familiar to her will no longer be part of her care.

For Ella's parents, their social networks have consisted mainly of the professionals attending to Ella's needs. With Ella being placed into residential care they will lose the social networks that were built around them. Because of their failing health and mobility it will be incumbent upon the social and medical personnel they have contact with concerning their own health needs to encourage and develop new networks to replace the support they have lost. In addition to the loss of social support they will also lose the use of Ella's car, which will impact greatly on their ability to venture far from their home and may restrict the frequency of their visits to Ella.

Activity 2

- Look at who is in Ella's and her parents' support networks.
- How are Ella and her parents socially excluded?
- In your opinion what ought to happen?
- How can Ella be supported?
- How can her parents be supported and encouraged to develop a larger social network?
- Who should be responsible for this – health and social care workers, family, friends, others?

HEALTH PROMOTION AND OLDER PEOPLE

Health care professionals should aim to ensure the social support needs of the older person are met and should encourage more social networking. An area of social support that is both useful to the professional and beneficial to the older person (as it encourages social networking) is that of health promotion. These social networks can help in learning new skills and behaviour and help people change unhealthy habits and promote healthier, more positive lifestyles. We have seen a number of health promotions in recent years, such as smoking cessation and healthy eating campaigns, which target social support or peer influence to alter habits considered to be detrimental to our health (Scottish Government Health Promotions, 2008). Many of the programmes implemented by health care workers rely on giving facts about health problems but it is rare to include social support in relation to this aspect of care. Examples of health promotion initiatives are listed below However, a more comprehensive list with links to useful sites can be found on **www.healthscotland.com** or **www.nhs.uk**

Smoking control

Smoking control is arguably the most crucial single preventative measure that someone can take, not only in relation to cardiovascular disease, but also for chronic respiratory disorder, cancer and osteoporosis. Attempting to reduce smoking among their clients is a daunting challenge for all primary health care workers. Success depends on convincing the individual of the benefits of not smoking, therefore creating strong incentives to stop the habit. It is necessary to identify the barriers to individuals giving up smoking, therefore making giving up easier, and to provide encouragement to persevere until the outcome is achieved (Heath and Schofield, 1999).

Diet and nutrition

Individuals usually require to be convinced of the benefits of healthy eating and the part diet and nutrition can play in the prevention of illness. Very low fat diets can bring down cholesterol levels, but this depends on how strictly the diet is maintained (Heath and Schofield, 1999). A report by Huffman (2002) suggests older people with unintentional weight loss are at higher risk of infection and depression and a specific cause is not identified in approximately one quarter of older people with unintentional weight loss.

Obesity

Most people are aware that obese individuals of any age are at high risk of mortality from cardiovascular disease and stroke. It is therefore important to identify those with a body mass index of 30 or more. These individuals can then be given appropriate information, dietary advice and supportive help, as requested (Heath and Schofield, 1999).

Blood pressure

The most effective ways of reducing blood pressure in older people appear to be:

- increasing levels of physical activity;
- taking fish oil supplements;
- reducing salt intake, alcohol consumption and smoking;
- increasing potassium intakes.

Heath and Schofield suggest there is strong evidence to support medical treatment of even mild degrees of hypertension up to 85 years, with a 25–33 per cent reduction in cardiovascular risk (Heath and Schofield, 1999).

Alcohol intake

Traditionally, health education on alcohol consumption has not been directed at older people. However, drinking behaviour should be identified and specific guidance given as required (Heath and Schofield, 1999).

Outdoor activities

There is growing interest among health and social care professionals in the social and therapeutic value of outdoor activities and, in particular, in horticulture to develop confidence as well as increase social networks. *Health, Well-being and Social Inclusion: Therapeutic Horticulture in the UK* (Sempik *et al.*, 2005a), highlights the value of horticulture and gardening for vulnerable groups, including older people, those with a learning disability and those with mental health problems. Sempik *et al.*, (2005b) have published a practical guide on how horticulture and gardening can help to promote social inclusion. The guide looks at ways in which social and therapeutic horticulture projects can help foster independence, build self-esteem and confidence and provide training and employment opportunities for people with health or social problems.

CONCLUSION

The importance of social support networks for older people cannot be overestimated. Experts agree that well-connected, user-friendly local services such as community transport, impartial advice, befriending and shopping schemes as well as older people's activity services can transform the lives of older people. Services such as these can help older people to maintain a good quality of life. The government believes that these types of services can offer a solution to tackling older people's exclusion from their community.

Involving older people at all levels of service planning and delivery is a key factor in social inclusion. Taking part will in itself provide meaningful activity and a role in the community for the service user. Inclusion of older people from minority communities will enable them to contribute their own knowledge, skills and experience and ensure their needs will not be overlooked. It is important for local authorities to ensure support is available to enable the development of skills and confidence to smooth the way for active participation.

Social exclusion means not being able to access the things in life that most of society takes for granted. It's not just about having enough money. It is a build-up of problems across several areas of people's lives. Focussing on social inclusion means emphasising things like access to services, good social networks, decent housing, adequate information and support, and the ability to exercise basic rights.

Despite all the relevant literature and media focus on older people being lonely, infirm and requiring the intervention of health care workers to assist in developing social networks, care should be exercised as many older people continue to enjoy a high quality of life, unimpaired by disability and would reject attempts to influence their choices.

Growing older is not always easy and the infirmities of ageing can be very limiting for some people, but it is important to remember that physical or mental limitation does not necessarily mean a limited life. It has been well documented that the number of older people in our population is rising and will continue to rise. This increase in older people will have a significant impact on our health care system and, arguably, on nurses most of all. Nurse leaders are in a position to help shape a health care system which will benefit older people.

FURTHER READING

Heath, H. and Schofield, I. (1999) *Healthy Ageing: Nursing Older People*. Oxford: Elsevier/Mosby
This book brings together gerontology and nursing to provide a comprehensive and valuable resource for professionals working with older people in a broad range of settings. This book is a significant contribution to the need to understand more about ageing and later life. It deals with many aspects rarely found in other nursing journals.

McCarthy, H. and Thomas, G. (2004) *Home Alone: Combating Isolation with Older Housebound People*. London: Demos
This book argues that users need to become 'co-producers' of personalised services and that policy makers must learn from the voluntary and community sectors to help older housebound people develop their own networks of support. This book can be downloaded through the link below.
http://books.google.com/books?id=BtgZA9sAJogC&printsec=frontcover &dq=Home+alone:+combating+isolation+with+older+housebound+peo ple#PPA2,M1 (Accessed 2 October 2008)

Sempik, J., Aldridge, J. and Becker, S. (2005a) *Health, Well-being and Social Inclusion: Therapeutic Horticulture in the UK*. Bristol: The Policy Press
This book analyses the processes involved in promoting and achieving health and well-being outcomes using gardening, horticulture and related activities.

Useful websites

www.scotland.gov.uk
Scottish Government

www.helptheaged.co.uk
Help the Aged

www.dementia.stir.ac.uk
Dementia Services Development Centre (DSDC)

www.scie.org.uk
Social Care Institute for Excellence

REFERENCES

André-Peterson, L., Engstrom, G., Hedblad, B., Janzon, L. and Rosvall, M. (2006) 'Social support at work and the risk of myocardial infarction and stroke in women and men'. *Social Science and Medicine*, 4: 830–41

Banerjee, S. and MacDonald, A. (1996) 'Mental disorder in an elderly home care population: associations with health and social service use'. *British Journal of Psychiatry*, 168: 750–6

Berkman, L. and Syme, S. L. (1979) 'Social networks, host resistance and mortality: A nine year follow up study of Alameda County residents'. *American Journal of Epidemiology*, 109: 186–204

Brandt, P.A. and Weinert, C. (1981) 'The Personal Resource Questionnaire (PRQ): a social support measure'. *Nursing Research*, Sep–Oct 30 (5): 277–80

Cabinet Office (2006) *A Sure Start to Later Life – Ending Inequalities for Older People*. **www.cpa.org.uk** (Accessed 19 May 2008)

Cabinet Office Social Exclusion Task Force (2006) *Reaching Out: An Action Plan on Social Inclusion*. Cabinet Office: London

Care Services Improvement Partnership (2006) *Partnership for Older People Project (POPP)*. **www.changeagentteam.org.uk** (Accessed 20 February 2008)

Combat Poverty Agency (2004) *Action on Poverty Today*. Galway Social Inclusion Strategy 2006–2009

Copel. L. (1998) 'Loneliness'. *Journal of Psychosocial Nursing*, 26 (1): 14–19

Del Bono, E., Sala, E., Hancock, R., Gunnell, C. and Parisi, L. (2007) 'Gender, older people and social exclusion. A gendered review and secondary analysis of the data'. ISER Working Paper 2007–13. Colchester: University of Essex

Department of Health (2006) *Our Health, Our Care, Our Say*. Department of Health White Paper. **www.dh.gov.uk** (Accessed 20 February 2008)

Fisher, M., Butt, J., Moriarty, J., Hoon Sin, C. and Brockmann, M. (2002) *Quality of Life and Social Support Among Older People from Different Ethnic Groups*. ESRC Society Today. **www.esrcsocietytoday.ac.uk** (Accessed 20 February 2008)

Heath, H. and Schofield, I. (1999) *Healthy Ageing: Nursing Older People*. Oxford: Elsevier/Mosby

Helgeson, V.S., Cohen, S., Schulz, R. and Yasko, J. (1999) 'Education and peer discussion group interventions and adjustment to breast cancer'. *Archives of General Psychiatry*, 56: 340–7

Helgeson, V.S., Cohen, S., Schulz, R. and Yasko, J. (2001) 'Group support interventions for people with cancer: Benefits and hazards' in Baum, A. and Anderson, B.L. (eds) *Psychosocial Interventions for Cancer*. Washington, DC: American Psychological Association

Huffman, G. (2002) 'Evaluating and treating unintentional weight loss in the elderly'. *American Family Physician*, 65 (4): 640–50

Kerr, B., Gordon, J., MacDonald, C. and Stalker, K. (2005) *Effective Social Work with Older People*. **www.scotland.gov.uk/Publications/2005/12/16104017/40183** (Accessed 13 May 2008)

Lewis, M.A., Rook, K.S. and Schwarzer, R. (1994) 'Social support, social control and health among the elderly' in Penny, G., Bennett, P. and Herbert, M. (eds) *Health Psychology: A Lifespan Perspective*. Philadelphia, PA: Harwood Academic Publishers

McCarthy, H. and Thomas, G. (2004) *Home Alone: Combating Isolation with Older Housebound People*. London: Demos

Norbeck, J., Lindsey, A. and Carrieri, V. (1981) 'The development of an instrument to measure social support'. *Nursing Research*, 30 (5): 264–9

Peterson, J. A. (2000) 'Nurses providing social support now and in the future'. *Kansas Nurse; Topeka*, Jun/Jul: 18–23

SCIE (2007) *Dignity in Care. Practice Guide*. **www.scie.org.uk** (Accessed 20 February 2008)

Scottish Executive (2005) *Better Outcomes for Older People*. **www.scotland.gov. uk/Publications/2005/05/13101338/13412** (Accessed 13 May 2008)

Scottish Executive (2005) *Effective Social Work with Older People*. **www.scotland. gov.uk/Publications/2005/12/16104017/40197** (Accessed 13 May 2008)

Scottish Government Health Promotions (2008). **www.scotland.gov.uk/ Topics/Health**

www.scotland.gov.uk/Topics/Health/health/Tobacco (Accessed 2 October 2008)

www.scotland.gov.uk/Topics/Health/health/19133 (Accessed 2 October 2008)

www.scotland.gov.uk/Topics/Health/health/Alcohol (Accessed 2 October 2008)

Sempik, J., Aldridge, J. and Becker, S. (2005a) *Health, Well-being and Social Inclusion: Therapeutic Horticulture in the UK*. Bristol: The Policy Press

Sempik, J., Aldridge, J. and Becker, S. (2005b) *Growing Together: A Practical Guide to Promoting Social Inclusion Through Gardening and Horticulture*. Bristol: The Policy Press

Squire, A. (2002) *Health and Well-Being for Older People: Foundations for Practice*. Edinburgh: Elsevier Science Limited

Stewart, M.A. and Tilden, V. (1995) 'The contributions of nursing science to social support'. *International Journal of Nursing Studies*, 32 (6): 535–44

Tilden, V., Nelson, C. and May, B. (1990) 'The IPR inventory: development and psychometric characteristics'. *Nursing Research*, 39 (6): 337–43

Victor, C. (1989) 'Inequalities in later life'. *Age and Ageing*, 18 (6): 387–91

Victor, C. (1991) *Health and Health Care in Later Life*. Buckingham: Open University Press

Wenger, C. A. (1995) 'A comparison of urban and rural support networks: Liverpool and North Wales'. *Ageing and Society*, 15: 59–81

Glossary

Dyscrasia: 'Bad mixture'. Specifically it is defined in current medicine as a morbid general state resulting from the presence of abnormal material in the blood, usually applied to diseases affecting blood cells or platelets.

Hawthorne Effect: An increase in productivity prompted by the psychological stimulus of being singled out and made to feel important. Originated in a factory called Hawthorne Works, where a series of experiments on factory workers were carried out between 1924 and 1932.

Homeostasis: The ability of a person (or organism) to regulate the state of their internal environment so as to maintain a stable, constant condition.

Iatrogenic: Any good or bad effect resulting from the activity of physicians or another health care professional. It is almost exclusively used to refer to a state of ill-health or adverse effect or complication caused by or resulting from medical treatment.

Life-limiting illness: An incurable illness which could potentially shorten the life of its sufferer.

Mechanistic: Automatic and impersonal.

Palliation: Derived from the Latin word *pallium* (meaning a cover or cloak) is an approach intended to relieve or remove symptoms rather than effect a cure.

Psychosis: A generic psychiatric term relating to loss of contact with reality.

Salutogenic: A term used to describe a health promotion approach in which the focus is on the factors that support health rather than the factors that cause disease. The term was first used by Aaron Antonovsky in 1979, when he studied the influence of a variety of sources of stress on health and was able to show that relatively unstressed people had much more resistance to illness than those who were more stressed.

Social exclusion: Describes marginalisation from employment, income, **social networks** such as family, neighbourhood and community, decision making and from an adequate quality of life.

Social inclusion: The position from where someone can access and benefit from the full range of opportunities available to members of society.

Social networks: The means through which **social support** is distributed and which consists of family, friends, neighbours and other contacts.

Social support: A network of family, friends, neighbours, and community members that is available in times of need to give psychological, physical, emotional and financial help.

Systematic: Methodical in procedure, characterised by thoroughness and regularity.

Tautology: In this case tautology refers to a series of statements that are constructed in such a way that the truth of the proposition is guaranteed. Consequently the statement conveys no useful information regardless of its length or complexity.

Index for The Care and Wellbeing of Older People

Added to the page number 'f' denotes a figure, 'g' denotes the glossary and 't' denotes a table.

Index